P9-CTP-079

B. Horney

# First Aid Principles and Practices

Andrew Carnegie Library
Livingstone College
701 W. Monroe St.
Salisbury, N.C. 28144

# First Aid Principles and Practices

Edited by

## ANDREW J. BROWN

State University of New York
College at Brockport

**MACMILLAN PUBLISHING COMPANY**
New York

**COLLIER MACMILLAN PUBLISHERS**
London

128572

*Development Editor*/**Mary Hoff**
*Manuscript Editor*/**Leslie Reindl**
*Production*/**Morris Lundin, Pat Barnes, Jean R. Starr**
*Design*/**Jean R. Starr**
*Illustrations by*/**BioGraphics, Inc., Visual Communications for the Life Sciences, Fort Collins, Colorado, and Gene Kohler, Edina, Minnesota.**

Copyright © 1987 by Macmillan Publishing Company, a division of Macmillan, Inc.

All rights reserved. No part of this book may be reproduced or transmitted, in any form or by any means, electronic or mechanical, including photocopying, recording, or any information storage and retrieval system, without permission in writing from the Publisher.

Macmillan Publishing Company
866 Third Avenue, New York, New York    10022
Collier Macmillan Canada, Inc.

Library of Congress Cataloging-in-Publication Data

First aid principles and practices.

Includes bibliographies and index.
1. First aid in illness and injury.    I. Brown
Andrew J.    [DNLM: 1. First Aid. WA  292 F5287]
RC86.7.F58    1987          616.02'52          86-28368
ISBN 0-02-327150-7

ISBN 0-02-327150-7

Printed in the United States of America

Printing  1  2  3  4  5  6  7 8        Year  7  8  9  0  1  2  3  4  5  6

*To Mary Hoff*
*for service above and beyond*
*the call of duty*

# CONTRIBUTORS

**Andrew J. Brown**     is Professor and Chairman of the Department of Health Science/Recreation and Leisure, State University of New York College at Brockport. He is also the author of *Community Health: An Introduction for the Health Professional*.

**Rick Barnes**     is Associate Professor and Coordinator of Health Education at East Carolina University. He is an American National Red Cross certified instructor in cardiopulmonary resuscitation and standard first aid and has taught emergency care/first aid for a number of years.

**David L. Bever**     is Associate Professor of Health Education at George Mason University. He is the author of *Safety: A Personal Focus* and the developer of the *Illness-Injury Severity Index*, a computerized patient assessment scale used by emergency medical personnel.

**Neal R. Boyd, Jr.,**     is Chair and Associate Professor of the Department of Health Education at Southern Mississippi University. He has been active in both health education and accident prevention, with research in both areas.

**Iris G. Brown**     is Head/Professor, Department of Health Education, Norfolk State University. He is the author of a number of health education publications.

**John L. Echternach**     is Professor and Chairman of the Department of Community Health Professions and Director of the Program in Physical Therapy at Old Dominion University. He is the author of a diverse group of publications, primarily in the field of physical therapy.

**Gene Ezell**     is Professor of Health Education at the University of Tennessee at Chattanooga. He is the author or coauthor of six college textbooks on various aspects of health and safety education and has had over twenty articles published in state, regional, and national professional journals.

**Gerald C. Hyner**     is Assistant Professor of Health Promotion at Purdue University. He is the author of numerous articles on health risk appraisals, work site health promotion, and program evaluation.

**Sandra J. Levi**     was formerly Associate Professor of Physical Therapy at Old Dominion University. She is a licensed physical therapist and an American National Red Cross certified instructor in cardiopulmonary resuscitation.

**Judith McLaughlin**     is Assistant Professor in the Department of Health and Safety Education at the University of Georgia. She teaches community health education courses and conducts research in the ethnographic study of self-care behavior and coping with chronic illnesses, qualitative evaluation of programs, and the scientific development of measurement instruments.

**Christopher L. Melby**     is Assistant Professor of Health Promotion at Purdue University. He has published numerous research articles regarding the influence of diet, exercise, and stress on blood pressure and other health parameters. He is also an affiliate childbirth educator with the American Academy of Husband-Coached Childbirth.

**Richard S. Riggs**     is Associate Professor and Unit Coordinator of Health Education at the University of Kentucky. He has taught safety education and emergency care/first aid for a number of years and has published a variety of health education articles.

**Frank Schabel**     is Assistant Professor of Physical Education and Leisure Studies and Coordinator of the Health Studies Program at Iowa State University. He has specialties in health teacher education, substance abuse, and emergency health. He is currently an American National Red Cross certified instructor trainer for cardiopulmonary resuscitation and first aid.

**Stephen H. Stewart** is Associate Professor and Assistant Department Head of the Department of Physical Education and Health Science at James Madison University. He is a member of the National Examination of Cardiovascular Knowledge Task Force for the American Heart Association.

**David M. White** is Assistant Professor of Health Education at East Carolina University. He is a regional consultant for the American National Red Cross and an instructor trainer in standard first aid, cardiopulmonary resuscitation, and basic first aid.

**Ara Zulalian** is Professor Emeritus of the Department of Health Science/Recreation and Leisure at the State University of New York College at Brockport. He is an American National Red Cross certified instructor trainer in first aid and a certified instructor in cardiopulmonary resuscitation.

# CONTENTS

# PREFACE

After a long hard struggle, we have finally entered an era in our approach to health in the United States that can be characterized as one of health promotion and disease prevention. Despite the continued disproportionate flow of resources into reactive, acute care within the American health care system, support is increasing for commitment to a proactive, preventive orientation. In truth, most efforts in this area today are directed toward mortality reduction, as a cursory review of the ten leading causes of death in the United States would quickly bear out. Health professionals and lay public alike are continuously exposed to health education messages designed ultimately to reduce the incidence of such chronic diseases as cancer, heart disease, cerebrovascular disease (stroke), and diabetes. Significant public and private resources are also being committed to the prevention of alcoholism, suicide, and homicide, all leading sources of mortality with psychosocial roots. Regardless of how effectively we are utilizing available information and resources, most of us are cognizant of the preventive efforts under way.

There is, however, a glaring omission in the current focus on prevention. Accidental death, which has ranked throughout the twentieth century as one of the ten leading causes of death in the United States, is being overlooked. To appreciate fully the severity of the threat to quality of life posed by accidents, we must think not only of the 100,000 plus American lives lost annually, but of the millions of individuals who are incapacitated either permanently or temporarily by accidents. We must begin to take the steps necessary to prevent accidents.

Emphasis on accident prevention will not alter the critical need for individuals properly trained in first aid principles and practices. Emergencies will always arise despite the best preventive actions. Indeed, accidents are not the only source of emergencies. Sudden illness, too, can strike, despite preventive action. The life-style we have adopted in the United States, with its inherent risks to well-being, necessitates the training of millions of citizens in first aid. These Americans should be prepared to assist the injured or suddenly ill, whether in a school or factory, on the highway, or in the home.

**First aid is, in all actuality, preventive in nature.** It is not primary prevention, in that it is not designed to avert the occurrence of an emergency. It is, however, clearly a secondary level of prevention. Timely and properly administered first aid care can prevent a life-threatening situation from becoming a life-taking situation. The skilled application of first aid care can *prevent* further injury or aggravation of a given condition. The competent practitioner of first aid care can *prevent* undue pain and suffering.

Properly administered first aid care can *prevent* long-term disability, extended hospital stays, and unnecessarily long recuperative periods. In short, first aid care can *prevent* not only loss of life but loss of quality of life for those emergency victims fortunate enough to receive competent care from a well-prepared practitioner.

The purpose of this text is to give the reader the opportunity to become a skilled, competent first-aider. Prepared basically for use in college-level classes, the text can also be used effectively by other community-based groups (e.g., firemen, police, and scout and campfire leaders). Individuals interested in acquiring a first aid care delivery capability will find this text a most useful resource. *First Aid Principles and Practices* may be used either as the single text in a first aid course or as a more in-depth text to complement the American National Red Cross publication. A first aid text should be available in every home for quick reference. This text is designed also to serve that purpose.

The text that follows represents the first aid care perspectives of fifteen contributing authors from college and university campuses across the nation. They propose to provide the reader with the best possible first aid care strategies based on the most current information. To this end, the revised standards and guidelines emanating from the National Conference on Cardiopulmonary Resuscitation and Emergency Cardiac Care (first published in the June 6, 1986 edition of the Journal of the American Medical Association) have been incorporated into this text. The first aid care practitioner, however, must continuously remain alert to new developments as they occur in this field. First aid is a dynamic area of practice, subject to change as our understanding of the human organism and means for responding to it in crisis expands. First aid practitioners must continuously refresh their knowledge and skill base to maintain optimum competence. The first-aider should periodically reread this or any other first aid text and regularly practice the skills described. We would all want this to be true of any first-aider who might come to our assistance in an emergency, and we also owe this to anyone whom we might be called on to assist.

Many individuals have made significant contributions to the preparation of this text. First and foremost among these dedicated professionals has been Mary Hoff, our development editor at Burgess Publishing, who has nurtured this project from beginning to end. There are four others whose comments, suggestions, and constructive criticisms have also been greatly appreciated:

Ms. Debra Ann Ballinger
Arizona State University, Tempe

Professor Barry Ochockmel
University of Wisconsin—La Crosse

Dr. Sherman K. Sowby
California State University, Fresno

Dr. Jayne Troyer
St. Cloud State University, St. Cloud, Minn.

A.J.B.

# 1

# Introduction to First Aid and Its Practice

ANDREW J. BROWN, ED.D., M.P.H.

After completing this chapter the student will be able to
- Define first aid care.
- Identify the general responsibilities of the first-aider.
- Describe the fundamental benefits associated with timely, properly rendered first aid care.
- Demonstrate awareness of the need for follow-up medical care for many injured or suddenly ill persons who receive first aid care.
- Discuss the need for formal study of the body of knowledge and skills that underlie the practice of first aid.
- Demonstrate realistic understanding of the legal aspects of first aid care.
- Explain the meaning of the "reasonable and prudent care" concept in liability cases.
- Demonstrate awareness of the need for continuous updating and applied practice of first aid knowledge and skills.
- Explain the purpose and scope of documentation in first aid care delivery.

## ____INTRODUCTION

For many people, the term *first aid* conjures up images of splints and bandages, broken bones and lacerations, and the trauma of automobile and other accidents. But situations requiring first aid and the skills needed for its safe, effective practice range far beyond accidents and the ability to stop bleeding and immobilize the skeleton.

The American National Red Cross (1979) defines first aid simply as "the immediate care given to a person who has been injured or suddenly taken ill." Beyond this simple definition, however, the Red Cross views the scope of first aid and the responsibilities of the deliverer of first aid care as much broader in nature:

> [First aid] includes self-help and home care if medical assistance is not available or is delayed. It also includes well selected words of encouragement, evidence of willingness to help, and promotion of confidence by demonstration of competence. (P.17)

The first-aider may be required to perform many functions, depending on the condition of the victim and the setting in which he or she is encountered. All or any combination of the following activities may be necessitated:

**1** Identify the condition of the victim(s) in the emergency situation and set a plan of action for caring for the injury or illness.

**2** Assess the circumstances and the safety of the setting in which the victim(s) has (have) been encountered and move the person(s) only if necessary.

**3** In the case of multiple victims, prioritize (triage) the order for treatment of each on the basis of the severity of the threat to life, as follows:
**a** Possibility of immediate death
**b** Possibility of death within hours
**c** Nonsevere injury
**d** Already dead

**4** In the case of multiple injuries or conditions, prioritize the order for treatment of each on the basis of the severity of the threat to life and provide care. Highest priority needs are:
**a** Restoration of breathing
**b** Restoration of cardiac functioning
**c** Control of severe bleeding
**d** Prevention or control of shock

**5** Control any crowd that may have gathered.

**6** Record accurately the condition of the victim, evidence of circumstances surrounding the emergency incident, specific first aid care rendered, and the response (any change in condition) of the victim. Transmit this information to the medically qualified individuals who subsequently assume responsibility for care.

**7** Provide physical and psychological reassurance to the victim and any others involved in the emergency situation.

**8** Spontaneously improvise implements for bandages, splinting, and (if the situation requires) moving or transporting the victim.

**9** Arrange for or possibly carry out transportation of the victim to an appropriate medical care source.

In essence, the first-aider is expected to exercise judgment under conditions that may be severely stressful. He or she should be prepared to provide a wide variety of emergency assistance. The first-aider should be able to provide both physical and psychological comfort to the victim and psychological reassurance to any others affected by the emergency situation. Last, but not least, he or she must make provision for the continued safety of the victim, for the safety of any others who come upon the emergency scene, and for personal safety.

## ——THE VALUE OF FIRST AID

Clearly, the early arrival at an emergency scene of someone skilled in the principles and techniques of first aid is of great value. Early administration of quality first aid care has many benefits besides the obvious one of preserving life. Timely, effective care often can prevent further injury or aggravation of a condition. It can reduce pain and suffering; it can shorten the length of time required for recuperation from an injury or illness; and it can alleviate the anxieties of those involved in the emergency situation. All of these lead to a better outcome for the victim; more considered, effective decision making by all parties, including the first-aider; and less likelihood of a stress-induced outcome for any of those involved (e.g., loss of emotional or intellectual control, or both; cardiovascular seizure). Properly administered first aid care can, at times, even lead to a briefer in-patient stay if the injured or ill person requires hospitalization.

**First aid care is not meant to replace medical care**. When an injury or sudden illness requires medical attention, the role of the first-aider is basically to stabilize the condition until skilled medical personnel arrive or the victim can be safely moved. Still, most minor episodes of illness or sudden injury can be satisfactorily managed with first aid care (often in the form of self-care) alone. Thus, knowledge of basic first aid principles and the ability to apply first aid skills allow individuals to care for themselves or to assist others in the case of most minor injuries or sudden illnesses. As a general rule, however, *qualified follow-up medical advice should be sought if there is any question in the mind of the first-aider, victim, friends, or family regarding the need for further care.*

## ___THE NEED FOR SPECIAL TRAINING

Everyone, at some point in life, is likely to witness or come upon an emergency situation requiring first aid. As previously indicated, timely delivery of appropriate first aid care can mean as much as the difference between life and death or simply the alleviation of pain or discomfort. The uninitiated tend to perceive first aid training as just so much common sense, requiring little in the way of studied preparation. Such a perception is invalid. True, first aid does not involve the delivery of "medical" treatment. Nonetheless, the potential first-aider must acquire a considerable body of knowledge and master a multitude of skills before being considered competent. First aid knowledge and practices that border on the realm of common sense are of little value without formal study.

First aid based only on common sense rather than on studied preparation leads to the prospect of assistance rendered on the basis of presumption rather than on knowledge and skills. Clearly this is not acceptable in situations involving life and death. Nor should it be acceptable in less severe emergencies in which improperly administered first aid care may, among other outcomes, lead to brain damage, disfigurement, loss of limb, excessive pain, or prolonged recovery or any combination of these. By abstracting the common sense elements of first aid and formally studying them as a body of knowledge and skills, the first-aider acquires the capability of applying these elements in any emergency in which they might be of use. Further, training in first aid leads to an understanding not only of the first-aider's potential but also of his or her limitations in a given emergency situation.

*First-aiders must remember that they are neither physicians nor emergency medical technicians.* They act instead as buffers between the injured or suddenly ill individual and a potentially harmful outcome. This buffer role lasts until the more sophisticated medical care needed is available. First-aiders who have, to the best of their ability, competently and conscientiously applied their knowledge and skills to stabilize a life-threatening condition, to prevent further injury or deterioration, to prevent undue pain and suffering, and to provide psychological comfort to the victim (and any others involved) have successfully met their obligation.

## ___LEGAL ASPECTS OF FIRST AID

Fear of the potential legal consequences of becoming "involved" in an emergency situation often hinders people from offering assistance. This fear is unfortunate, and in most emergency situations is exaggerated. First-aiders who stay within the limits of their competencies and render assistance consistent with the best interests of the suddenly ill or injured victim need not fear legal action or its outcome, even if the person assisted should bring suit. Generally speaking, the conditions under which the deliverer of first aid might be held liable include

1 An act or omission that causes unintended harm, which harm should have been foreseen and prevented.
2 An act that is itself contrary to law or an omission of a specific duty, which act or omission causes unintended harm.
3 An act that is intended to cause harm and does so (National Education Association 1982, p.4).

Two concepts embodied in these conditions are of significance to the first-aider from a legal liability perspective. First, a person may be held equally as liable for the failure (omission) to provide care that could (i.e., was within the capability of the person) and should have been provided, as for the provision of inappropriate care. Second, under the legal concept of *foreseeability*, the first-aider is required to think ahead, particularly in terms of expected outcome for the victim as a result of application of or omission of a particular first aid technique.

Physicians coming unexpectedly upon an emergency situation were once in a most difficult position. They faced the double risk of legal action for the care delivered or legal action for failure to provide care. This double risk is believed to have led physicians often to avoid involvement in emergency situations. Partly to relieve physicians of this burden, but also to protect others who might be in a position to render assistance in an emergency, many states have passed Good Samaritan laws. *The first-aider or any other individual who comes to the aid of an injured or suddenly ill person is generally considered covered by Good Samaritan laws.* The care provided must be consistent with the care a reasonable, prudent individual with a similar background would provide under similar circumstances. Successful legal actions are not likely against first-aiders whose assistance meets this "reasonable, prudent" test.

Some states have gone beyond Good Samaritan laws and have passed "bystander laws," laws that typically require bystanders to provide assistance to those in distress (if this can be accomplished without the bystanders endangering themselves). Bystander laws have been relatively ineffective, however, and are seldom enforced. A legal obligation to assist in an emergency situation also exists if there is a preexisting relationship between the victim and the first-aider (e.g., parent-child, driver-passenger).

Trying to force one person to come to the aid of another in distress is not realistic, however. In truth, an emergency situation poses an ethical rather than a legal dilemma. Despite Good Samaritan laws or the legal requirements of bystander laws and preexisting relationships, it is the first-aider who must decide whether to provide assistance. The first-aider makes the decision to come to the assistance of an injured or suddenly ill person not because he or she is legally required to do so but because that is the morally appropriate course of action.

The purpose of this discussion of the legal aspects of first aid is to place the issue in an objective light. The first-aider is legally bound to provide care and is morally obligated to do so if capable. *The first-aider must not let fear of possible subsequent legal action obstruct the effort to assist.* Clearly, however, good judgment and conscientious foresight must be employed in determining what first aid techniques will or will not be applied. The victim of an injury or sudden illness deserves no less.

## THE NEED FOR MAINTAINING KNOWLEDGE AND SKILL LEVELS

Thousands of Americans are trained annually in the practice of first aid through schools, colleges, and community agencies. Unfortunately, many of those trained never update their knowledge or refresh their skills. Equally unfortunate is the fact that their potential for offering assistance to injured or suddenly ill persons will eventually be lost.

Individuals trained in first aid must periodically participate in short courses, workshops, or other continuing education activities for two basic reasons. First, as previously indicated, advances occur over time in knowledge of the human organism and the manner in which it functions. With these advances frequently come parallel changes in our understanding of how to provide care when that organism and its subsystems are threatened by injury or illness. The second reason is the "use it or lose it" aspect of skill development and maintenance. Applied (i.e., hands-on) skills are best learned and most competently utilized when practiced regularly. Lack of practice inevitably leads to a decline in skill. Although everyone can expect to encounter a situation requiring first aid sooner or later, no one can determine when or how often the demand (emergency situation) will occur or what skills will be needed. *First-aiders must, therefore, make a conscientious effort to reinforce their competence periodically through self-study and organized continued training opportunities.*

## DOCUMENTING THE FIRST AID CARE DELIVERED

As evidenced in the discussion to this point, the fundamental responsibilities of the first qualified individual who comes upon an emergency situation are to:

1 Identify the condition(s) of the victim(s) and apply the concept of triage in determining the order of care.
2 Assess the safety of the setting in which the victim(s) is (are) found and move the victim(s) only if essential to ensure continued safety.
3 Attempt to stabilize life-threatening situations and minimize further injury and complications until more medically skilled personnel are reached or they arrive on the scene.

Embodied within the third responsibility is the requirement that the first-aider provide all information possible to the medically trained personnel who subsequently assume responsibility for the injured or ill victim (Figure 1.1). At a minimum, this information should include

1 The exact time the victim(s) was (were) found.
2 A detailed condition of the victim(s) as found.
3 The specific first aid care rendered, including the order in which it was provided and the response (changes in condition) of the victim(s).
4 The circumstances (if known) contributing or leading up to the onset of the injury or sudden illness.

Gathering and recording this information for subsequent transmittal can be a formidable task. In many emergency situations there is no time to put such information in writing before medically trained personnel arrive. This places even greater responsibility on the first-aider to remain calm and make considered decisions. He or she will often have to recall from memory the observations made and first aid actions taken.

First-aiders should make every reasonable effort to gather information regarding the circumstances leading up to the injury or sudden illness and changes that may have occurred in the person's condition before their arrival. The conscious victim is asked to provide any information he or she can, and witnesses are interviewed, as circumstances permit. Appropriate personal information is also gathered, if possible. Useful information includes (1) victim's name, address, and phone number, (2) names of friends or

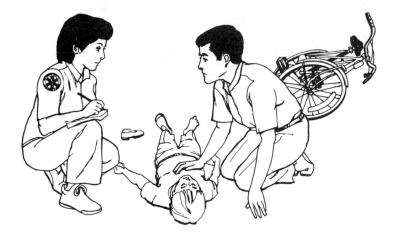

**FIGURE 1.1**

The first-aider must be prepared to transmit all pertinent information to the skilled medical personnel assuming responsibility for the victim.

family to notify, and (3) names of the victim's personal physician or other principal source of primary care. The quality of the information relayed by the first-aider to those responsible for further care can play a critical role in the victim's ultimate recovery.

## _____MATERIALS USED IN FIRST AID

First-aiders cannot carry with them all of the first aid materials that might be needed in a given situation. They can, however, establish first aid inventories at different sites, including the home, workplace, and principal recreation settings. Despite such foresight, emergency situations often occur where first aid materials are not available. The ability of the first-aider to improvise materials then becomes an important skill, creative ingenuity a needed talent. Handkerchiefs can become bandages. Shirts, ties, and loose boards can be combined to make padded splints. The extent to which clothing and other articles can be pressed into service as first aid supplies is limited only by their availability at the emergency scene and the creativity of the first-aider.

## ———————————————————— SUMMARY ————————————————————

First aid care is the initial care provided to an individual who has been injured or suddenly taken ill. Its purpose is to prevent death or further injury or complication, to prevent shock, to relieve pain and suffering, and to provide necessary care until more qualified medical assistance is available. First aid principles and practices need organized study. The responsibilities of the first-aider and the legal implications of the provision of first aid care are significant. Generally, first-aiders are considered covered by Good Samaritan laws in states in which such laws have been established. The basic condition that must be met is that the care be rendered in good faith and be consistent with what any reasonable, prudent individual with similar training would provide under similar circumstances. First aid care is not meant to replace medical care. If there is any question concerning the prognosis of an injured or suddenly ill victim, follow-up medical care should be promptly sought.

## ———————————————— CHAPTER MASTERY: TEST ITEMS ————————————————

**True and False**                                                                                          **Circle One**

1. The practice of first aid is limited to the control of life-threatening            **T**      **F**
conditions.
2. The victim should never be moved from the position in which he or            **T**      **F**
she is found.
3. Most minor episodes of illness or sudden injury can be satisfactorily          **T**      **F**
cared for with first aid alone.

4. Properly administered first aid care eliminates the need for subsequent more sophisticated medical care regardless of the victim's condition.   T   F

5. Mastering the knowledge and skills that comprise first aid practice does not require formalized study.   T   F

6. The quality of assistance rendered by the first-aider is judged by both the care provided and the care not provided.   T   F

7. First aid skills must be practiced regularly for the first-aider to maintain competence.   T   F

8. The quality of the information relayed by the first-aider to medical personnel responsible for further care of the victim can play a crucial role in the victim's recovery.   T   F

9. The first-aider is responsible for assessing conditions in the emergency setting and assuring the safety of everyone in the immediate area.   T   F

## Fill In the Missing Word(s)

1. The American National Red Cross defines first aid as _____.
2. The term used to identify the process of classifying the ill or injured in priority order for care is _____.
3. Should a victim subsequently undertake legal action, the first-aider will not be held liable if it is determined that the care delivered was consistent with the care a _____, _____ individual with similar training would have given under similar circumstances.
4. The first-aider should be prepared to provide as much information as possible in each of the following areas to those who will subsequently care for the victim: _____, _____, _____, and _____.

## Multiple Choice (Circle the Best Answer)

1. In rendering first aid care to the multiply injured victim, which of the following would have the highest priority?
   a. Write down the condition of the victim as found.
   b. Arrange for getting the victim to appropriate medical care.
   c. Provide psychologic reassurance to the victim.
   d. Restore breathing if respiration has ceased.
   e. Immobilize any fractures present.
2. When timely appropriate first aid care is administered, it can
   a. preserve life.
   b. prevent further injury, complications, or both.
   c. reduce pain and suffering.
   d. reduce recuperation time.
   e. All of the above.

3. An individual who provides assistance in emergencies is generally protected from legal action by
   a. the American National Red Cross.
   b. Good Samaritan laws.
   c. the legal concept of foreseeability.
   d. a preexisting relationship between victim and first-aider (e.g., teacher–student).
4. The term that is defined as the extent to which a first-aider should have expected the outcome realized by the victim is
   a. triage.
   b. foreseeability.
   c. liability.
   d. negligence.
   e. none of the above
5. Materials that might be used by a first-aider should be
   a. stockpiled in accessible sites in which the potential is high for their use.
   b. carried with the first-aider at all times.
   c. only those that are medically approved.

**Discussion Questions**

1. On what bases can the need for continued updating of training in first aid be justified?
2. What is meant by the term "buffer" in describing the role of the first-aider?
3. What potential benefits can the injured or suddenly ill individual realize from the provision of timely, competent first aid care?
4. Under what conditions does a first-aider have a legal obligation to assist a person in distress?
5. Explain what is meant by the concept of "reasonable and prudent" care.

_____ **BIBLIOGRAPHY** _____

American National Red Cross. *Advanced First Aid and Emergency Care*. 2d ed. Garden City, N.Y.: Doubleday, 1979.

National Education Association, Research Division for the National Commission on Safety Education. *Who is Liable for Pupil Injuries*? Washington, D.C.: National Education Association, 1982.

# 2

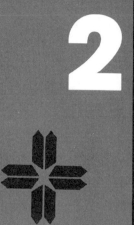

# Assessing the Emergency Situation

ANDREW J. BROWN, ED.D., M.P.H.

## OBJECTIVES

After completing this chapter the student will be able to
- Identify and perform the tasks involved in assessing an emergency situation in preparation for the administration of first aid care.
- Identify and check for conditions that pose an immediate threat to life to an injured or suddenly ill person.
- Identify and categorize emergency conditions according to three priority levels for response:
  - Immediately life threatening
  - Potentially life threatening if not responded to promptly
  - Not life threatening but requiring assistance
- Identify the components of the emergency situation and conduct a satisfactory secondary assessment, including
  - A subjective interview
  - An objective examination including
    - Determination of vital signs.
    - Head-to-toe physical assessment.

## ____INTRODUCTION

The first few moments after the first-aider encounters an emergency situation are critical. For many, the greatest initial challenge is overcoming the natural human responses to an emergency (e.g., confusion, anguish, fear, and intellectual shock) that can interfere with good judgment and negate potential for providing appropriate assistance.

In an emergency situation, decisions made and actions taken during the stressful initial moments of contact generally determine the success or failure of the first-aider's efforts. Besides mastering and maintaining control of innate reactions, the first-aider must perform many tasks, ranging from situational and victim assessment, through application of first aid, to stabilization of the suddenly ill or injured individual. Many of these tasks (and their individual steps) must be performed sequentially. This chapter specifies and discusses the procedures the first-aider should follow when first arriving on the scene. These procedures assist in assessing the emergency situation and the condition of the victim. Assessment in turn determines the order, type, and amount of assistance to be delivered.

# GENERAL DIRECTIONS

The old adage that "haste makes waste" appropriately applies to the efforts of the first-aider in an emergency situation. Undue haste leads to much more than waste in this circumstance. Failure of the first-aider to evaluate the safety of the setting in which the emergency is encountered may expose the first-aider and possibly bystanders to an unacceptably high level of risk of injury or even death. Rushing to treat the first injury noticed in a victim may allow the person to die from an unnoticed life-threatening condition. Hurrying to care for the first victim encountered in an emergency may allow another more severely injured victim to die.

This discussion about haste is not intended to discount the desirability of swift response to an emergency. The speed with which the first-aider responds can be crucial to the survival of people involved or the severity of outcome. But a speedy response without consideration of the appropriateness of the action taken may not benefit anyone and may even aggravate the situation.

On arriving at an emergency scene, the first-aider must carefully assess the status of the victims as well as the setting. Quickly but carefully the first-aider determines if the setting is a safe one in which to provide assistance. If not, it may be necessary to move the victim (and possibly bystanders) to a safer setting. (Techniques for lifting and moving injured persons are discussed in Chapter 18.) Concurrently, the first-aider determines the nature of the injury or sudden illness as well as the immediacy and severity of the threat it poses to life.

The conditions that might be encountered in an emergency situation can be categorized as follows:

1 *Conditions that immediately threaten life.* These must be identified during the initial examination and given priority.
2 *Conditions that potentially threaten life.* These must be identified during the extensive secondary assessment of the victim and the emergency scene.
3 *Conditions that do not threaten life but necessitate assistance for the victim.* These are also identified during the extensive secondary assessment of the victim. These conditions produce discomfort or pain or both and interfere with the victim's ability to function. They are the "routine" injuries or sudden illnesses for which timely, appropriately administered first aid relieves anxiety and suffering and improves recuperative outcome.

The purposes of examining the victim and of inspecting the emergency scene are to identify and rank order, by perceived threat to life, those conditions for which the first-aider is qualified and prepared to respond. Assessment allows for the orderly administration of appropriate assistance at the emergency scene. Inadequate assessment can lead to an unfortunate outcome for the victim, the first-aider, and bystanders.

# INITIAL ASSESSMENT

As a general rule, the first-aider should not attempt to move a suddenly ill or injured person unless essential. Circumstances may, however, pose an immediate threat to those

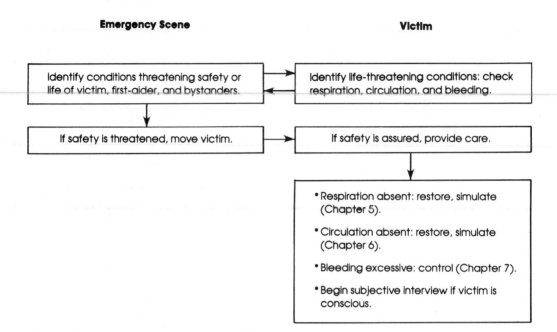

**Emergency Scene**  **Victim**

| Identify conditions threatening safety or life of victim, first-aider, and bystanders. | → ← | Identify life-threatening conditions: check respiration, circulation, and bleeding. |

If safety is threatened, move victim. → If safety is assured, provide care.

- Respiration absent: restore, simulate (Chapter 5).
- Circulation absent: restore, simulate (Chapter 6).
- Bleeding excessive: control (Chapter 7).
- Begin subjective interview if victim is conscious.

**FIGURE 2.1**

Summary of initial assessment.

present at the emergency scene. The first-aider must thus give priority to protecting his or her own life and the lives of bystanders as well as of the victim.

In the discussion that follows, the procedures to be observed by someone rendering first aid care are cited in a logical step-by-step progression. In a real emergency situation, however, speed of reaction to life-threatening conditions is critical. Therefore, the first-aider frequently must carry out a number of tasks almost simultaneously. Initial assessments of both victim and emergency scene may have to be done concurrently. Figure 2.1 summarizes the initial assessment sequence.

## —Emergency Scene Inspection

The purpose of the initial emergency scene inspection is detection of high-risk circumstances that could place the lives of the victim, the first-aider, and bystanders (if any) in jeopardy. The first question to be asked is, "Is this a safe area in which to begin first aid care?" In the case of an automobile wreck, a ruptured fuel tank creates the serious risk of fire or explosion or both. Gaseous fumes from an accidental chemical spill pose a serious threat. In the relatively rapid emergency scene inspection, the first-aider's attention should be directed to any life-threatening conditions that require clearing the area.

If the setting poses an immediate threat to life, the first-aider must (1) take steps to ensure the safety of everyone in the area (e.g., move the injured person) and then (2) respond to the victim's needs, dealing in priority order with the conditions most threatening to life. *There is little justification for further jeopardizing the victim. There is no justification for placing at risk the lives of the first-aider and other possible emergency scene bystanders.*

## ― Victim Examination

The purpose of the initial examination of the victim of an emergency situation is to assess functional status for immediately life-threatening conditions and to apply appropriate first aid care as needed. Three conditions are of primary concern and require a response, in the order indicated:

**1** Absence of or interference with respiration
**2** Loss of circulation
**3** Extensive uncontrolled bleeding

When more than one of these conditions exist, the first-aider must respond as concurrently as possible. Indeed, the cardiopulmonary resuscitation (CPR) technique presented in Chapter 6 provides for simultaneous response to respiratory and circulatory emergencies. The time required to restore cardiopulmonary functioning may preclude waiting until this is accomplished before an attempt is made to control bleeding. This attempt may be necessary even while the victim's cardiopulmonary status is being assessed. The first-aider may attempt to "draft" a volunteer bystander to assist under his or her direction and supervision. The first-aider working alone will find responding to the needs of a victim with multiple life-threatening conditions a severe challenge. Nonetheless, he or she must give first priority to an open airway and adequate breathing.

### Absence of or Interference with Respiration
The adequacy of the victim's breathing is determined immediately. Absence of breathing will cause death or brain damage in minutes. Inadequate exchange of air poses a severe threat. To ascertain breathing status, the first-aider watches the chest movements associated with breathing while placing the face near the victim's mouth and nose and listening and feeling for movement of air for at least five seconds (Figure 2.2).

Absence of breathing may be due to a relatively simple blockage of the airway. **The existence of an open airway is thus the next condition to be checked.** Appropriate first aid care for airway damage is provided if needed. (Techniques for alleviating blockage of the airway are presented in Chapter 5. A special technique is used if spinal cord injury is suspected.) If the victim does not breathe after the airway is cleared, the first-aider begins artificial respiration (see Chapter 5).

### Loss of Circulation
The first step in checking circulation is to palpate for the pulse (Figure 2.3). The rhythmic beating of the heart pushes blood through the arteries in surges that are perceptible to the touch (the pulse). The thumb is not used in feeling for the pulse because it has its own pulse which will obscure the victim's pulse. Palpation requires a gentle touch: Too much pressure can cause the pulse to fade. The pulse is most readily detected in an

**FIGURE 2.2**

The victim's breathing status is determined by watching chest movements and listening to and feeling for the movement of air from the nose and mouth.

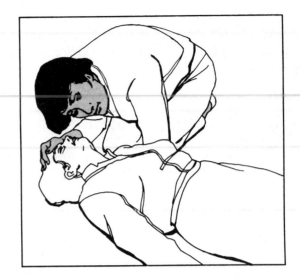

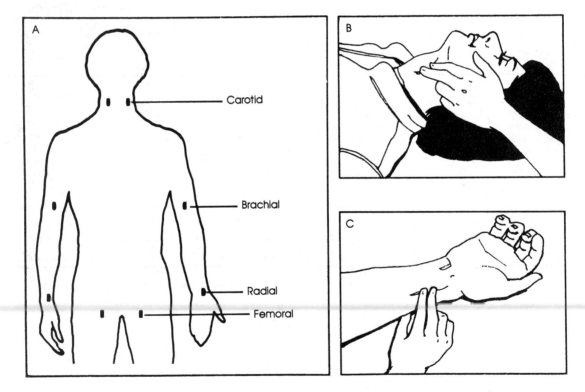

**FIGURE 2.3**

Location of arteries where pulse can be felt (*A*). Index and middle fingers are used to take the carotid pulse in the neck (*B*) or the radial pulse in the wrist (*C*).

artery that lies close to the surface of the skin (e.g., carotid artery), or passes over a bone (e.g., radial artery) (Figure 2.3*A*).

A *carotid pulse* is found by gently placing the tips of the index and middle fingers on the Adam's apple or center of the throat and then slowly moving them off center toward the side of the neck (Figure 2.3*B*). A carotid artery lies on either side of the neck. The pulse is preferably taken from the side nearest the first-aider.

The *radial pulse* is found by placing the tips of the index and middle fingers on the palm side of the hand in the approximate center of the wrist (Figure 2.3*C*). With the index finger as anchor, the fingers are turned toward the outer edge (thumb side) of the wrist and gently pressed. This technique should assure that at least one finger will locate the radial artery and sense the pulsations.

If the victim's injury or position precludes feeling for the carotid or radial pulse, the femoral or brachial pulse may be checked. The *femoral pulse* is found by pressing gently with the index and two middle fingers on the femoral artery, located in the groin between the thigh and the trunk. Though this is considered the second most reliable artery (after the carotid) for measuring the pulse, a variety of problems are associated with its use. One is the necessity of removing or disturbing the person's clothing. **Clothing should not be disturbed if spinal cord injury is suspected.** It may be possible to cut or tear clothing without moving the victim. Protection of privacy is another problem in femoral pulse measurement, particularly for females. As a general rule, a first-aider should not disturb the clothing of a victim of the opposite sex without a witness being present.

Regardless of the victim's sex, the first-aider uses a combination of caution, common sense, and respect for the privacy of the individual. If clothing must be disturbed, the first-aider explains what is going to be done and the reason to the victim (or to a reliable witness, if available, if the victim is unconscious). Only those parts of the victim's body that must be inspected or checked are exposed, and actions may have to be justified later as consistent with sound principles of first aid.

The *brachial pulse* is found by placing all four fingers on the upper inside portion of the arm, approximately midway between the elbow and the shoulder, with the thumb to the outside of the arm. By applying pressure with the fingers, the first-aider should be able to locate the brachial artery between the biceps and triceps muscles (Figure 2.3*A*). *The brachial artery is recommended as the primary location for measuring the pulse of infants.* This is due both to difficulty in locating or sensing the carotid pulse in the infant neck and the threat of excess pressure interfering with the infant's air flow.

To summarize, the presence of a pulse indicates that the heart is functioning and blood is circulating. If no pulse is detectable, the first-aider begins cardiopulmonary resuscitation (CPR) immediately (see Chapter 6). If the initial examination shows, or first aid care provides, an open airway, respiration, and a discernible pulse, the first-aider checks for bleeding.

### Extensive Uncontrolled Bleeding
Extensive uncontrolled bleeding threatens life in two ways. First is the obvious threat of bleeding to death. Second is the threat of severe shock. In emergencies involving serious bodily injury, either outcome can occur within a relatively brief time, even minutes.

When attempting to assess the extent of bleeding, the first-aider must take a variety of factors into account. First, many bleeding wounds appear more severe than they actually are. Gross soft-tissue injuries in particular can appear life threatening. Unless bleeding is profuse, however, soft-tissue damage is usually more psychologically distressing than life threatening.

Second, though severe bleeding from open wounds could be expected to be readily observable, it often is hidden by the position of the victim or by absorption into clothing. (This is especially true during colder months when several layers of clothing are worn.) To eliminate the possibility of severe external bleeding going undetected, the first-aider examines the injured person's entire body. Again, clothing may have to be disturbed for this examination, and again the privacy of the victim must be protected. Examination for bleeding in a person who should not be moved requires careful inspection by hand for tell-tale signs.

Internal bleeding is less readily detectable than external bleeding but is not necessarily less life threatening. Serious internal bleeding is very likely in crushing or penetrating injuries of the chest or abdomen (e.g., as might occur in a motor vehicle accident or a shooting or stabbing). Serious internal bleeding can also be suspected when significant external bleeding is absent but the injured person begins to exhibit signs and symptoms of shock. (First aid care for control of shock and internal bleeding are dealt with in Chapters 4 and 7, respectively.) Detection of internal bleeding is usually carried out as part of the secondary phase of examination.

### Subjective Interview

Although the subjective interview is discussed as part of the secondary assessment of the victim, it should be noted that this interview begins with the initial assessment *if the person is conscious.*

## __Initial Assessment: Summary

The purposes of initial assessment of someone suddenly injured or ill are identification of immediate life-threatening conditions and prompt application of appropriate first aid care. The purpose of initial inspection of the emergency scene is determination of its safety. Under most circumstances the injured or ill person should be moved only by the trained medical personnel who eventually replace the first-aider. However, if conditions at the emergency scene pose a threat to life or safety or both, moving the victim may be necessary before aid can be administered.

The first priority of care must go to an open airway and the maintenance of adequate respiration. The second priority is maintenance of blood circulation. Third is the need to control severe bleeding. *The status of the injured or ill person may require simultaneous response to all three conditions.* The CPR techniques discussed in Chapter 6 provide a mechanism for simulating/stimulating the victim's own heart action and respiration. A concurrent need to control severe bleeding will add to the difficulties faced by the first-aider. He or she may have to ask bystanders, if any, for assistance.

# ___SECONDARY ASSESSMENT

The purpose of the secondary assessment is to identify all other conditions that require corrective action. Concern is on two levels. The first level is conditions that may not threaten life initially but may do so if care is not given promptly and properly. The second level is conditions that are unlikely to threaten life but may be further aggravated or result in undue pain and suffering, or both, without timely and effective first aid care.

The secondary assessment is carried out in a systematic, orderly fashion. It includes reappraisal of the emergency scene; detailed reexamination of the injured person; gathering of pertinent data from this person, from other appropriate sources, or from both (this may have been started during the initial assessment); formulation of a plan of action and its implementation; and finally, continued monitoring of the person's condition (and adjustment of care as needed) until more sophisticated medical care becomes available. The secondary assessment is summarized in Figure 2.4.

When properly conducted, the secondary assessment serves to reassure the victim and concerned bystanders that qualified assistance is being provided. This in turn significantly reduces the emotional stress experienced by all parties, including the first-aider.

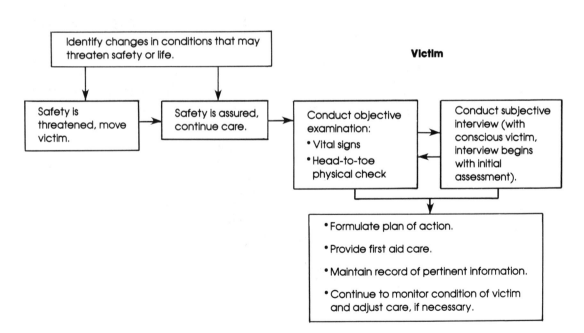

**FIGURE 2.4**

Summary of secondary assessment.

## ___Emergency Scene Reappraisal

During secondary assessment, the safety of the emergency scene is reappraised, because circumstances may have changed considerably since the initial assessment. This is particularly true if the first-aider has devoted extensive time to correcting immediately life-threatening conditions. Increasing numbers of bystanders may threaten the collapse of a platform or landing on which a person injured in a fall is lying. Leakage of hazardous substances, minimal at first, may have increased to the point of placing everyone in the vicinity in jeopardy. Traffic around a motor vehicle accident may have become dangerously congested.

In the case of such an accident, and depending on the circumstances (e.g., availability of flares or other signals and of helpers), placing markers to alert oncoming traffic may be called for. These markers should be positioned at regular intervals to the rear of the accident scene (and ahead, if the traffic pattern warrants) to allow a safe stopping distance for approaching vehicles (Table 2.1). The minimum distance from the accident scene for the markers is determined by adding the posted speed limit to the safe stopping distance at that speed (Grant, Murray, and Bergeron 1983). Thus, if the posted speed limit is 50 miles per hour, the maximum safe stopping distance is 186 feet; and the markers should be placed at regular intervals up to a total of 236 feet (50 plus 186) to the rear and, if necessary, ahead of the accident (National Safety Council 1975).

Ensuring a safe environment may require further responses by the first-aider during the secondary assessment. When safety has been assured, the next step in secondary assessment, detailed reexamination of the victim, can be performed.

## ___Victim Reexamination

Secondary assessment is much more extensive and systematic than initial assessment. As stated previously, its purpose is to identify conditions that are not immediately life

**TABLE 2.1**

Minimum Distance Markers Should Be Placed to Warn Oncoming Traffic of a Traffic Accident

| Speed Limit (mph) | Stopping Distance Range* (ft) | Minimum distance markers should be placed (ft) |
|---|---|---|
| 25 | 53–59 | 84 |
| 30 | 69–78 | 108 |
| 40 | 108–124 | 164 |
| 45 | 132–153 | 198 |
| 50 | 160–186 | 236 |
| 55 | 193–226 | 281 |

*This column adapted from *Student Workbook and Defensive Driver's Manual* (Chicago: National Safety Council, 1975).

threatening but require corrective action. Some can become life threatening, others can cause unnecessary pain and suffering if not cared for.

Reexamination has two parts: *subjective interview* and *objective examination*. The subjective interview is conducted with the injured or ill person if the person is conscious, or with witnesses (if available) if the person is unconscious. The questions to ask, the order in which to ask them, ways to ask them, and how to utilize the information thus gathered are discussed subsequently.

### The Subjective Interview

The interview with a conscious victim can, and probably should, begin when the first-aider arrives on the emergency scene. An interview consists of more than a simple series of questions. It can also serve as a calming exchange of dialogue. The potentially stress-reducing reassurance provided by the interview for the frightened, apprehensive victim can be an important factor in a first aid encounter.

**First Steps in the Interview**     The first steps in a subjective interview may appear rather fundamental when written out. In the heat of an emergency situation, however, fundamental principles and guidelines are often forgotten. It is advisable for the first-aider to follow a consistent pattern of information sharing and questioning in developing subjective interviewing skills. Learning such a pattern will facilitate the gathering of necessary information in the actual situation. Being organized and composed in asking questions reassures the victim that the first-aider is competent. It is recommended that the subjective interview of a conscious victim be initiated in the following manner:

1 Take a position so as to be seen by the victim.
2 Introduce yourself and ask the victim's name.
3 Reassure the victim. Use his or her name while conversing or asking questions. Make eye contact whenever possible (Figure 2.5). Don't be afraid to touch (e.g., a hand, the back, a shoulder); touch is comforting and reassuring. Do not use empty phrases of reassurance (e.g., "Nothing to worry about," "Everything's OK"); the person's confidence will probably be diminished by such comments.
4 Begin by asking simple, direct questions. A good starter set of questions includes
  a *What happened?* Ask for specific information; simply finding out that the person fell is not sufficient. Find out, for instance, what the distance was and how the person landed. The former can provide insight into the extent of injuries and the latter into the likely (though not necessarily the only) area of the body that is injured.
  b *Are you in pain? Where?* The answers to these questions can also give directions to injuries. It is always possible, however, for some injuries to be masked by the pain of others. The objective examination should uncover these. With an illness-related emergency, the questions can be rephrased or extended: How long have you felt ill? Have you had this problem before?

**FIGURE 2.5**

During the interview, the
first-aider tries to take a
position where eye contact
with the victim is possible.

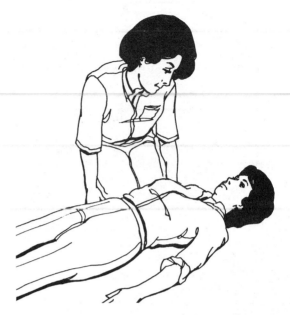

What medication (if any) do you take or have with you for this problem?
Have you taken it as prescribed?

c *Can you move your arms, legs, fingers, toes?* Inability to do so may indicate
injury to the spinal cord. Be careful about asking the person to actually
move an extremity. If it is broken, moving it can cause additional damage.
Ask about numbness, tingling, or burning sensations in the extremities—
these symptoms also indicate possible spinal cord damage. **In any instance
of suspected spinal cord injury, do not move the person unless essential.**

These first four steps in the subjective interview need not be delayed until the initial
assessment has been done. If the victim is conscious, the interview should begin immediately and be carried out simultaneously with the examination for immediate life-
threatening situations. The interviewer must take care, however, not to appear dis-
tracted or not listening. A perception of lack of attention will seriously erode the victim's
confidence in the first-aider. This is another reason the first-aider should develop a
relatively consistent pattern for conducting the subjective interview.

The information gathered during the interview must be retained for transmittal to
the medical personnel who relieve the first-aider. When working alone and dealing with
a life-threatening condition requiring continuous care, the first-aider may have to rely
on memory alone. Under other circumstances, however, it may be possible to take notes
(or have a bystander do this). In any case, the first-aider must retain some form of
"record" of the information gathered from the victim and/or witnesses, the specific care
delivered and the individual's response to that care, and relay this information to arriving medical personnel.

5 Beginning with the first exchange and throughout the subjective interview
with the conscious victim, maintain a calm, directed, "emergency-side"
manner. Ask questions that elicit answers about how the person feels. Do not

ask leading questions (e.g., "Do you feel pain radiating from your chest down your arms?"); such questions can place fear-arousing symptoms and conditions into the person's mind. Remember that one of the most important benefits of a well-handled subjective interview is the reassurance the injured person receives that he or she is not alone in this crisis—that a concerned, competent first-aider is there to help.

**Continuing the Interview**     The following questions may be viewed as comprising the second stage or phase of the subjective interview. In reality, the interview continues uninterrupted. As it progresses, the first-aider may also begin or continue the secondary assessment of physical condition.

1 *How old are you?* The answer tells whether the injured person is a minor, and it may be needed for other reporting purposes. If the person is indeed a minor, ask how his or her parents can be contacted. Arrange to have the parents notified as soon as possible, and inform the person that this has been done.

2 *What is your current medical status?* Knowledge of previously existing conditions related to the current emergency is clearly of importance. Previous sudden illnesses of this nature, and even medical problems not related to the current emergency, may be important in determining what first aid care and subsequent medical care should be provided or avoided.

3 *What medication(s) are you currently taking?* This extends beyond medication that may be directly related to the emergency. It includes all medicines. The information gathered serves the same purpose as the medical status data.

4 *Do you have any allergies?* A sudden illness may have its basis in an allergic response (e.g., anaphylactic shock after a bee sting). Information related to medicinal allergies will be of particular importance to the medical personnel who take subsequent responsibility for the victim.

5 *Do you wear any type of emergency medical care symbol (or carry a card of this nature)?* Generally the answer to this would surface in response to one or more of the previous questions. A confused or disoriented person, however, may fail to volunteer this information. The presence of a "medical alert" type of bracelet, necklace, or wallet card signals that this person has a particular medical problem that must be taken into account in any emergency (Figure 2.6).

6 *Do you want any particular persons contacted regarding this emergency?* As indicated previously, the parents (or legal guardian) of minors should be contacted. The adult victim may want a spouse, relative, or close friend notified. Regardless of his or her age, the person may want the family physician notified. Arranging for notification of persons identified by the victim further contributes to reassurance.

**Subjective Interview: Summary**     As repeatedly indicated, the subjective interview is not conducted in a vacuum. Initial and secondary assessments of the victim's condition need to be done almost simultaneously. If a consistent pattern of questioning and information sharing is followed by the first-aider, the interview should take only a few minutes. Conducted concurrently with other examinations, the interview will not delay the administration of necessary first aid care.

**FIGURE 2.6**

Medic Alert bracelet.
(Photo used with permission of Medic Alert Foundation International, Turlock, Calif.)

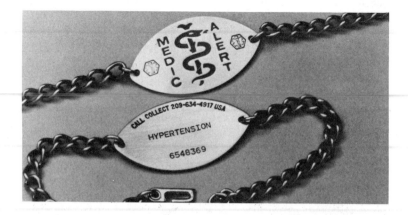

When properly conducted by a competent, confident first-aider, the subjective interview can be a source of much needed reassurance for the victim and of information necessary for decisions about the first aid care to be delivered. The interview of witnesses because of unconsciousness or incoherence of the victim requires judgment on the part of the first-aider. Witnesses who are relatives or friends may, because of their emotional involvement, prove poor choices. The first-aider who has to rely on witnesses for the subjective interview may need to approach them as psychological victims of the emergency.

Finally, the information gathered may prove invaluable to the first-aider and subsequent personnel responsible for the victim's care. The completion of the subjective interview is a required aspect of first aid care unless prohibited by the conditions found at the emergency scene.

**The Objective Examination**

The objective examination involves checking for signs and symptoms that indicate the existence or effects of an otherwise not readily observable injury or illness. *Signs* are objective evidence of dysfunction. *Symptoms* are subjective in nature, depending on personal experience or on the observer's judgment. Signs are definitive, while symptoms are speculative. Chief among the signs or definitive indicators of dysfunction are changes in *vital signs*: pulse, respiration, skin temperature, and occasionally skin color. Many other signs and also symptoms can help identify dysfunction and point the way toward the appropriate first aid response. Following the assessment of a victim's vital signs the second phase of the objective examination involves a head-to-toe physical assessment of the victim's body integrity. The latter is principally needed in emergencies involving trauma.

On completing the objective examination, the first-aider must develop a plan of action for meeting the first aid needs identified and then deliver the indicated first aid care in an organized, logical sequence. It is possible to proceed in a deliberate manner during secondary assessment because any immediately life-threatening conditions have already been addressed in the initial assessment. As indicated above, the objective examination itself is divided into two sequential parts: (1) determination of the victim's vital signs and (2) the head-to-toe examination.

**Determination of Vital Signs**     Vital signs include the pulse, respiration, and temperature. Some authorities also include skin color, but a variety of difficulties limit its usefulness as a sign for the first-aider. Vital signs provide definitive, quantifiable data related to the strength and stability of three of a victim's basic life-sustaining functions: heart action (pulse), breathing (respiration), and equilibrium between heat production and heat loss in the body (temperature).

During the initial assessment, the first-aider has quickly checked for the presence or absence of respiration and a pulse and has undertaken immediate resuscitation if one or both were not found. The purpose of checking the pulse and respiration during the secondary assessment goes beyond mere determination of presence or absence: It is to determine the perceived strength, consistency, and precise rate of each. Body temperature is not checked during the initial assessment but is given high priority during the secondary assessment. Abnormal body temperature can signal the presence of a variety of conditions, some of them life threatening and requiring immediate attention (e.g., shock). In the conduct of the objective examination, vital signs are checked as follows:

*PULSE*     Three characteristics of the pulse are assessed: rate, consistency/regularity, and strength. As during the initial assessment, the carotid artery is the preferred site, but the radial or femoral artery (the brachial in an infant) may be used if the carotid artery is not accessible.

1 *Rate.* Pulse rates vary from person to person. As a general rule, an adult's pulse rate with the body at rest is usually between 60 and 80 beats per minute. The pulse rate in children tends to be higher—80 to 100 beats per minute—and of infants generally between 100 and 120 beats per minute. The first check of pulse rate during the objective examination preferably encompasses two or three readings of fifteen seconds each (one-fourth of a minute). Each reading is then multiplied by four to determine the number of beats per minute. The rationale for this is rather simple. Given the number of distractions that can occur in any emergency situation, maintaining an accurate count over a sixty-second period of a beat as rapid as that of a pulse is very difficult. More than one initial fifteen-second reading is necessary to protect against interpreting a momentary deviation as representative of the pulse rate. (At this stage of the assessment, the victim is indeed breathing and has a pulse. If not, the first-aider would be administering CPR and would not be spending fifteen seconds measuring pulse rate) (see Chapter 6).

2 *Consistency/regularity and strength.* Determining pulse consistency/regularity and strength requires a subjective judgment by the first-aider. Because blood is forced through the arteries by the rhythmic beat of the heart, the surges felt when pressure is applied to the artery should occur at constant intervals. The strength of the pulse is essentially dependent on the ease with which it can be detected by the fingertips. Strength is a difficult characteristic to determine because it varies from person to person under normal circumstances.

In attempting to take a victim's pulse, regardless of the anatomic site, some general rules apply. As noted in the initial assessment section of this chapter, the thumb should not be used to measure a pulse because it has a pulse of its own that will mask the pulse being measured. Concentration and the proper amount of pressure are required to locate and sense a pulse. Locating and measuring a weak pulse usually require more concentration. Finding the femoral pulse in a very fat or muscular person may require considerable pressure. Again, too much pressure is not advisable as it can cause the pulse to fade and may interrupt blood flow. Excessive pressure on the carotid pulse may interfere with respiration.

Variations in pulse can be interpreted in many ways. Some of these interpretations require further verification through continued assessment. Others may point to specific first aid measures to be taken (e.g., no pulse—CPR). The meanings of specific findings and appropriate first aid responses are discussed later in this text. Here, the reader might review the techniques presented earlier in this chapter for checking the pulse in the carotid, radial, femoral, and brachial arteries.

*RESPIRATION*    During the initial assessment, the first-aider is concerned only with the presence or absence of breathing or of an obstruction in the airway. During the secondary assessment, attention is directed to the quality of respiration. Quality is assessed by measuring the rate and determining respiratory characteristics through a complete respiration cycle.

*Respiration rate* is measured in units of complete respiration cycles. One full respiration cycle includes both inhalation and exhalation. Respiration rate slows with age. Infants normally breathe from thirty-five to fifty times a minute. The respiration rate in children can vary considerably, though it is normally above twenty per minute. *Taber's Cyclopedic Medical Dictionary* lists the respiration rate for children during the second year of life as twenty to thirty per minute, and during the fifteenth year as fifteen to twenty per minute. Grant and colleagues (1983) indicated that the condition of a 1- to 5-year-old child is serious if the respiration rate exceeds forty-four per minute, and that medical care should be sought for children 5 to 15 years of age if the respiration rate is above thirty-six per minute. Likewise a respiration rate below twelve per minute is cause for seeking medical care.

*Measuring the respiration rate involves counting the number of full respiration cycles,* usually by observing the rise and fall of the chest wall. Typically this is done in fifteen- or thirty-second time frames and multiplied by four or two, respectively, to arrive at the number of respirations per minute. Some factors can complicate the accurate measurement of respiration. The victim's rate can be affected by his or her awareness of being observed. A simple trick for avoiding this is to appear to be monitoring the pulse (e.g., the first-aider remains in position and continues gentle pressure on the artery) while actually counting respiration cycles. Additionally, for various reasons it may not be possible to discern chest movements. In such a case, if the person is lying on the back and does not have apparent chest or abdominal injuries, the first-aider attempts to feel for chest movements by lightly resting the hand near the base of the sternum (xiphoid process). Another technique is for the first-aider to drape the victim's arm over his or her chest, hold the wrist, and observe the up and down movements of the arm (Thygerson 1982).

Respiration is assessed by observing the respiratory characteristics of rhythm, depth, difficulty of breathing, and associated noises. In addition to an appropriate rate, the *rhythm* of respiration should be consistent, each cycle occurring at regular intervals. The *depth* of breathing and the *difficulty* the person seems to encounter during it can be of particular significance. When breathing is intermittent, difficult, and gasping in nature, airway obstruction may persist and appropriate clearing procedures should be followed. *Noises* unnatural to the breathing process should also be noted.

Abnormalities in any of these respiratory characteristics can be indicative of a wide variety of conditions. The first-aider's job is to clear the airway, restore or artificially supplant the breathing cycle, and notify the proper medical authority of observations when he or she is relieved of responsibility for the victim.

*BODY TEMPERATURE*     Normal body temperature is considered to be 98.6° F; however, a difference of one degree plus or minus may be found depending on the body site where temperature is measured. Typically, body temperature is measured by placing an oral thermometer under the tongue for three to five minutes. This is the site that produces the 98.6° F reading. Measurement of body temperature rectally typically yields a temperature one degree higher. The rectal thermometer should be left in place for three minutes. Axillary temperature measurement (e.g., in the armpit) is less reliable and typically produces a temperature one degree lower. Five to ten minutes are needed to record an axillary temperature. In young children and infants, body temperature is preferably measured rectally. In all other individuals, temperature should be measured orally. Axillary temperature recording is a measure of last resort. New disposable thermometers that provide "rapid" digital readouts are receiving favorable response from medical authorities. As a final note, the first-aider should be aware that body temperature no matter where it is measured, even in healthy people, can range from 97° to 99° F. Thus, variations from the norm should be noted, but are not cause for alarm unless the deviation is greater than 1.5° F.

*SKIN TEMPERATURE AND COLOR*     A more rudimentary way to assess the state of equilibrium between heat production and heat loss is to "measure" *skin temperature*. Simplistically this involves placing the back of the hand against the person's skin. The first-aider will often be able to detect differences in the coolness or heat of the skin, an indication that excessive heat is being retained or lost.

Determination of skin color is not a particularly useful diagnostic technique, principally because of difficulty in identifying the victim's normal skin tone for comparison. Cyanosis, resulting from a deficiency of oxygen (and therefore an excess of carbon dioxide) in the blood, produces one of the most marked changes in skin color. The reduced presence of hemoglobin typically causes a bluish or grayish discoloration, often first noted in the toes and fingers. Even this change may be difficult to identify, particularly among Blacks and those with darkly pigmented skin. Nonetheless, there may be times when changes in skin color can be effectively determined and illness or trauma consequently identified. These situations are discussed in subsequent chapters.

**The Head-to-Toe Examination**     During the head-to-toe examination the first-aider examines the victim's entire body in a systematic fashion. The person's condition is determined in an anatomic stepwise process beginning with the head and neck and culminating with the toes. Before discussing the head-to-toe examination, a few general points are worth considering. First, not all accident or sudden illness situations require such an examination. In some instances, the emergency condition and the first aid care needed will be self-evident. In other instances, the need to maintain first aid care for life-threatening conditions may preclude engaging in the secondary assessment altogether. **Finally, the head-to-toe examination is more applicable to injuries involving trauma than to sudden illness.**

The conscious victim should be alerted to the potential discomfort or pain that may be experienced during the examination. Necessarily, the first-aider exercises great care in the conduct of the head-to-toe examination until he or she has confirmed the absence of neck and spinal cord injuries. Indeed, the severity of the threat posed by spinal cord injuries requires assessment of the neck as the first step in the examination. Should the presence of spinal cord injury be suspected, the head and neck must be immobilized before proceeding with the examination (see Chapter 9).

*THE NECK*    If the first-aider is unsure whether a neck injury has occurred, the victim should not be asked to move the head. The anterior neck is carefully exposed and checked for cuts, bleeding, and deformities. The windpipe is examined for proper alignment in the middle of the neck. Victims of throat cancer or other conditions that have resulted in surgery to the upper airway often have an opening in the front or side of the neck for taking in air. This opening is called a *stoma.* If a stoma is present, the first-aider makes sure it is open. (Artificial respiration for a person with a stoma is discussed in Chapter 5.) If the victim is wearing a medical device, the information on the device is noted but the device is not removed.

The *cervical spine* is that section of the spinal column that passes through the neck. The cervical spine is checked for deformity, pain or tenderness, cuts, or bleeding. This is done by first steadying the person's head by cradling the chin in one hand, then, with the other hand on the lower portion of the back of the neck, gently applying fingertip pressure along the cervical spine to the point where the head and neck meet. The hands are switched and the examination is repeated on the other side of the neck. If pain, tenderness, or deformity is present, the head is immobilized before the head-to-toe examination is continued.

*THE HEAD*    Examination of the head involves checking the condition of the scalp, skull, eyes, ears, nose, and mouth. In general, the first-aider attempts to determine the presence or absence of pain, tenderness, deformity, cuts, and bleeding. Additionally, the level of consciousness is continuously monitored.

The *scalp* is checked by placing the fingers behind the neck and gently moving them across the scalp toward the top of the head. This can be done even when the person is supine, without moving the person.

The *skull*, including facial bones, is checked for deformities, fractures, and swelling and examined for discoloration. Particular care is taken to avoid further contamination of skull wounds with dirt or possible bone fragments.

The *eyes* are examined to see if they respond appropriately to changes in light. Bright light should cause the pupils to constrict, while removal of that light should result in dilated pupils (Figure 2.7). Certain accident or sudden illness situations can result in uneven pupils, that is, in one being constricted and one being dilated. Failure of the

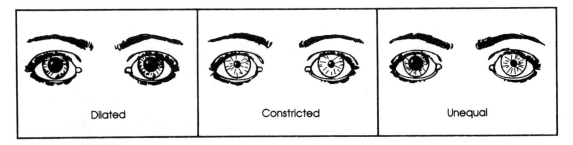

Dilated          Constricted          Unequal

**FIGURE 2.7**

The eyes are examined for the proper response to changes in light.

pupils to respond to changes in the amount of light entering the eyes indicate a number of problems. Dilated pupils are a sign of cardiac arrest, stimulant drug reaction (e.g., overdose of amphetamines), or any number of other conditions resulting in unconsciousness. Constricted pupils are associated with disorders of the central nervous system and with depressant drug reaction (e.g., codeine, heroin). Unequal pupils are generally associated with head injury or stroke. The first-aider should not attempt to diagnose a specific condition from examination of the eyes. This is the role of a skilled medical care provider. The first-aider simply checks (and subsequently monitors) the eyes, principally to ascertain the consciousness of the victim.

To check the victim's pupils, the first-aider shines a penlight into one eye at a time and observes the pupil for dilation. Initially the light should not be directed into the pupil. Rather it is aimed at one corner of the eye and moved toward the pupil, while the first-aider watches for gradual constriction. If a penlight is not available, in daylight or in a brightly lighted environment the test can be made by placing a hand alternately over each eye and then removing it, watching for pupillary response. If the person is unconscious, the eyelids should be kept closed to prevent the corneas from drying out. Each eyelid can be drawn back to test for light response.

*If the victim is wearing contact lenses, he or she should remove them if possible, or at least move them off the cornea.* The latter is also recommended for an unconscious victim. Otherwise serious eye damage can result.

The *ears and nose* are observed for the presence of fluid or blood. The person's head should not be turned to inspect the ears. Clear fluid draining from the ears may indicate injury involving the loss of cerebrospinal fluid. This clear, waterlike fluid can also be lost through the nasal passages. Whenever such fluid drains from the ears, nose, or both, the possibility of a skull fracture is strong.

The *mouth* is again examined to assure the maintenance of a clear airway. The mouth is gently opened to check for bleeding or accumulation of blood from other sources (e.g., nose or lungs). If any foreign objects in the mouth were missed during the initial assessment, or if others have since accumulated (e.g., vomitus), they are removed at this time.

**FIGURE 2.8**

The first-aider examines the rib cage by placing his or her hands at each side of the victim's chest and gently pressing toward the sternum.

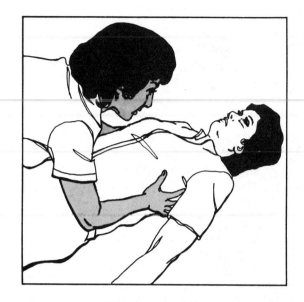

*THE SHOULDER GIRDLE*    The shoulder girdle is examined for possible fracture of the clavicle or scapula. The clavicle (collarbone) is gently palpated and checked for any deformities from the point where it joins the sternum to the point where it joins the scapula. The scapula is seldom involved in an injury (as opposed to the clavicle) except in cases of severe back blows. Fracture or dislocation of the clavicle or scapula should be suspected if the shoulder on the injured side appears clearly lower than that on the noninjured side.

*THE CHEST*    In the head-to-toe examination, the area of the body being checked often must be exposed. When the injured person is female and the first-aider is male, or vice versa, this can be embarrassing and uncomfortable for both. The first-aider must simply remember the purpose of the objective examination and cope with the embarrassment. The conscious victim, however, should be reassured. He or she should be fully informed about what is to take place and why it is necessary. A witness of the same sex as the injured person should be present, if possible. Finally, the privacy of the person being examined is carefully maintained to the extent feasible under the emergency conditions.

The chest is examined for pain, deformity, open or closed wounds, penetrating objects, and bleeding. Gentle pressure is applied starting at the clavicle, moving on to the sternum, and then to the rib cage. The rib cage is examined by placing the hands at each side of the chest and then compressing the ribs (Figure 2.8). The person must be alerted to the possibility of pain associated with these procedures. The chest is observed for unequal expansion during respiratory cycles. Unequal chest expansion (i.e., alternately one side expanding while the other contracts) can be life threatening because of potential for interfering with the respiratory cycle.

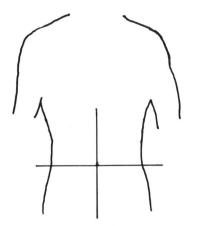

**FIGURE 2.9**
Division of the abdomen
into quadrants. The lines
bisect at the umbilicus.

*THE ABDOMEN*    The first-aider examines the abdomen for pain, tenderness, deformity, rigidity, lumps, wounds, penetrating objects, and bleeding. The palm portion of the fingers is used to carefully palpate the entire abdomen, after alerting the victim to the possibility of pain. The abdomen should be perceived as divided into four quadrants (Figure 2.9), and then the specific quadrant(s) noted in which pain, rigidity, or any other abnormality is identified.

*THE LOWER BACK*    The back is examined in two stages. First the lower back is checked. Then, *before the upper back is examined, all other steps in the head-to-toe examination of the supine victim are carried out.* As with the cervical spine inspection, the first-aider examines the lower back principally for pain, tenderness, and deformity. In the supine person, the curvature of the spine leaves a gap (small of the back) that allows the hand to be slid gently under the person to the spine. Applying gentle point pressure with the fingertips, the first-aider moves the hand up and down the spine as far as possible (without necessitating movement by the victim), searching for pain, tenderness, and deformity. If any of these is encountered, the patient's spine should be immobilized before the examination proceeds further (see Chapter 8).

*THE PELVIS*    The pelvis is gently compressed to check for pain. The presence of pain may indicate a fracture. The victim should be alerted beforehand to the possibility of pain from this procedure.

*THE LOWER EXTREMITIES*    Both legs are examined from the hips to and including the feet. The first-aider checks for pain, tenderness, deformity, wounds, bleeding, protruding bones, swelling, dislocation, and sensation. Gentle palpation for pain can identify possible fracture sites.

The lower limbs should not be moved, because the possibility of spinal cord injury has still not been eliminated. The *distal pulse* (Figure 2.10) is checked to determine whether circulation to the lower extremities is impaired. The first-aider checks also for nerve pathway injury by asking the victim to flex the feet. Additionally, he or she presses

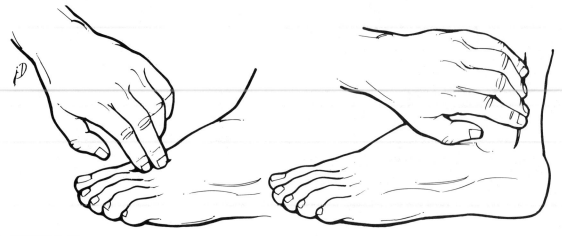

**FIGURE 2.10**

The distal pulse, a sign of circulation in the lower extremities, can be checked in two ways.

gently on a toe, asking the person to identify which toe is being touched. With a pencil or other pointed object, the first-aider presses against the sole of the victim's foot to test for sensation. Finally, the victim is asked to push the foot against the palm of the first-aider's hand (Figure 2.11). Inability to do so can indicate spinal cord injury. To adequately examine the lower extremities it may prove necessary to cut or tear pants legs. The person is alerted to this, and it is done without moving the extremity to be examined.

*THE UPPER EXTREMITIES* The first-aider checks the arms for pain, tenderness, deformity, swelling, discoloration, protruding bones, wounds, and bleeding. Each arm is

**FIGURE 2.11**

The spinal cord may be damaged if the person cannot press his or her foot against the first-aider's palm.

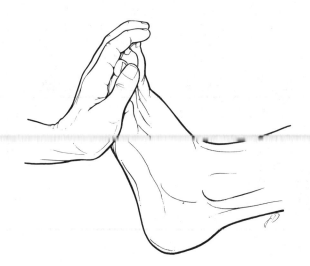

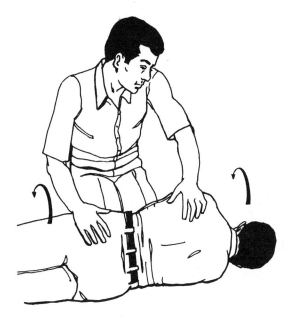

**FIGURE 2.12**
The upper back is examined by rolling the victim as a unit onto the side. This is not done if neck, spinal cord, chest, or abdominal injuries are suspected.

examined from clavicle to fingertips. Suspected fracture areas are gently palpated. The pulse is again checked (as during the initial assessment) to assure continuation of adequate circulation. The victim is asked to flex the hand. The first-aider touches the person's fingers and asks him or her to identify each contact. In addition, the victim is asked to grip the first-aider's hand firmly. Inability to flex the hand, sense the fingers being touched, or grip firmly are indications of spinal cord injury. These procedures are repeated on the other arm and hand.

*THE UPPER BACK*    If spinal cord injury has not been indicated during the head-to-toe examination to this point, examination of the upper back is appropriate. The person is rolled onto his or her side (unless injury to the extremities, chest, or abdomen prevents this). Kneeling on the victim's side toward which he or she will be rolled, the first-aider slides his or her hands well under the victim's shoulder and hip and turns the body as a unit toward the first-aider's knees (Figure 2.12). *If any uncertainty exists about the presence of a neck injury, examination of the upper back is not attempted unless there is no other way to stop severe bleeding.*

*THE UNCONSCIOUS PERSON*    The head-to-toe examination should be carried out even if the person is unconscious. **The first-aider should always assume the presence of a spinal cord injury when working with an unconscious victim.** Testing for nerve pathway damage in the extremities of an unconscious person requires the pressing of a pointed instrument (e.g., pencil, small stick, even a pin if nothing else is available) against the bottom of the foot and the palm of the hand. The first-aider must be very sensitive to subtle reactions to pain in testing for tenderness or other conditions. A

**TABLE 2.2**

Sequential Summary of the Objective Examination

**Determine vital signs.**

Assess characteristics of pulse.
Assess characteristics of respiration.
Determine body temperature.
Check skin color and temperature.

**Conduct head-to-toe examination of**

Neck: windpipe, cervical spine
Head: scalp, skull, eyes, ears, nose, mouth
Shoulder girdle: clavicle (collarbone), scapula
Chest: sternum, rib cage
Abdomen (note condition by quadrant)
Lower back: spine
Pelvis
Lower extremities: hip, upper leg, lower leg, ankle, foot, toes
Upper extremities: upper arm, forearm, wrist, hand, fingers
Upper back

sequential summary of the objective examination is presented in Table 2.2. Subsequent chapters of this book cover specific first aid measures for each condition suspected to be present as a result of the initial and secondary assessments of a suddenly ill or injured person.

## SUMMARY

How the first-aider responds during the first moments after coming upon an accident or sudden illness situation can be crucial. The victim's life can hang in the balance. Long-term disabling conditions may be prevented. The first-aider's reaction depends on how well prepared he or she is and how systematically he or she is able to utilize this preparation in the emergency situation. Conditions that pose an immediate threat to life must be responded to first, then those that potentially threaten life if not treated, and finally those that do not threaten life but do require assistance. An initial assessment is done to determine immediately life-threatening conditions. The three major areas of concern are

1 Absence of or interference with respiration.
2 Loss of circulation.
3 Extensive uncontrolled bleeding.

When these conditions have been either excluded or adequately responded to (i.e., respiration and circulation stabilized and bleeding controlled), a secondary assessment is done to inventory all possible conditions requiring first aid care. The secondary assessment comprises a subjective but systematic interview and an objective examination. The latter is divided into two parts:

**1** Determination of vital signs
**2** Head-to-toe examination

The objective examination should be conducted regardless of the victim's state of consciousness. Slightly different procedures are indicated if the person is unconscious, and the first-aider must be more sensitive to involuntary responses.

The first-aider must relay to medical personnel who subsequently take responsibility for the victim all pertinent information gathered from the victim and witnesses, details regarding the care delivered, and the person's response, and any other changes in the person's condition since being discovered.

_____ **CHAPTER MASTERY: TEST ITEMS** _____

**True and False**

Circle One

1. A victim of a life-threatening emergency should be given first aid care immediately, regardless of the safety of the setting.   T   F
2. The most immediately life-threatening emergency is severe bleeding.   T   F
3. The femoral artery is located in the groin.   T   F
4. The first-aider should move the suddenly ill or injured person to a place where assistance can be conveniently administered.   T   F
5. Loss of large amounts of blood can cause shock.   T   F
6. Severe external bleeding is always readily observable.   T   F
7. Internal bleeding can be life threatening.   T   F
8. The safety of the emergency scene is reappraised during the secondary assessment.   T   F
9. Signs are subjective in nature and represent personal or observed perceptions of body dysfunction.   T   F
10. A victim of accident or illness is reassured if the first-aider discounts the seriousness of the emergency by making statements such as, "There is nothing to worry about."   T   F
11. If the victim is conscious when found, determining his or her prior state of consciousness is not necessary.   T   F
12. With a conscious victim, the subjective interview should begin immediately and be conducted simultaneously with the initial examination.   T   F
13. If the victim is a minor, the first-aider must obtain parental or guardian consent before administering first aid care.   T   F
14. The first-aider must try to identify what medications, if any, the ill or injured person is currently taking.   T   F
15. Witnesses who are related to the victim may need to be cared for as psychological victims of the emergency situation.   T   F

16. The pulse rate of adults at rest usually ranges between 100 and 120   **T**   **F**
    beats per minute.
17. If the victim's clothing must be disturbed, it is advisable to have a   **T**   **F**
    witness present who is of the same sex as the victim.
18. Respiration rate is measured in units of respiration cycles.   **T**   **F**
19. Rectal temperature typically is one degree lower than oral temperature.   **T**   **F**
20. The head-to-toe examination has greater applicability for emergencies   **T**   **F**
    involving sudden illness than for those involving trauma.
21. Shining a bright light in the eye should cause the pupil to dilate.   **T**   **F**
22. In treating an unconscious person wearing contact lenses, the lenses   **T**   **F**
    should not be disturbed.
23. Uneven chest expansion may indicate a life-threatening respiratory   **T**   **F**
    condition.
24. Asking the victim to grip the hand of the first-aider is a test for spinal   **T**   **F**
    cord injury.
25. An objective examination is **not** conducted on an unconscious person.   **T**   **F**

## Fill In the Missing Word(s)

1. Conditions that do not threaten life but do require first aid care are identified during the _____.
2. The purpose of the initial assessment is to determine the presence or absence of conditions that are _____.
3. A first aid technique for responding simultaneously to a combined circulatory and respiratory emergency is _____.
4. In a respiratory emergency, artificial respiration should continue to be provided until _____.
5. During the secondary assessment, symptoms of injury or sudden illness that are not readily observable are identified while conducting the _____.
6. An objective piece of evidence indicative of an illness or other dysfunction of the body is called a _____.
7. The head-to-toe examination has greater applicability to emergencies involving _____ than to those involving _____.
8. Medical alert devices typically come in the form of _____, _____, or _____.
9. The objective examination has two sequential components: _____ and _____.
10. Quantifiable data related to the strength and stability of three of a victim's basic life-sustaining functions are obtained by checking a victim's _____.
11. The three characteristics of a victim's pulse and respiration that are checked during the objective examination are _____, _____, and _____.
12. The artery recommended as the primary source for measuring the pulse of an infant is the _____.
13. Because it has a pulse of its own that will mask the victim's, the first-aider should not palpate a pulse using his or her _____.
14. A single respiration cycle includes one _____ and one _____.
15. The respiration rate per minute for infants typically ranges from _____ to _____.

**Multiple Choice (Circle the Best Answer)**

1. A condition that would **not** be considered immediately life threatening is
   a. severe bleeding.
   b. cardiac arrest.
   c. spinal deformity.
   d. respiratory cessation.

2. The order in which the first-aider must respond to the conditions listed in question 1 is
   a. B, A, D, C.
   b. D, B, A, C.
   c. A, B, C, D.
   d. B, D, C, A.

3. The preferred first step in checking circulation is to palpate the
   a. carotid pulse.
   b. radial pulse.
   c. brachial pulse.
   d. femoral pulse.

4. The secondary assessment should
   a. identify all remaining injury or sudden illness conditions requiring first aid.
   b. be carried out in a systematic, orderly way.
   c. serve to reassure the victim and concerned bystanders.
   d. all of the above.

5. A procedure that is not a part of the secondary assessment is
   a. an interview of the victim or other appropriate parties.
   b. identification of conditions that are an immediate threat to life.
   c. formulation of an appropriate plan of first aid action.
   d. a detailed reexamination of the victim.

6. The information gathered by the first-aider during the subjective interview **need not always**
   a. be retained in some form of "record."
   b. specify the first aid care delivered.
   c. be in written form.
   d. be relayed to the skilled medical personnel who replace the first-aider.

7. In determining the status of vital signs, the measure that is the least effective is
   a. pulse characteristics.
   b. skin color and temperature.
   c. body temperature.
   d. respiration characteristics.

8. In the head-to-toe examination, the first body part examined is the
   a. scalp.
   b. skull.
   c. eyes.
   d. neck.

9. The presence of a clear, waterlike discharge from the ears or nose or both may indicate

   a. skull fracture.
   
   b. lung damage.
   
   c. cardiac arrest.
   
   d. fractured clavicle.

10. A distal pulse is taken in checking the status of circulation to

    a. the extremities.
    
    b. the neck.
    
    c. the abdomen.
    
    d. the eyes.

11. A procedure that is **not** done during examination of the lower extremities is

    a. palpation for pain or tenderness.
    b. pressing of a pointed object against the sole of the foot.
    c. straightening of bent legs before the examination.
    d. requesting the victim to press the foot against the palm of the first-aider's hand.

12. The first-aider should always assume that he or she is dealing with spinal cord injury when

    a. the victim is unconscious.
    b. the victim is unable to flex the foot or feet.
    c. the victim is unable to grip the hand of the first-aider.
    d. all of the above.

## Discussion Questions

1. What is the purpose of the initial victim and emergency scene assessments? Why should they be conducted concurrently? Give a simple example of how this might be accomplished.

2. The first-aider has a responsibility to protect the privacy of the victim. How can this best be achieved?

3. When should the first-aider consider palpating a brachial pulse?

4. Explain how the checking of respiration and circulation during the secondary assessment differs from the checking of these same functions during the initial assessment.

5. Under what circumstances might it **not** be appropriate to conduct the head-to-toe examination?

## BIBLIOGRAPHY

Grant, H. D., R. H. Murray, and J. D. Bergeron. *Emergency Care,* 3d ed. Bowie, Md.: Robert J. Brady, 1983.

National Safety Council. *Student Workbook and Defensive Driver's Manual.* Chicago: National Safety Council, 1975.

*Taber's Cyclopedic Medical Dictionary.* 14th ed., s.v. "respiration."

Thygerson, A. L. *The First Aid Book.* Englewood Cliffs, N.J.: Prentice-Hall, 1982.

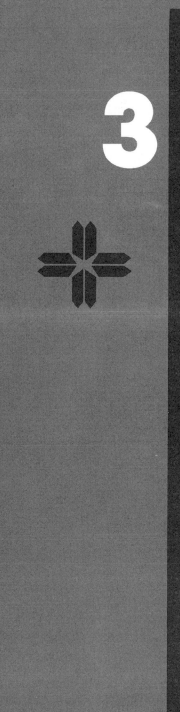

# 3

# Psychological First Aid

JUDITH MCLAUGHLIN, PH.D.

After completing this chapter you will be able to

- Define psychological first aid, rape, psychiatric emergency, suicide, and violent behavior.
- Describe the most important points in dealing with a psychological emergency.
- Explain why it is important to control personal negative emotions, to the extent possible, in administering psychological first aid.
- Describe the behavior, and the reasons behind it, of accident victims, bystanders, and family and friends present at the scene.
- Discuss the goal of psychological first aid for accident victims, family, friends, and bystanders; rape victims; disturbed persons; suicidal persons; violent persons.
- Describe the range of emotions that occur in the aftermath of a rape.
- Explain the role of fear in abnormal behavior.
- Describe the guidelines for judging which behavior is normal or abnormal.
- Explain what to do for a person who appears disturbed.
- Demonstrate recognition of the characteristics of the suicidal person, and factors that contribute to the decision to commit suicide.
- Identify the clues of suicidal intent.
- Explain what to do to prevent suicide, and what to do if suicide is in progress.
- Cite some causes of violent behavior.
- Describe characteristics of the violent individual, and what to do when someone becomes violent.
- Describe community health resources involved in the prevention, treatment, and follow-up of various mental health crises.

## _____INTRODUCTION

Anxiety and fear are natural reactions when threats to health suddenly appear. Anyone who receives a physical injury in an accident will suffer emotional trauma. It clearly is of great value when someone skilled in the techniques of psychological first aid is among the first on the scene of an accident or illness. Because the mind has a dramatic effect on the eventual outcome of the victim, the act of providing comfort and reassurance (essentially the definition of psychological first aid) helps recovery start almost immediately. Similarly, if the first-aider recognizes the fear and anxiety inherent in psychiatric emergencies, the calming effects he or she elicits may enable the disturbed person to trust the care givers who follow.

The most important point in handling any psychological emergency is to be calm, direct, purposeful, and confident. Panic is communicable. If the first-aider behaves in a composed, assured manner, often the individual, bystanders, and family members also calm down. A second important point is the fact that first-aiders, like everyone else, have their own prejudices and limitations, and successful intervention with psychological first aid techniques demands the ability to control these prejudices well. The first-aider may encounter a situation in which an individual's aberrant behavior is causing the individual personal difficulty and also difficulty for others, and the first-aider must take control and act. The first-aider may witness behavior that is shocking, frightening, or degenerate and may not be able to avoid feelings of anger or disgust. The first-aider should not stifle these reactions, but should develop ways of channeling them and turning them to good use. Involvement with the disturbed person may be unavoidable, but emotional reactions can be controlled. By anticipating personal feelings, as well as the feelings of others, the first-aider reduces the number of unknowns in the situation and thus enhances his or her own effectiveness in attending to physical first aid needs.

The sections that follow are for persons not trained in psychological counseling or law enforcement but who may be on the scene when an individual requires psychological first aid.

## ——PSYCHOLOGICAL EMERGENCIES

### ——The Needs of the Injured Person

Persons who have just been in an accident have many mixed emotions and feelings. Victims may fear they are going to die, or that they will be disfigured. They may experience a distortion of reality, especially when faced with the possibility of amputation or body mutilation. Fears of disfigurement may often be greater than the situation indicates. They may feel helplessness or loss of control, especially when they are totally dependent on the help of someone they do not know. They may show signs of regression, reverting to childlike behavior because they are fearful and in need of comfort. They may attempt to deny or minimize their injuries; they may be angry or confused. To a great extent, the way a particular person copes with a traumatic event such as an accident depends on his or her psychological makeup, but it is important for the first-aider to respect and recognize the spectrum of behavior that can occur. *The goal of psychological first aid is to reduce stress, fear, and embarrassment and to preserve the victim's dignity as much as possible.*

Steps to take with the injured person:

**1** Identify yourself and specify what is going to happen. While attending to physical needs, explain what is being done, even if the person seems dazed or incoherent. The victim may be uncomfortable accepting care from a stranger, and explanations of procedure help develop a relationship.

2 Have and communicate the attitude that the situation can be coped with. There is no need to deny that a given situation is serious, but convey a positive attitude that the victim will recover.

3 Each person responds differently to stress and anxiety. Thus, respect the victim's right to behave as he or she does, even if the behavior is not understood or condoned. Never tell an accident victim to "shape up." Never show blame, resentment, or ridicule. Such judgments interfere with the ability to be helpful.

4 Do not say anything in the presence of a semiconscious person that it is undesirable for the person to hear. Even people who appear unconscious can often relate events and conversations later (Riehl 1970). Avoid statements like "I've never seen such a bad injury," or "He isn't going to pull through." Do not be responsible for instilling unnecessary fear and anxiety through careless words.

5 Protect the person's dignity by covering naked parts of the body. The victim may be embarrassed and shamed by being unclothed. If clothing was burned off or has been removed to facilitate care, and the condition of the person allows, drape the body with towels, clothing, or blankets.

6 Do not take angry or hostile outbursts personally. The accident victim is most likely extremely frightened and anxious, and is directing inner turmoil at those closest. Remain calm and continue to reassure the person.

7 If the victim asks about injuries, be honest about explaining their extent, but use tact and sensitivity.

8 If the victim asks about the condition of family members or friends who were also in the accident, it is generally a good idea to tell the truth about the extent of the injuries as known (Schultz 1983). There is some disagreement about this, however; some emergency medicine specialists feel it is not in the best medical interests of a badly injured person to have to deal in addition with shock and grief over a loved one's condition (Russell and Biegel 1982). Still, most people fear the worst, and whatever information is provided may not be nearly as bad as they had imagined. Hiding the truth may increase fear, especially if the person knows the seriousness of the accident. If information about the condition of others involved in the accident is not at hand, try to obtain it; otherwise, if appropriate, tell the victim that care is being provided for friends and family members by others and they are doing the best they can. It is best to let someone in authority disclose the deaths of others in the accident (Schultz 1983).

The American Psychiatric Association (1964) has identified five possible behaviors in disasters that involve multiple casualties. Because anyone, including bystanders, victims, and family members, may exhibit these behaviors in even a minor accident, they are given here.

• *Normal reaction.* Fear and extreme anxiety, expressed as shakiness, sweating, and nausea, are hallmarks of the normal reaction.

• *Panic.* In addition to the symptoms and signs of the normal reaction, judgment and reasoning disappear and the person appears hysterical and may run from the scene. This kind of behavior can lead to mass panic in others. Care should be taken to isolate a person in panic and provide reassurance.

- *Depression.* The person moves slowly, appears numb and dazed, and seems unable to respond. He or she is in danger of walking in front of dangerous equipment or into the path of oncoming cars. A person in depression is helped by establishment of rapport, being allowed to ventilate feelings, and being given a small task to do.
- *Overactive reaction.* The person begins markedly increased physical activity, talks rapidly, jokes inappropriately, or makes useless suggestions. He or she may be argumentative and may interfere with other activities. The best help is giving the person something to do and allowing him or her to ventilate feelings.
- *Severe physical reaction.* This may include severe nausea or hysterical blindness or paralysis. The symptoms are very real to the person and should not be denied. The person should be made comfortable and medical aid summoned.

## —The Needs of the Family and Bystanders

Bystanders can be assigned tasks at the scene if this is appropriate. Having something to do reduces their anxiety and helps them feel useful. They can help direct traffic, act as messengers, obtain something warm to drink for family members, help clear debris, or help contain any crowd that gathers, among other activities. If people stop to help, the first-aider can make use of this sometimes unexpected resource. Bystanders, rather than just being in the way, can be extremely helpful and useful.

The first-aider may have to provide psychological first aid to uninjured family members or friends of the accident victim at the scene. They may be emotionally disabled by what has happened; their behavior can range from numbness and disbelief to hysteria and flight. Emotional stress secondary to an accident situation is as disabling as any physical injury. Family members fear for their loved ones and may be extremely anxious, frightened, and distressed. In some cases their anxiety may be so extreme that they become angry, demanding, and hostile and interfere with the emergency care being given to the victim. Family members commonly lash out at care givers, implying or stating incompetence and demanding that their own physician be called. However upsetting this may be, the first-aider must realize that the behavior arises from concern and distress and should not be taken personally. Understanding this enables the first-aider to accept and acknowledge family anger. Family members will remember later any kindness and understanding shown to them at the scene and will be grateful for efforts on their behalf. *The goal of psychological first aid for family members is reassurance and concern for their needs.*

Steps to take with family members:

1 If lifesaving measures are in progress, have someone act as a communication link to the family and provide as many details as possible of the extent of the injuries and what is being done. It does not help family members to withhold

information because "they can't handle it." Be positive, but by all means be truthful. Convey the facts with care, concern, and tact.

2 Try giving the individual a small task; having something to do channels the emotional energy into action, rather than reaction.

3 Offer something warm to drink if it is available. This does not necessarily take the individual's mind off what is happening, but it conveys caring and concern.

4 Try sitting quietly with the person (if this is possible), touching the forearm or holding the hand. This communicates humanness and personal concern. Doing this makes it possible for the family members to ventilate feelings and fears.

5 Monitor personal feelings. Do not allow resentment of the behavior of the family member to surface. It is important to understand the range of behavior that occurs with acute emotional reactions to stress situations. Telling someone to "snap out of it" only increases the person's feelings of inadequacy.

6 If the accident victim dies at the scene, do not try to prevent the family from viewing the body if they so request. Many family members have later stated their anger at being advised not to view the body because the injuries were "too severe" (Schultz 1983). In reality, the injuries may not be as bad as they fear, and may be less than what they imagined. Seeing and touching a lifeless body at the scene of an accident makes death hard to deny; acceptance of the reality of death helps the family gain the courage to do what must be done—planning the funeral, burying the loved one, and eventually letting go. As Schultz (1983) noted, families who do not see the body have a difficult time believing that it was their loved one who was on the train when it crashed, or whose body was dredged from the river. The family member may cry out, hug the body, try to breathe life into it, or sit quietly and talk to the dead person. Let this happen; it will help immeasurably later.

7 Suggest that the family and friends contact their minister, priest, rabbi, or counselor to be with them now. Many families do not want to bother this very important resource person, but often the person is a valuable part of the family's support group, and the value of his or her presence as an anchor now and in the future is great.

## ___ASSISTING THE RAPE VICTIM

Rape is forcible sexual intercourse. It is a crime of violence and aggression, not of lust or passion, though it takes place in a sexual context. The weapon in rape is the penis, which is used to attack, humiliate, and subordinate the victim, usually a woman (Strong and Reynolds 1982). The actual incidence of rape is probably four to ten times higher than what is reported, and it is estimated that approximately one woman in every thousand will be a rape victim each year (Reed-Flora and Lang 1982).

A rape victim often suffers great psychological damage as well as physical trauma. She may have been brutally beaten, forced into bizarre sexual acts, and psychologically assaulted. She may fear reprisal from the rapist or believe she caused or could have prevented the rape, a belief that is also held by many men. She may be reluctant to obtain needed medical care because she does not want her parents or friends to know (Strong and Reynolds 1982).

*The goal of immediate care after a rape is to reduce the victim's stress state, preserve evidence, care for shock or minor bleeding, and arrange for transportation to a facility that can collect evidence of the assault as well as provide medical treatment.*

Steps to take with a victim of rape (Foley and Davies 1983):

1 Communicate empathy, warmth, and respect. Studies have shown that rape victims remember vividly the remarks made to them shortly after the rape assault (Holmstrom and Burgess 1978). Therefore it is particularly important that care be nonjudgmental and reassuring; anything else can impede the person's resolution of the rape experience.

2 If talking with the victim by telephone, calmly suggest that she lock all doors and windows to protect her safety until someone can reach her. This is a first step in conveying that someone cares, and helps the person initiate something herself to reduce her fear and anxiety. If unable to go to her, suggest that she call a rape crisis center, the police, or at least a friend for support. If the victim is not in a safe place, call the police or a rape crisis center for someone to go to the victim.

3 Make sure the victim is dressed warmly. Physiological and psychological stress can cause a person to go into shock. Control any minor bleeding.

4 To help preserve the evidence that can later identify and convict the assailant, advise the victim **not** to change clothing, straighten the scene, wash herself, or douche, gargle or rinse her mouth, eat, drink, urinate, or defecate. If she insists on changing clothes, have her bag each item separately in a paper bag to carry to the hospital. *It is crucial to collect rape evidence according to legal protocols developed by the emergency care facility and police crime laboratories.*

5 Some victims who are very anxious may perceive immediately subsequent physical contact as a threat and may withdraw from anyone's touch. Others are comforted and reassured by touch, and may accept a hand to hold if offered. Do not be afraid to try, and do not take any rebuff personally.

6 Resist any impulse to blame the victim for the assault. The first-aider's role is to provide comfort and help the victim to a place where she can obtain care.

7 Some women respond to rape with furious anger. These feelings may frighten them, because they were brought up to be gentle. It helps to explain that this is a normal response. Rape is a terrible experience, and victims respond in all kinds of ways, from calm to hysteria to fierce anger. Reinforce for the victim that her feelings, whatever they are, are okay.

8 Guilt is one of the most destructive emotions in the aftermath of a rape attack. Be sure to explain to the victim that she is not responsible for another's violent behavior.

A rape victim has just survived an assault in which power and control were the key issues. She has been humiliated, degraded, and abused. An advocate from a rape crisis center can help a fearful and anxious victim through the crisis and explain the upsetting events that often occur in the aftermath of a rape. Increasingly, hospitals and emergency departments are developing guidelines for sensitive care of rape victims and protocols for a rape examination. Nurses are being trained to respond to the special psychological and medical needs of the rape victim (Foley and Davies 1983). Many police departments now provide extensive training for their officers in handling rape victims. Sensitive care can help the victim immeasurably in coping with the immediate crisis, and can go a long way toward facilitating physical and psychological healing.

# ___PSYCHIATRIC EMERGENCIES

A psychiatric emergency exists when an individual suddenly exhibits unusual, disordered, or socially inappropriate behavior (Weiss 1974). Abnormal behavior and mental illness often cause fear, repugnance, and misunderstanding in the public. Social attitudes toward them are shaped by popular stereotypes and the movies rather than by direct experience or sound information. However, most episodes of abnormal behavior are temporary and transient, and in some cases self-limiting. The most bizarre, grotesque, or socially unacceptable behavior may be short-lived. Also, most change in behavior is toward improvement and regaining of self-control, no matter how grotesque the behavior may seem at the moment (Weiss 1974).

## ___The Disturbed Person

Several general and specific characteristics of abnormal behavior, regardless of cause, help in deciding whether a person requires help from mental health professionals (Matthews and Rowland 1974). These characteristics are illustrated in the following questions:

1 Have sudden, big changes in the person's life-style and behavior taken place? The first-aider should inquire about present behavior compared with past action. If a man was a homebody, loved his wife and children, never quarreled with anyone, and never missed a day of work and then suddenly began drinking excessively, abusing his wife, and not showing up for work, he might have a mental disorder or a brain tumor.

2 Is there memory loss? All people have memory loss at one time or another, but if the person cannot remember even simple things like name, location, or the day, month, or year, the possibility of brain damage or psychological dysfunction is high.

3 Does the person have feelings of persecution? People actually do plot against others, but some disturbed persons *imagine* that someone is going to cause them serious harm or even kill them, and their reasons for believing this are often bizarre or not readily understood.

**4** Does the person have grandiose ideas? Some disturbed people may believe they are very important and this alone explains why they act as they do. For example, they may believe they are Christ.

**5** Does the person talk to himself or herself? All people talk to themselves on occasion, especially when they are upset. People with psychological dysfunctions, however, can carry on entire conversations with imaginary people for long periods of time.

**6** Does the person hear voices? It has been speculated that these voices are the person's own thoughts, though the person may deny knowing where they come from. Alternatively, the person may claim they are coming from the television set, or act as if listening to someone else.

**7** Does the person have visions, smell strange odors, or have a peculiar taste sensation? Sometimes physical illness, such as brain tumor or the effects of alcohol or drugs, can be responsible for changes in senses.

**8** Does the person think he or she is being watched or talked about?

**9** Does the person have unrealistic physical complaints? Some disturbed people believe that something is wrong with their body that is not medically possible, such as that their brain is decaying or their fingers have turned into snakes. These symptoms are very real to the person and cause as much suffering as any actual physical complaint.

**10** Does the person exhibit extreme fright? The person may tremble or glance over the shoulder in terror, and may incur injury or cause injury to others in getting away from what is feared.

The term "psychotic" should not be an important term to the first-aider. For many reasons psychosis cannot be precisely determined, and whether a person is mentally competent is ultimately a judicial question. More important to the first-aider is the ability to recognize symptoms that indicate the kind of care needed. Most mentally ill people are neither violent nor dangerous, although the possibility exists. *However bizarrely they act, people with mental illness are afraid.* They are afraid of the world in which they live, the people around them, and what is happening to them. If their behavior is the outcome of fear, steps can be taken to reduce the fear. An offer of help and protection from the first-aider gives the disturbed individual a means to trust someone. *The goal of psychological first aid for the disturbed person is to reduce the person's fear and emotional distress while arranging his or her transportation to a facility where appropriate referral can be made.*

Steps to take with a disturbed person (Matthews and Rowland 1974):

**1** Because of the many causes of bizarre behavior, the person should be evaluated by a trained mental health professional. Call the office of a mental health facility and ask about its referral procedures. In most cases it will have a qualified counselor meet with the person, evaluate the cause of the behavior, and begin treatment. (Not all cases of unusual behavior require a call for emergency help, but the person definitely should be evaluated by a professional who can tell if the cause is an organic illness, alcohol or other drug abuse, or "mental illness.")

**2** If the person is dangerous to himself (herself) or others, call or have someone else call the police and an ambulance. Do not try to handle the situation alone. Police officers are or should be trained to handle mentally disturbed persons, can physically restrain a violent person, and can control any crowd that gathers. Ambulance personnel can provide medication for sedation, if necessary, and transport the person to an emergency facility or a mental health facility. Make sure the caller requests that sirens and bullhorns not be used. A disturbed person's sensory awareness may be heightened, and loud or shrill noises can increase fear.

**3** While waiting for help, be gentle, calm, and nonthreatening. Do not display force. Mental confusion and perceptual disturbances increase distrust.

**4** Stay some distance away from the person at first, to preserve his or her sense of personal space. Do not make the person feel controlled or pressured. Move closer as rapport is established, but do not touch the person.

**5** Actively listen to the person. Not being listened to is a common reason for violent outbursts. Paraphrase the individual's words and feed them back: "I hear you saying that...." This corrects misunderstandings and lets the person know that someone is listening.

**6** Decide on a plan of action, then stick firmly to it. Surprisingly, the disturbed person will often find this firmness reassuring, but being in an ambivalent mental state, the person may argue about whatever is suggested.

**7** Do not argue about delusions, and do not agree with them. Do not convey the impression that the person is crazy. If asked, "Do you believe me?," say something like "I believe that your feelings are true and that you are telling me the truth as you see it."

**8** **Never** try to physically restrain an adult singlehandedly. Physical restraint should be used only as a last resort, and is most effectively done in a coordinated team effort directed by a trained person such as a police officer or an emergency medical technician. Physical restraint is most often needed to transport someone likely to cause personal harm or harm to others, when sedation of the person is not possible, or while waiting for sedating medication to take effect.

**9** Do not leave the person alone.

**10** Do not lie or in any way try to deceive the disturbed person. This will erode any trust built up in the disturbed person and will make it difficult for the person to accept future help.

**11** It is natural to react in a hostile manner to verbal abuse. Try instead to remain calm and ask why the person is afraid or angry. Ventilating these feelings may help the person calm down.

**12** Take careful note of the person's symptoms, as well as what is being said. Is the person hallucinating or talking about plots? Does he or she mention any particular person or group?

## ___The Suicidal Person

Although suicide deaths are underreported because of the stigma attached to them or because the circumstances of death are equivocal, suicide is on the increase, especially among young persons. Around 35,000 deaths annually are attributed to suicide in the United States (Hatton, Valente, and Rink 1977).

It is generally accepted that a combination of factors contributes to the decision to commit suicide; the act does not result from one simple problem. Some common themes include

- Inability to cope with lost relationships or the death of someone important
- Overwhelming depression, a sense of helplessness
- A crisis/impulse response to a major life change, such as loss of a job
- The influence of drugs or alcohol
- Revenge, or an attempt to punish another
- Success, promotion, or an increase in responsibilities
- Sickness, serious illness, surgery, accident, loss of limb, or inability to withstand physical pain
- No sources of support, or inability of friends and family to help
- An attempt to regain contact with a loved one who died
- A feeling that no one, anywhere, cares
- One or more almost successful attempts in the past

Most people who commit suicide give clues to their intentions. Danger signals include

- Statements revealing a desire to die (e.g., "you'd be better off without me")
- Open talk of suicide
- Sudden changes in behavior (withdrawal, apathy, moodiness)
- A sudden improvement in mental attitude, as if a decision has been made
- Giving away cherished possessions
- Buying or updating insurance
- Putting personal affairs in order, such as paying longstanding bills, making a will
- Purchase of a rope, gun, or other weapon
- Excessive drug or alcohol use
- Insomnia, crying spells

The risk of suicide is greatest in men over the age of 40, young persons between the ages of 14 and 22, and anyone with a history of suicide attempts. However, all kinds of people die by their own hand—young and old, rich and poor, male and female, of all races and creeds. *The goal of the first-aider relating to suicide is to recognize clues and warnings that a person is contemplating suicide and to obtain professional help for the person; or to provide immediate first aid care to the person who has attempted suicide and to arrange transportation to an emergency facility where appropriate care can be given and referral to mental health professionals can be made.*

Steps to take in preventing suicide*:

1 Speak to the individual regarding concern about his or her welfare (e.g., "I've been worried about you lately.").

2 Give nonjudgmental feedback about the individual's behavior (e.g., "I've noticed that you aren't sleeping much; you're losing weight and seem withdrawn from people.").

3 Do not be afraid to ask the individual directly if he or she has been contemplating suicide. It is a pervasive myth that talking about suicide may give the person the idea; suicidal people already *have* the idea. Normalize the thought of suicide by acknowledging that it is common for people to feel helpless and hopeless enough to think about ending life, and that everyone has those thoughts from time to time.

4 Emphasize that the crisis will only last a short time, and ask if the individual would be willing to postpone the decision and explore other choices about solving the problem. Suggest that there might be a different solution (not better, but different).

5 Share confidences, if it seems appropriate, but only if it is possible to be truthful (e.g., "I have a counselor whom I call when I need to be taken care of, who gives me support when I feel hopeless.").

6 Take charge in a firm, confident, caring manner. Most people in a crisis want someone to do this. Formulate a plan of action, then say, "For now we are going to do this...."

7 Do not scoff or laugh at the individual's reasons for feelings of despair (e.g., "Don't you realize he is a worthless person anyway?"). Conditions that may seem improbable to you are very real and painful to one contemplating suicide.

8 Do not attempt to shock the person out of action by saying, "Go ahead!" Impulsively he or she may do just that. In many cases people contemplating suicide feel they have gone too far and therefore must go through with the act, or they will be blamed or punished. Emphasize that nothing has been done that cannot be undone.

9 Do not leave the individual alone, not even for a moment, no matter how urgently the person pleads. If it is necessary to leave the room, have someone else come in.

10 Accompany the individual to a mental health center or a hospital where an appropriate referral to a mental health professional can be made. Professional help can show new approaches, improve the person's situation, suggest alternatives, help raise the person's self-esteem, and provide appropriate drug therapy if necessary. Give active emotional support, but be aware of your limitations regarding the care of the suicidal person.

---

* Adapted from "Suicide: Intervention Guidelines" (pamphlet) (Atlanta: Link Counseling Center, 1983), with permission.

Steps to take if a suicide is in progress:

1 If a victim of poisoning is conscious, induce vomiting if the poison is a drug but not if it is a strong acid, strong alkali, or petroleum product (see Chapter 10). Stop any bleeding caused by slashing of wrists or other parts of the body, using direct pressure and pressure points; then apply a clean bandage (Chapter 7). If a substance such as carbon monoxide has been inhaled, get the person to fresh air at once and administer mouth-to-mouth resuscitation if necessary (Chapter 5). In any case, call for help or go to the nearest hospital immediately.

2 If the individual is unconscious, and the cause of unconsciousness is not apparent, keep him or her warm and lying on the side to prevent choking (see Chapter 15, coma position). Administer mouth-to-mouth resuscitation if breathing stops. Call an ambulance immediately.

3 If talking by telephone to someone who has attempted suicide, firmly ask the individual to give his or her location. This is an essential step, because the person may lose consciousness during the call. Ask for the street address, the apartment number, and the telephone number and area code. If the person appears confused or does not know the number, ask him or her to read aloud the number from the center of the dial.

  At this point there may be several alternatives. If it is possible to have someone call an ambulance from another telephone, tell the individual to unlock the door and leave it open, and keep the person on the line until help arrives. Keep reassuring the person that everything is being done to help. Do not become judgmental or hostile—remain calm and affirmative. Alternatively, ask the individual if anyone is there or nearby. If so, firmly tell the individual to bring that person to the phone **now**. Be assertive; press on the individual the need for someone to be there. Ask whether that person can drive him or her to the nearest emergency facility. If very close to where the victim is calling from (e.g., within five minutes), consider hanging up the telephone, calling an ambulance, and then going to the person to administer assistance.

4 If the individual requests that someone in the family be notified, do so promptly.

5 Understand that the ultimate decision to live or not to live is the individual's. The suicide attempt may be successful. A first-aider may experience feelings of guilt, anger or betrayal. Try instead to take credit for having tried to help. Obtain personal support through counseling—it is important to talk the crisis through.

People who attempt suicide are not usually psychotic or mentally ill, and most of them do not want to die. Often a suicide attempt is a means of communication and indicates intense despair and pain; some people feel unable to make their point any other way. It is important for the first-aider to be aware of the problem of suicide, to learn about available resources in the community, and to give persons considering suicide the support and direction that might shift the balance toward the decision to live.

## __The Violent or Homicidal Person

Violent people are assaultive and exhibit destructive behaviors or threats. Violence often accompanies medical or psychiatric illnesses, and may be recurrent. Violent individuals exhibit such behavior as shouting, pacing, shaking the fist, slamming doors, swinging a chair, or displaying a weapon such as a knife or gun. They may destroy their own or their family's property and may commit violent assault with any weapon. It is well known that a person with homicidal tendencies is more likely to attack family members than strangers (Eisenberg and Copass 1982).

The great majority of persons who perpetrate violent acts, especially homicide, do not have a psychiatric or medical condition as strictly defined, but have personalities that are characterized as antisocial or sociopathic. Also, those who are most likely to commit such acts tend to have histories of criminal activity, such as a juvenile record, a number of previous arrests, or conviction for a violent crime. Age is related to violence, almost 80% of violent acts being performed by those under 50 years of age (Slaby, Lieb, and Tancredi 1981). Some of the causes of violent behavior include alcohol intoxication, temporal lobe epilepsy, drug intoxication from PCP (phencyclidene, also known as angel dust) or amphetamines, antisocial personality, organic brain syndromes such as brain tumor, paranoid states, schizophrenia, catatonic excitement, and interpersonal stress, such as a family quarrel (Slaby, Lieb, and Tancredi 1981). *The goal of psychological first aid for the violent or homicidal person is to keep the situation from becoming worse.*

Steps to take with a homicidal person:

1 The first task is to obtain help for the person and those whom he or she might be threatening. Be empathetic and nonthreatening, but call the police. They can help see to it that violence does not escalate into a tragedy and can determine if an ambulance is needed for transportation to a hospital or mental health facility.
2 In some cases, a person threatening violence verbally can be given time to calm down and cool off. Many loud-mouthed people will cease their assaultive behavior, especially if there is no threat. *If unsure, call for help immediately.*

## ___THE MENTAL HEALTH CARE SYSTEM: WHERE TO SEEK ADDITIONAL HELP

Many communities have federal and state supported mental health care facilities that are involved in the prevention, treatment, and follow-up of psychological and psychiatric problems. They are particularly useful in providing counselors to individuals who have not coped well in the aftermath of an accident or disaster or to those suffering from the psychological trauma of rape, a suicide attempt, or an actual suicide. They usually offer individual and group therapy, and families of victims can discuss with trained professionals their concerns and questions. These agencies, as well as hospital emergency facilities, can make referrals to private psychiatrists and psychologists in the community.

Some communities also have rape crisis centers and suicide crisis centers; these agencies provide community education about the problems of rape and suicide, offer preventive strategies, and have available advocates for a rape victim or a suicidal person.

Voluntary, private, and self-help groups or agencies, such as Alcoholics Anonymous and drug treatment centers, offer support and therapy when an underlying problem such as alcohol and drug abuse can be identified. They also give help to family members and make referrals to other mental health professionals in the community.

Some emergency departments and mental health departments offer brief counseling for families who have lost a loved one in an accident or by homicide or suicide. Ministers, rabbis, and priests are also an important resource for help with adjustment after a traumatic episode or loss. These community resources exist to assist people through the stages of grief, to help them avoid crippling emotional problems, and to aid in their healing.

## SUMMARY

Psychological first aid is the comfort and reassurance provided to accident victims, their family and friends, and bystanders; to rape victims; to disturbed persons; and to suicidal persons or their survivors. Knowledge of psychological first aid techniques is invaluable at an accident or illness scene, where attention to the victim's psychological needs can help speed physical recovery. Additional goals are prevention of embarrassment and shame, preservation of dignity, and provision of a means for appropriate referral for additional psychological help. Many victims can resolve the crisis state within a relatively short time after the episode. For those who cannot, a number of mental health agencies exist that can provide resources and professional support. With care and personal concern, victims of psychological and psychiatric crises can be helped to recover.

## CHAPTER MASTERY: TEST ITEMS

### Discussion Questions

1. Discuss the emotions and feelings of a person who has just been in an accident.
2. Why is it important for the first-aider not to say anything in the presence of a semiconscious person that he or she would not want the person to hear?
3. List and discuss the five possible reactions identified by the American Psychiatric Association that people experience in disasters involving multiple casualties.
4. Define rape. What factors contribute to the psychological trauma of the rape victim?

5. Why is it important to advise a rape victim to dress warmly?

6. Why should the rape victim not change clothing or wash?

7. What is the most destructive emotion following a rape attack?

8. Which factors shape our attitudes of fear and misunderstanding toward the mentally ill?

9. Why should the term "psychotic" not be important for the first-aider?

10. When is physical restraint used to control a mentally disturbed person?

11. Define suicide. Why are suicide deaths underreported?

12. Which age groups are most vulnerable to suicide?

13. What are the danger signals of an impending suicide?

14. What are some of the causes of violent behavior?

15. Why is it important to call the police when dealing with a violent person?

16. While driving in a rural area, a car some distance ahead inexplicably crosses the centerline and hits an oncoming car head-on. The driver of one car is dead, the other driver is severely injured, and the first-aider is alone on the scene as yet. In addition to attending to physical needs, what should he or she do to attend to the psychological needs of the injured person?

17. David has been very depressed lately. He sleeps a lot and is missing his classes. He has given his much beloved stereo set to an acquaintance, and last night a handgun was discovered hidden in his closet. From the standpoint of psychological first aid, what is an appropriate course of action?

18. A student driving through a park on the way to a night class sees a young woman suddenly stumble from the bushes, half clothed. Her face and body appear bruised, and cuts on her face are bleeding. When the student stops to help, she hysterically explains she has been raped. What should the student do to assist her?

———————————————— **BIBLIOGRAPHY** ————————————————

American Psychiatric Association. *First Aid for Psychological Disasters.* Washington, D.C.: American Psychiatric Association, 1964.

Eisenberg, M. S., and M. K. Copass. *Emergency Medical Therapy.* Philadelphia: W. B. Saunders, 1982.

Foley, T. N., and M. A. Davies. *Rape: Nursing Care of Victims.* St. Louis: C. V. Mosby, 1983.

Getz, W. L., D. B. Allen, R. K. Myers, and K. C. Lindner. *Brief Counseling with Suicidal Persons.* Lexington, Mass: Lexington Books, 1983.

Hatton, C. L., S. M. Valente, and A. Rink. *Suicide: Assessment and Intervention.* New York: Appleton-Century-Crofts, 1977.

Holmstrom, L. L. and A. W. Burgess. *The Victim of Rape: Institutional Reactions.* New York: Wiley, 1978.

Matthews, R. A., and L. S. Rowland. *How to Handle and Recognize Abnormal Behavior.* New York: National Association of Mental Health, 1974.

Reed-Flora, R., and T. A. Lang. *Health Behaviors.* St. Paul: West Publishing, 1982.

Riehl, C. S. *Emergency Nursing.* Peoria, Ill.: Charles A. Bennett, 1970.

Russell, H. E., and A. Biegel. *Understanding Human Behavior for Effective Police Work.* New York: Basic Books, 1982.

Schultz, C. A. "Grief and Loss." In T. Dravis and C. Warner, eds. *Emergency Medicine: A Comprehensive Review.* Rockville, Md.: Aspen, 1983.

Slaby, A. E., J. Lieb, and L. Tancredi. *Handbook of Psychiatric Emergencies.* New York: Medical Examination Publishing, 1981.

Strong, B., and R. Reynolds. *Understanding Our Sexuality.* St. Paul: West Publishing, 1982.

Weiss, J. M. "Evaluation and Treatment of Psychiatric Emergencies." In H. E. Stephenson, ed. *Immediate Care of the Acutely Ill and Injured.* St. Louis: C. V. Mosby, 1974.

# 4

# Shock

ARA ZULALIAN, PH.D.

After completing this chapter the student will be able to
- Cite the signs and symptoms of shock.
- Describe the basic body changes that occur during shock.
- Perform the first aid necessary to care for shock.

## ___INTRODUCTION

One of the most challenging experiences for any first-aider is the need to respond to shock or to help a victim at risk to shock. Shock can occur immediately and without warning or can be delayed. Shock is best defined as a circulatory deficiency within the body associated with the depression of essential organ functions.

Shock results from lowered cardiac output, not from lowered arterial pressure. Early shock can be present and arterial pressure still be "normal," owing to nerve reflexes that maintain arterial pressure within the normal range even when cardiac output is diminished. The victim may feel fine, be coherent, and act uninjured. The best precautionary measure for the first-aider is to care for all injuries as if shock were suspected. **Preventive first aid for shock can save a life.**

## ___OVERVIEW

Several types of shock may be encountered by a first-aider, and each is considered serious. The most common type, traumatic or physical shock, results from injury and loss of blood. Other types of shock include respiratory, septic, anaphylactic, neurogenic, psychological, metabolic, cardiogenic, brain, and electrical.

In shock, the entire body assumes a defensive physiologic posture. There is generalized disruption of the blood flow. The heart beats faster and superficial blood vessels constrict, forcing more blood to vital organs (the nerve centers of the brain, the heart, the kidneys, and the liver). Some blood that cannot pass through the constricted vessels is lost through seepage into surrounding tissue.

Body cells fail to receive the proper amount of blood and thus do not receive adequate amounts of oxygen and nutrients. Additionally, removal of cellular end products is severely curtailed by the reduction in blood flow. Eventually the blood vessels themselves fail to receive sufficient nutrients and lose their ability to constrict. Following the path of least resistance, the blood rushes back to fill these dilated vessels, and the vital organs are thereby deprived of a sufficient blood supply. The functional capacity of the vital organs gradually begins to diminish and death occurs if shock is not reversed (Figure 4.1).

**It is crucial to begin first aid for shock or for its prevention promptly.** The longer the condition is untreated, the more difficult the victim's recovery. There is a point beyond which death cannot be prevented. In general, any injury or psychological insult that disrupts the blood volume and flow can produce shock. Currently there is no standard measure that can be used to determine the likelihood of shock occurring. People react differently to body tissue damage: What is serious for one person need not be serious for another. Shock can result from blood loss, heart damage, dehydration, internal hemorrhage, venous pooling, injury to the autonomic nervous system, fainting, fractures, burns, poisoning, pain, concussions, excessive heat or cold, and psychological trauma. In view of the numerous emergency situations in which shock may be encountered, the best rule to follow is to **provide first aid for shock in all incidences of sudden injury or illness.**

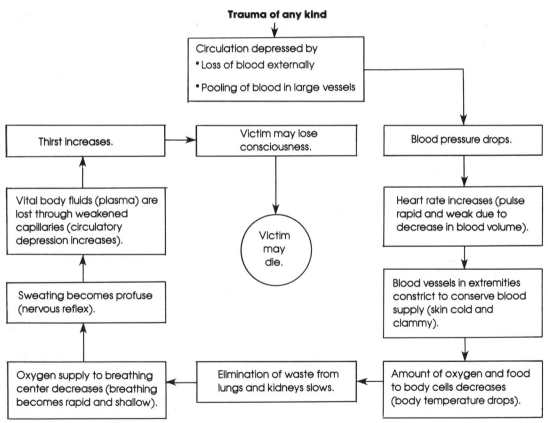

**FIGURE 4.1**

Traumatic shock cycle. (Adapted from Brennan, William T., and James W. Crowe, *Guide to Problems and Practices in First Aid and Emergency Care*, 4th ed. © 1971, 1976, 1981 by Wm. C. Brown Publishers, Dubuque, Iowa. All rights reserved. Reprinted by permission.)

## ___TYPES OF SHOCK

The types of shock identified below result from injuries and insults to the body or psyche that necessarily demand first aid measures beyond care for shock. Each of these emergencies and its related first aid care, however, are discussed in other chapters of this text (e.g., controlling trauma-induced bleeding, Chapter 7). The focus of this chapter is on the shock-related dimensions of such emergencies.

### ___Traumatic

Trauma with subsequent hemorrhage is probably the most common cause of shock. Even contusions can cause traumatic shock, because they often damage the capillaries, thereby allowing loss of plasma into surrounding tissues.

### ___Respiratory

Whenever an injury damages the lungs, the oxygen level in the blood is reduced. This sets in motion the shock process. For obvious reasons this is identified as lung or respiratory shock.

### ___Septic

In the past this condition was commonly called "blood poisoning." Simply stated, it is an infection disseminated throughout the body. The infection travels by way of the blood stream, affecting and causing extensive damage to tissue.

### ___Anaphylactic

Anaphylactic shock is a severe allergic reaction caused by an insect sting, food, medication, or inhalants. It can occur immediately after contact with the allergic substance or can be delayed for several hours. (For a more extensive discussion of anaphylactic shock, see Chapter 10 under the heading Injected Poisons.)

### ___Neurogenic

Neurogenic shock results from an injury to the spine or brain or both. In neurogenic shock the amount of blood reaching the brain is reduced. Control of the diameter of the blood vessels is lost owing to damage to the nervous system, and thus blood circulation is disrupted.

### ___Psychological

Psychological shock occurs when fear or other emotional trauma causes a nervous system reaction, which in turn dilates the blood vessels, interrupting normal blood flow to the brain. At this point fainting may occur. This type of shock is often mild and self-correcting, enduring only temporarily. Psychological shock can, however, be as deadly as any other type of shock. The possibility of psychological shock should be considered in any emergency and preventive first aid carried out.

## __Metabolic

Metabolic shock is usually caused by dehydration after severe diarrhea, vomiting, or other body fluid loss.

## __Cardiogenic

Cardiogenic shock is caused by inadequate functioning of the heart. It develops when the heart muscle cannot pump blood in a balanced and rhythmic manner to all parts of the body.

## __Burn

Burns are classified according to severity. Third- and fourth-degree burns are of primary concern. All such burns can result in shock, because there is complete loss of all layers of the skin, destruction of deeper structures, and loss of body fluids from the burned area.

# ___SIGNS AND SYMPTOMS

Shock has numerous manifestations (Figure 4.2). A person with the following signs and symptoms is experiencing or is susceptible to shock:

- Pulse rapid (usually over 100 per minute) but weak
- Facial skin pale or cyanotic (in individuals with dark skin pigmentation, check the mucous membranes in the mouth or under eyelids and the color of the nails)
- Extremities cool and skin pale and usually moist
- Eyes vacant and lackluster, pupils dilated
- Respiration shallow and irregular
- Inability to remain in an upright or erect position
- Nausea, possibly vomiting
- Perspiration and thirst
- Restlessness or dizziness
- Visible amounts of blood or fluid loss
- Internal bleeding
- Skin dull or chalklike
- Expression anxious or dull
- Eyelids closed or partially closed
- Arms or legs shaking as though chilled
- Partial or total unconsciousness
- Slow responses or answers unrelated to questions
- General weakness

**FIGURE 4.2**

Signs and symptoms of shock.

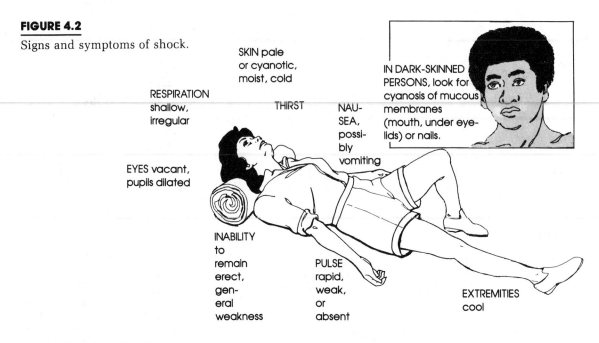

## ＿FIRST AID CARE

Certain general first aid care must be considered before a person is evaluated and treated for shock. The following should be done:

1 Whenever possible keep the victim in the supine position.
2 Assess and provide care as needed for breathing, circulation, and excessive bleeding, and continue to monitor these.
3 Loosen clothing, avoiding unnecessary or rough handling.
4 Do not give fluids or foods.
5 Call for medical assistance.

Whenever a first-aider is caring for a possible shock victim, three words should come to mind—position, heat, and fluids—though not always in this order.

## ＿Position

A victim of an injury or sudden illness is best kept lying down (Figure 4.3). This position aids the return of venous blood to the heart. Figure 4.3 shows four possible positions. The following are guidelines for the use of these positions:

1 The primary function of the position chosen is to maintain an open airway.
2 Whenever possible, keep the person supine (on the back).
3 Elevate the person's feet between eight and twelve inches, except in the case of head injury.

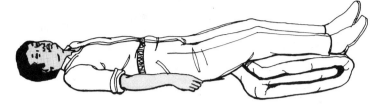

Raise feet slightly to improve circulation.

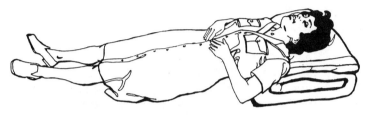

Elevate head and shoulders for head injury, etc.

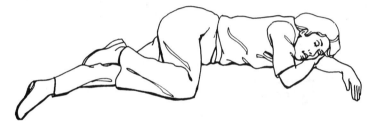

Place unconscious person on side (coma position).

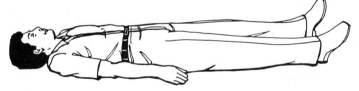

Keep person flat if in doubt.

**4** If on elevation of the feet the person complains of pain, lower the feet.
**5** In the event of a neck or spine injury, do not move the victim.
**6** If the person has difficulty breathing, elevate the head and chest as a unit.
**7** In the event of a head or chest injury, elevate the head and chest as a unit.
**8** If the person is unconscious, place him or her on the side if there is no spine or neck injury.
**9** In the event of vomiting, turn the victim's head to the side using a technique consistent with any other injuries present.
**10** If in doubt as to what to do, keep the person flat on the back.

**FIGURE 4.4**

A blanket, coat, or other covering helps maintain body temperature.

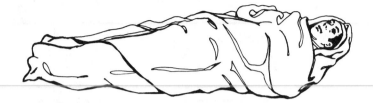

## —Heat

In caring for shock, the victim's body heat must be maintained. The following lists procedures to follow.

1 Maintain body heat as close to normal as possible. Excessive heat causes dilation of superficial blood vessels of the skin, leading to a reduction in the amount of blood in circulation. Cold can lead to shock; if not controlled, hypothermia (Chapter 13) and death may ensue.
2 If body temperature must be raised, be careful not to burn the person. Examples of external sources of heat are hot water bottles, heated bricks, and heated sand. When placing a heat source next to the skin, be sure to cover it with protective material.
3 If the victim's clothing is wet, remove it.
4 Place a blanket, coat, or any other light covering over the person to maintain body temperature and aid comfort (Figure 4.4). If movement will not cause further injury, place a blanket under the person.

## —Fluids

Fluids are necessary for body balance. However, *when caring for shock, give no fluids to the injured person unless essential.* The following are guidelines for giving fluids in relation to shock.

1 Do not give fluids to an unconscious or semiconscious person, one who is experiencing convulsions or vomiting, or one who has abdominal or head (brain) injuries.
2 If it is likely that the person will undergo surgery on arrival at the hospital, do not give fluids.
3 There is no harm in moistening the person's mouth and lips, if requested. Moisten a piece of cloth, squeeze it to extract as much water as possible, and then hold it to the mouth and lips.
4 When medical assistance is delayed for an excessive time (at least one hour at a disaster scene), give small amounts of lukewarm water or juice at fifteen-minute intervals, if needed. The water mixture should preferably include baking soda and salt—one level teaspoonful of salt and half a level teaspoonful of baking soda to a quart of water. Adults and teenagers can be given up to half a glass, children (age 1 up to age 12) a fourth of a glass, and infants, an eighth of a glass.

5 *Never substitute alcoholic beverages for water or any other fluids.* Alcohol increases the blood supply to the surface of the body, thereby diminishing the supply to the vital organs.

6 Seriously burned persons need fluids. If the person is conscious, give water, fruit juices, or sugar water.

## __Pain Reduction

Pain may increase the severity of shock. The corollary is that reducing pain can impede the development of shock or diminish its severity.

Measures that reduce pain include bandaging open wounds, immobilizing suspected and recognized fractures, avoiding rough handling and excessive movements, loosening tight clothing, and others.

## ____ELECTRICAL SHOCK: A SPECIAL EMERGENCY*

Electrical shock results from electricity passing through the body. It can paralyze the respiratory center in the brain. Electrical shock can result from contact with any of a number of sources of electric current, in the home, in the workplace, and outside. The severity of shock depends on the voltage and amps of the current and the duration of contact. The greater these are, the greater the severity. Other factors that affect the severity of electrical shock are the amount of moisture on the person's body surface and the amount of body surface that comes in contact with water during the contact with the source of electricity. Water is an excellent conductor of electricity. A further determinant of severity is the path taken by the current through the body. A path through the trunk and head greatly increases the severity compared with a path through the extremities only.

The electric current going through the victim's body will be transmitted to a rescuer's body if the rescuer touches the victim. Therefore, before a first-aider touches a victim of electrical shock, he or she must shut off the current, if possible. If this cannot be done, the first-aider tries to remove the individual from the source of the current by standing on a dry board and using a dry, nonconductive probe such as a wooden pole (Figure 4.5). The first-aider either rolls the victim away from the current or pulls or pushes the wire away from the victim.

* See also Chapter 11 for a discussion of electrical burns.

---

**Working Safely with Electricity**

Take all necessary precautions when working around electricity. The best safeguard is to shut off the current at the main power box before beginning work. Rubber gloves, rubber-soled shoes, or other appropriately insulated clothing should preferably be worn to reduce the likelihood of electrical shock.

**FIGURE 4.5**

If the current cannot be cut off immediately in a case of electrical shock, the rescuer stands on a dry board and uses a wooden pole or some other nonconductive probe to pull the live wire away from the victim or the victim away from the wire.

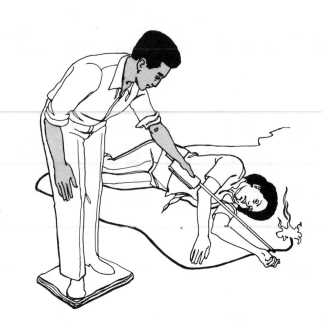

The breathing and circulation status of the victim are assessed. Artificial respiration is begun immediately if the person is not breathing (see Chapter 5). If there is neither a pulse nor respiration, CPR is begun (see Chapter 6). Medical assistance is summoned. If the electrical shock is associated with trauma, heavy bleeding, if present, must also be brought under control.

After the initial life-threatening conditions have been responded to, first aid for shock is completed. This includes maintaining proper body heat, proper position of the victim, giving fluids only if appropriate, and calling for medical help or getting the individual to a hospital.

## SUMMARY

Shock can be a life-threatening condition. The first-aider should be knowledgeable about the physiology of traumatic shock. Shock results from disruption of normal blood flow in the body. Abnormal circulation causes a decrease in the amount of oxygen and nutrients reaching the vital organs and body tissues.

The first-aider performs necessary assessment tasks first and responds to immediately life-threatening conditions (loss of respiration, interrupted circulation, severe bleeding), keeping the possibility of shock in mind. The three key words in caring for shock are position, heat, and fluids. The person should be kept supine (but not moved if spinal cord injury is suspected), kept warm, and given no fluids.

_____ **CHAPTER MASTERY: TEST ITEMS** _____

## True and False                                                                              Circle One

1. Shock results when cardiac output is lowered.                                          T        F
2. When the body goes into shock, blood flow is disrupted throughout the   T        F
   body
3. Individuals react differently to body tissue damage.                                   T        F
4. Alcohol, in a diluted state, may be substituted for water to comfort an   T        F
   accident victim, in the event medical assistance will not be available
   for some time.
5. At present there is a standard measure that is used to determine the      T        F
   likelihood of shock occurring.
6. The proper first aid procedure is to care for all injuries as if shock were   T        F
   present.

## Fill In the Missing Word(s)

1. The most common type of shock, resulting from loss of blood, is known as _____
   shock.
2. When the body is in shock, the removal of cellular end products is severely
   curtailed because of _____ flow.
3. A first-aider can reduce the pain experienced by an accident victim by such acts
   as _____, _____, and _____.
4. Shock that results from an allergic reaction to a foreign protein is called _____.
5. Whenever a first-aider administers care to a shock victim, three words—_____,
   _____, and _____—should come to mind.
6. Four signs or symptoms seen in or experienced by a person in shock are _____,
   _____, _____, and _____.

## Multiple Choice (Circle the Best Answer)

1. Metabolic shock is a condition usually resulting from
   a. inability of the heart to pump blood.
   b. injury to the brain.
   c. emotional trauma.
   d. severe diarrhea.
2. Which of the following is an injury to the spine or brain or both that causes a
   decrease in the amount of blood supplied to the brain?
   a. respiratory shock
   b. physical shock
   c. psychological shock
   d. neurogenic shock

3. Shock can best be defined as
    a. trauma.
    b. vacant eyes.
    c. shallow respiration.
    d. circulatory deficiency.
4. When an individual goes into shock, the body becomes physiologically unbalanced. Which of the following does **not** occur?
    a. Heart beats faster.
    b. Superficial blood vessels dilate.
    c. Blood flow becomes disrupted.
    d. Body assumes a defensive physiologic posture.
5. Septic shock in the past was commonly called
    a. neurogenic shock.
    b. cardiogenic shock.
    c. blood poisoning.
    d. respiratory shock.

**Discussion Questions**

1. Discuss the physiologic changes that take place in the body during shock.
2. A neighbor's young son has come into contact with a live wire downed as a result of a severe wind storm. How should he be separated from contact with the current source? What assessment procedures should be followed? What first aid care may be needed?
3. The single victim of an automobile accident is showing signs and symptoms of traumatic shock. The person is conscious and does *not* have a spinal cord injury. Bleeding has already been brought under control. What first aid care should be provided for the shock?

———————————— **BIBLIOGRAPHY** ————————————

Aaron, J. E., A. F. Bridges, D. D. Ritzel, and L. B. Lindaver. *First Aid and Emergency Care.* 2d ed. New York: Macmillan, 1979.
American National Red Cross. *Advanced First Aid and Emergency Care.* 2d ed. New York: Doubloday, 1082.
Bergeron, J. D. *First Aid and Emergency Rescue.* Beverly Hills, Calif.: Glencoe Press, 1970.
Brennan, W. T., and D. J. Ludwig. *First Aid and Civil Defense.* Dubuque, Ia.: William C. Brown, 1971.
Erven, L. W. *First Aid and Emergency Rescue.* Beverly Hills, Calif.: Glencoe Press, 1970.
Guyton, A. C. *Functions of the Human Body.* 2d ed. Philadelphia: W. B. Saunders, 1971a.
Guyton, A. C. *Textbook of Medical Physiology.* 4th ed. Philadelphia: W. B. Saunders, 1971b.

Hafen, B. Q. *First Aid for Health Emergencies.* 2d ed. St. Paul: West Publishing, 1981.

Henderson, J. *Emergency Medical Guide.* 2d ed. New York: McGraw-Hill, 1969.

Parcel, G. S. *Basic Emergency Care of the Sick and Injured.* 2d ed. St. Louis: C. V. Mosby, 1974.

Stephenson, H. E. *Immediate Care of the Acutely Ill and Injured.* St. Louis: C. V. Mosby, 1974.

Thygerson, A. L. *The First Aid Book.* Englewood Cliffs, N.J.: Prentice-Hall, 1982.

Winkelman, J. L. *Essentials of Basic Life Support.* Minneapolis: Burgess Publishing, 1981.

# 5

# Respiratory Emergencies

ROBERT C. BARNES, ED.D., M.P.H.

After completing this chapter the student will be able to
- Explain the relationship between the likelihood of recovery and the time lapse between respiratory arrest and resuscitation efforts.
- Demonstrate the methods used to determine respiratory arrest.
- Demonstrate the methods used to perform adult resuscitation.
- Demonstrate the methods used to perform infant resuscitation.
- Demonstrate the methods used to open an obstructed airway.

## ___INTRODUCTION

The average adult breathes twelve to twenty times a minute. The average child breathes twenty to thirty times a minute. These ranges can differ slightly, depending on the source used, but are generally acceptable. Cessation of breathing for as short a time as thirty seconds will involuntarily focus a conscious person's attention on the need to breathe.

The process of breathing is controlled by the respiratory center in the brain. Without an oxygen supply to this center, the cells begin to die in four to six minutes. Death is the most common outcome after six minutes, although revival has occurred in many cases beyond this time. The American National Red Cross has reported the odds for recovery on the basis of time lapse between respiratory arrest and the beginning of artificial respiration (Table 5.1). The absence of breathing is a number one priority of the first-aider. Breathing (and circulation) must be restored before lesser injuries receive attention.

## ___THE BREATHING/RESPIRATION PROCESS

For breathing to take place, the chest cavity must increase in size. This occurs when the muscles attached to the rib cage contract, pulling the ribs outward. At the same time the diaphragm pushes down and out. The expanded space in the chest means there is less pressure per cubic centimeter, which means that pressure in the chest is lower than atmospheric pressure. Air rushes in to equalize the pressure. For air to be exhaled, the rib cage muscles relax, the ribs move inward, and the diaphragm moves upward and inward. The reduced space creates increased pressure, and air moves outward from the lungs.

**TABLE 5.1**

Chances for recovery according to amount of time lapsed between respiratory arrest and beginning of artificial respiration

| Time to Resume Respiration | Recovery Rate |
|---|---|
| Within 1 minute | 98 in 100 |
| Within 2 minutes | 92 in 100 |
| Within 3 minutes | 72 in 100 |
| Within 4 minutes | 50 in 100 |
| Within 5 minutes | 25 in 100 |
| Within 6 minutes | 11 in 100 |
| Within 7 minutes | 8 in 100 |
| Within 8 minutes | 5 in 100 |
| Within 9 minutes | 2 in 100 |
| Within 10 minutes | 1 in 100 |
| Within 11 minutes | 1 in 1000 |
| Within 12 minutes | 1 in 10,000 |

Source: Adapted from American National Red Cross, Mid-American Chapter. *Artificial Respiration.* St. Louis, Mo.: American National Red Cross, November, 1964.

During respiration, body tissues are supplied with oxygen, and carbon dioxide, the main waste product of oxidation in the tissues, is eliminated from the body. The gas exchange between the blood and cells in the body is known as *internal respiration*. The gas exchange between the blood and air in the lungs is known as *external respiration*. The major organ of respiration in the human body is the lungs, and the major muscle of respiration is the diaphragm. The diaphragm separates the abdominal cavity from the chest cavity.

As air enters the body it passes through the nose, mouth, or both; the pharynx; the larynx; the trachea; the bronchi or bronchial tubes; and the bronchioles and finally reaches 700 million or so small sacs called alveoli (Figure 5.1). In these sacs oxygen is exchanged for carbon dioxide. Inhaled air contains approximately 20% oxygen and 80% nitrogen. Exhaled air contains approximately 16% oxygen, 4% carbon dioxide, and 80% nitrogen.

# ____TYPES OF RESPIRATORY EMERGENCIES

A respiratory emergency arises when breathing ceases completely or when breathing does not supply enough oxygen for the demands of the body. The most common causes of respiratory emergency are outlined here.

**FIGURE 5.1**

The respiratory system.

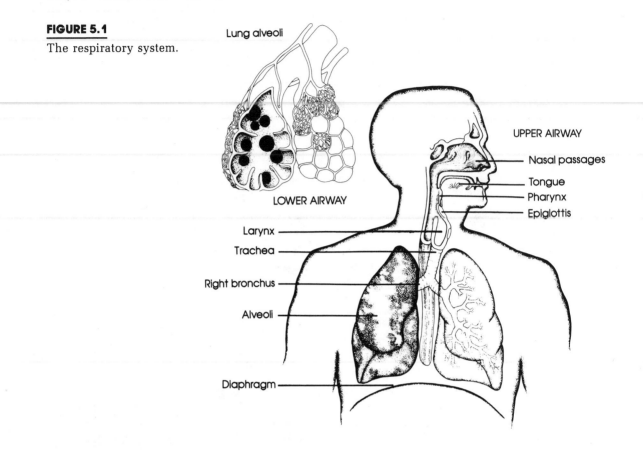

## ___Electrical Shock

Electrical shock is incurred from either lightning or a generator source. The effects of exposure to electricity depend on the amount and frequency of the current, the duration of exposure, and the pathway through the body. Many people have experienced mild electrical shock. In the case of electricity passing through the brain, a charge of 110 volts in a grounded victim (in such a victim the electrical charge passes through the body into the ground or floor and then returns to its source, completing the circuit) is sufficient to paralyze the respiratory center, causing cessation of breathing. Electrical shock is discussed in Chapter 4; electrical burn is discussed in Chapter 11.

## ___Gas Poisoning

Gas poisoning most typically involves carbon monoxide poisoning. Carbon monoxide is created by the incomplete combustion of fossil fuels. The immediate first aid procedure is removal of the victim from the source of poisonous gas, institution of artificial respiration, and if possible, an immediate call for assistance. Chapter 10 covers first aid procedures for gas poisoning.

## __Drug Poisoning

Overdoses of narcotic drugs depress the respiratory center of the brain. If breathing slows or stops completely, cardiac arrest occurs. Common symptoms of narcotic drug overdose include weak pulse, very relaxed muscles, cold and clammy skin, and deep sleep. CPR is started immediately if no pulse can be found (see Chapter 6). Artificial respiration should be given if the pulse is evident.

## __Compression of the Chest

Compression of the chest to the extent that chest muscles cannot expand to allow air to enter is a respiratory emergency. The cause can be a cave-in or other accident that puts a weight on or against the chest. The weight must be removed as soon as possible; however, artificial respiration should begin immediately and continue while removal efforts are under way.

## __Hanging

Whether planned or accidental, hanging blocks the air passage and leads to respiratory and cardiopulmonary arrest. Death usually results from this interruption in breathing and circulation rather than from a broken neck. Pressure on the throat should be removed at once and appropriate first aid care rendered as needed.

## __Drowning

Drowning is a form of suffocation. The air supply to the lungs is stopped by water or spasm of the larynx. Artificial respiration must begin immediately in a drowning situation. *Once begun, artificial respiration efforts must be continued until the victim resumes breathing unassisted or more sophisticated medical assistance becomes available* (see also Chapter 14 on drowning and in particular the mammalian diving reflex discussion).

# ____APPROPRIATE FIRST AID ACTION

## __Determining Airway and Breathing Status

**Consciousness**
The first information to be ascertained is whether the victim is unconscious. Consciousness can be determined by tapping the person on the shoulder while saying loudly, "Are you okay?" If there is no response, unconsciousness can be assumed. Whether the airway is open and the victim is breathing should be determined immediately. Figure 5.2 shows the sequence of steps used by the first-aider in caring for the unconscious person.

**Open Airway**
Establishing an open airway is the most important step in resuscitation. This measure alone results in spontaneous breathing in many cases. The first-aider kneels at the victim's side and tilts the person's head by putting the fingers of the hand nearest the

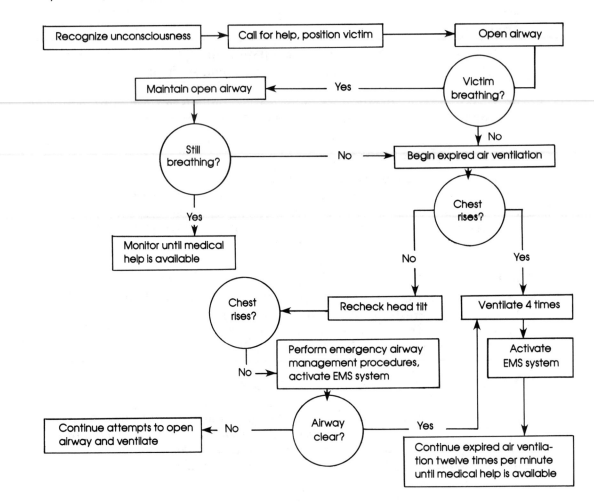

**FIGURE 5.2**

Steps in first aid care for a respiratory emergency in an unconscious person. (Adapted with permission from Kaiser, A.D., and G. C. Norman, *CPR*℠ Cardiopulmonary Resuscitation, Self-Instructional Workbook, p. 18. © 1975 by American Heart Association, Dallas.)

victim's feet on the boney structure below the chin and raising the chin while pushing the forehead back with the other hand. The chin is raised until the teeth are nearly together but some space remains (Figure 5.3). The thumb is normally not used but can be employed to pull back the lower lip, if necessary. In this position the tongue, a common cause of airway obstruction in an unconscious person, is moved away from the back of the throat, thus opening the airway. *Once the airway is opened, the airway must be maintained open by the first-aider, unless the victim regains consciousness.*

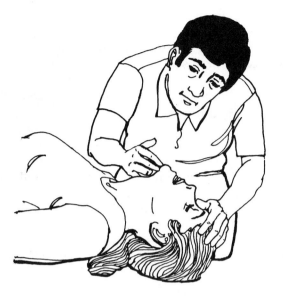

**FIGURE 5.3**
Head-tilt/chin-lift method to open airway. The chin is raised with one hand while the forehead is tilted back with the other. The airway must be maintained by the first-aider.

Some persons who have had partial or complete removal of the larynx breathe through an artificial opening in the lower part of the neck, called a *stoma*. The first-aider should check for the presence of a stoma by sliding the fingers from under the chin of the victim to the top of the breastbone. The stoma will be felt even if covered by clothing. This procedure is done during the breathing status check. (See subsequent discussion of mouth-to-stoma artificial respiration.)

**When spinal cord injury is suspected, all head and body movement should cease.** It is of the utmost importance to stabilize the head and trunk while still attempting to open the airway (see Chapter 9). In such an instance, the airway is opened with a jaw thrust performed without a head tilt. The first-aider supports the victim's head with both palms while placing the fingers behind the angles of the lower jaw. The jaw is then pushed forward while the head is not allowed to move (Figure 5.4).

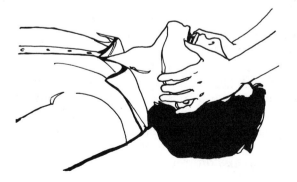

**FIGURE 5.4**
Jaw thrust without head tilt, used to open the airway when spinal cord injury is suspected. The head is supported with both palms and the jaw is pushed forward with the fingers.

**Breathing Status**

The presence or absence of breathing is determined by the LOOK, LISTEN, and FEEL method after the head is tilted to open the airway. **Caution: when spinal cord injury is suspected, the head tilt should not be used.** The first-aider looks to see if the victim's chest and abdomen are moving. He or she listens for air being inhaled and exhaled by placing the ear near the victim's mouth and feels for an exchange of air hitting the cheek. If the victim is breathing (or if spontaneous breathing occurs), the first-aider will see the chest and abdomen rise and fall, hear breathing, and feel air against the cheek. It is important that all three steps be performed to avoid misunderstanding the victim's breathing status. The chest and abdomen may move even when the airway is obstructed by foreign matter, but no air exchange will be heard or felt. Partial blockage of the airway generally produces noisy, insufficient breathing.

The combination of opening the airway and determining breathing status should take three to six seconds. Even if the victim has difficulty breathing, artificial respiration is not given until respiratory insufficiency develops. *Premature artificial respiration in a person who is breathing sufficiently may interfere with the person's normal breathing process.*

## __Initial Ventilations

If the victim does not begin breathing when the airway is opened, artificial respiration must begin IMMEDIATELY. It is critical that oxygen be delivered to the brain. While maintaining the airway open, the first-aider administers two full ventilations mouth to mouth (or mouth to nose, mouth to mouth and nose, or mouth to stoma), allowing 1 to 1½ seconds for each ventilation. For mouth-to-mouth initial ventilations, the procedure is as follows:

1 While maintaining an open airway, pinch the victim's nostrils shut with the thumb and forefinger of the hand on the forehead (Figure 5.5A). If the jaw thrust technique is being used, seal the victim's nostrils by pressing against them with your cheek (see subsequent discussion for ways to seal airways in all other situations).

2 Take a deep breath and create a seal by placing your mouth over and around the victim's mouth.

3 Blow two full breaths into an adult victim's lungs, short puffs into an infant's (the amount of air that can be held in the cheeks), and proportionately fuller breaths into a child's according to the child's size. Done correctly, this will effectively fill the collapsed alveoli in the lungs. Remove your mouth from the victim's only long enough to quickly take a breath. As air is blown into the lungs, watch the victim's chest. It should rise and fall if adequate ventilation is taking place.

4 After the initial two ventilations, turn your head, placing your cheek above the victim's mouth (but not sealing it) (Figure 5.5B). It should be possible to see the chest fall and feel passive exhalation from the victim.

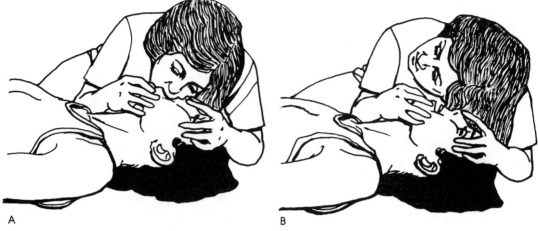

A    B

**FIGURE 5.5**

Mouth-to-mouth artificial respiration. While holding the victim's nose closed with the thumb and index finger and the head in tilt, the first-aider seals the victim's mouth with his or her own and forcefully blows into it (*A*). The first-aider then removes the mouth and listens and feels for exhaled air, at the same time watching for the chest to fall (*B*).

**5** If air is not seen and felt entering and leaving the victim's body, retilt the head (or repeat the jaw thrust action) to make sure the airway is open, and administer two full breaths as before. If air still does not enter the victim's lungs, use the obstructed airway maneuver (discussed subsequently in this chapter).

**6** After the two full breaths have been administered, check for circulation while observing the fall of the victim's chest and the passive expiration of air. [Circulation assessment techniques were discussed in Chapter 2. It is appropriate to review these at this time. Note again the preferred arterial pressure points for palpating the pulse of the adult (carotid) and infant (brachial).] Wait at least five seconds before deciding a pulse is absent.

**7** If the victim has a pulse, the airway is open, and the two full breaths have been effectively administered, begin artificial respiration (instructions follow).

**8** If the victim has no pulse and is not breathing, administer CPR (see Chapter 6).

If the victim's mouth cannot be opened, the mouth or jaw is severely injured, it is impossible to ventilate the victim by mouth, or it is impossible to make an airtight seal over the victim's mouth, the first-aider uses the mouth-to-nose technique. The head-tilt/chin-lift method is used to open the airway; however, the victim's mouth is completely closed (Figure 5.6). The first-aider takes a deep breath, seals the area around the victim's nose with his or her lips, and blows smoothly and firmly until the chest rises.

**FIGURE 5.6**

Mouth-to-nose ventilation. When ventilation by mouth is impossible, the first-aider opens the victim's airway with the head-tilt/chin-lift method, completely closing the victim's mouth *(inset)*. The first-aider then seals the victim's nose with his or her lips and inflates the victim's lungs.

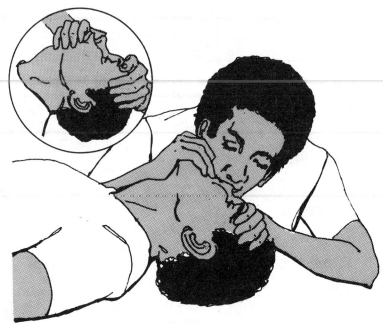

During the initial ventilation this is repeated two times; then the first-aider turns his or her head and listens and feels for exhalations while watching the victim's chest fall.

## Performing Artificial Respiration

### Mouth to Mouth

Mouth to mouth is the preferred method for administering air to another person. It is used whenever the mouth and jaw area are not severely damaged or a mouth-to-mouth seal can be assured. As during initial ventilations, the first-aider must ensure that the airway remains open. The victim's nostrils are pinched shut with the thumb and index fingers of the same hand holding the head in tilt. Again, if the jaw thrust technique is being used, it will be necessary for the first-aider to cover the nostrils with his or her cheek. The first-aider *blows into the lungs with pressure, yet smoothly, at the rate of one breath every five seconds, (ten to twelve breaths a minute for adults and children 4 years of age and over) or one puff every three seconds for infants and children under 4.*

To maintain an even cycle of ventilations, the first-aider counts between each breath using the method preferred by the American National Red Cross. To breathe once every five seconds, the rescuer counts "one one-thousand, two one-thousand, three one-thousand, four one-thousand, b-r-e-a-t-h-e." With this counting method, approximately five seconds will elapse between the start of each breath into the victim. Counting is adapted so that the first-aider breathes once every three seconds for infants.

### Mouth to Nose

The mouth-to-nose technique is used for the same reasons it is used for initial ventilations. The procedure remains the same and the breathing rates are the same as those used in mouth-to-mouth respiration.

### Mouth to Nose and Mouth

Mouth-to-nose-and-mouth respiration is used primarily with an infant or other victim whose mouth is too small for effective mouth-to-mouth breathing. Artificial respiration is initiated and maintained in essentially the same manner as already outlined. However, the mouth and nose of the victim are both sealed by the first-aider's lips and air passes through both.

### Special Situations

**Infants**    Infants and small children present a special situation in terms of artificial respiration. Their lungs are small, and as noted, the first-aider must blow gently and with small volume, using puffs (the amount of air held in the first-aider's cheeks). The ventilations are given at the rate of one every three seconds. The neck of an infant is very flexible; if it is overextended, the breathing passage may be obstructed. Consequently, the tilted position of the infant's head should not be exaggerated.

**Mouth to Stoma**    A second special situation in terms of artificial respiration is that presented by the laryngectomee, a person who has had partial or complete removal of the larynx and who breathes through a stoma. The artificial respiration procedure for a person with a stoma is essentially the same as that for other adults except for the head tilt. *In the laryngectomee, the head and neck must remain level.* The first-aider delivers air by mouth to stoma rather than by mouth to mouth. One of the first-aider's hands seals the mouth and nose (Figure 5.7), since air leakage from these organs is possible.

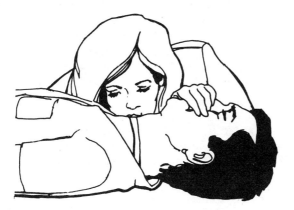

**FIGURE 5.7**

Mouth-to-stoma artificial respiration for a victim with a tracheostomy. The first-aider seals the mouth and nose with one hand. The victim's head is not tilted.

**Potential Problems**

**Fatigue**     Fatigue by the first-aider (or even simple loss of concentration) may result in failure to maintain a proper head tilt after artificial respiration is begun. Consequently, the air passage can become partially blocked, inhibiting and reducing the effectiveness of the first-aider's efforts. Fatigue often occurs because the first-aider does not breathe deeply enough. He or she must breathe for two people. Even when the head tilt is maintained, fatigue may cause slowing of the ventilation rate.

**Distention of the Stomach**     Distention of the victim's stomach can result from ventilations that overinflate the lungs or from partial blockage of the airway. Distention, if excessive, may elevate the diaphragm and reduce lung volume as well as promote vomiting. Vomiting presents the danger of aspiration of stomach contents into the lungs. There is disagreement whether pressure should be applied if the stomach is distended. The American National Red Cross does NOT recommend such an attempt by the first-aider. Too many other problems can arise as a result of the vomiting. If distention is severe, however, and the first aider believes relief is required, manual pressure may be applied over the upper abdomen. The victim should be turned, as a unit, onto the side (refer to Figure 2.12), light pressure applied to the upper abdomen, the mouth swept clean, and artificial respiration resumed. The first-aider should watch the rise and fall of the chest and adjust ventilations to avoid excessive pressure that can overinflate the lungs.

## __Choking and the Obstructed Airway

A uniquely different respiratory emergency occurs when an object lodged in the throat obstructs breathing and leads to asphyxiation. Approximately 3,000 people die from this condition each year. According to the American National Red Cross, two thirds of them are children under age 4. This condition in adults has been termed a *cafe coronary*. Adult victims often choke on food while eating. These victims typically are people who wear dentures, fail to cut food into reasonably small bites, or drink alcohol excessively before or while eating, or a combination of these. The victim is unable to speak because of the object in the throat, and onlookers typically assume the person is having a heart attack.

The obstructed airway emergency occurs when an object in the larynx holds the epiglottis (the valve guarding the opening from the throat to the trachea and lungs) over the trachea (Figure 5.8). This fully or partially prohibits the flow of air in and out of the lungs. Further, the muscles in the larynx may go into spasms, thus holding the object more firmly in place. This is a true respiratory emergency and the first aider must respond immediately.

The need to respond is complicated by the fact that the victim typically cannot speak and others may not immediately recognize the severity of the situation. The American Heart Association and the American National Red Cross are encouraging recognition and use of a universal distress signal for choking. This signal consists of the victim grasping the throat with one or two hands (Figure 5.9). The first-aider should recognize this signal. However, he or she should also remember that deaths due to choking occur most frequently among children too young to learn this signal or use it in an emergency.

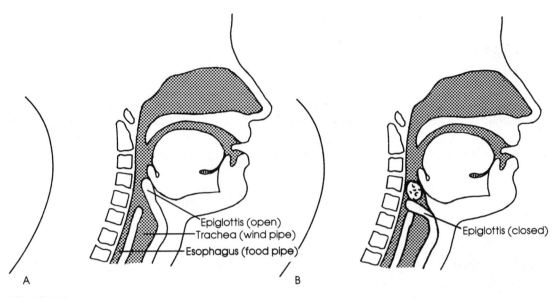

**FIGURE 5.8**

Mechanism of an airway obstruction by a foreign object. The epiglottis, which guards the opening to the trachea, is shown in its open position (*A*) and held closed by a bolus of food lodged in the esophagus (*B*).

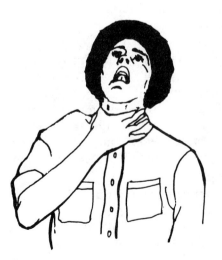

**FIGURE 5.9**

Recommended universal distress signal for choking. One or both hands may be used to clutch the throat.

An additional difficulty arises when the victim is discovered unconscious and not breathing. The first-aider may be unaware that the airway is obstructed until he or she attempts to administer ventilations.

### Determining the Presence of Obstruction

If an individual is suspected to be experiencing an obstructed airway, he or she is asked, "Can you speak?" If the victim can speak or cough, no attempt should be made to remove the obstruction! The person is kept calm and quiet and is observed while someone calls the rescue squad or summons medical attention. If the victim can breathe enough to speak or cough, the blockage is partial; any attempt to remove the obstruction may result in a complete blockage. In some cases of partial blockage, breathing efforts create a wheezing or high-pitched sound.

If the victim cannot speak or cough, the first-aider uses one or more of the following techniques to remove the object.

### Removing the Obstruction

**Manual Removal**     If the object can be easily seen and reached, the first-aider grasps it and gently pulls it out of the throat. Such objects include sucker stems, toys, and large bones. If the object cannot be easily grasped (it may be quite slippery), unsuccessful efforts to remove it waste valuable seconds. *The manual removal attempt does not work in most choking situations.* The recommended sequence for attempts to remove objects blocking the airway follows.

**Heimlich Maneuver or Manual Thrusts**     If the object cannot be removed manually, the first-aider next tries exerting pressure against it using the air remaining inside the blocked lungs. This pressure may pop the object out of the airway, just like air pressure causes a champagne cork to pop out. There are two types of manual thrusts. One is called the *abdominal thrust*. Originally recommended by Dr. Henry J. Heimlich, it is commonly referred to as the *Heimlich maneuver*. This maneuver is now recognized by both the American National Red Cross and the American Heart Association as an effective procedure for clearing an obstructed airway.

*ABDOMINAL THRUST*     The abdominal thrust is administered to the upper abdomen. It can be done with the choking victim standing or sitting. The first-aider stands behind the victim and circles the arms around the victim's waist while placing the thumb side of one fist in the middle of the abdomen between the navel and rib cage and grasping the fist with the other hand (Figure 5.10). He or she then presses the fist into the victim's abdomen with a quick inward and upward motion (Figure 5.10). This procedure is rapidly repeated until six to ten thrusts have been completed. A conscious person may perform this maneuver on himself or herself using his or her own fist or other firm object (e.g., a porch railing or chair back).

*CHEST THRUST*     The chest thrust can be substituted for the abdominal thrust if the victim's waist is too large to encircle with the arms or if the victim is in advanced pregnancy. The first-aider stands behind the victim and places the arms directly under the victim's armpits and around the lower portion of the rib cage. Positioning one fist

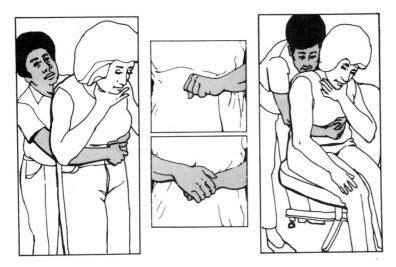

**FIGURE 5.10**

Abdominal thrust for a standing or sitting choking victim. Center illustrations show proper positioning of the hands: The thumb side of one fist is placed in the middle of the abdomen between the navel and the rib cage and grasped with the other hand for a quick inward and upward thrust.

with the thumb against the middle of the victim's sternum, he or she grasps the fist with the other hand and gives four quick thrusts by pulling straight back each time (Figure 5.11).

*SUPINE VICTIM*    If the victim is lying down, the abdominal thrust is performed by kneeling astride the victim's hips or thighs (or at the feet of small children). The heel of one hand is placed against the middle of the victim's abdomen with fingers pointed toward the person's head. The other hand is placed on top of the first. The first-aider's shoulders are directly above the victim's abdomen. The first-aider then presses inward and upward with six to ten quick thrusts (Figure 5.12).

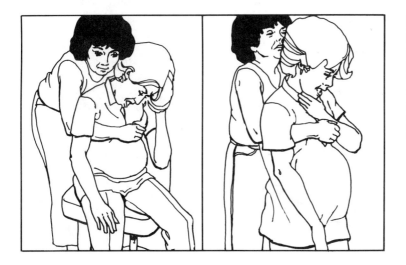

**FIGURE 5.11**

Chest thrust for a choking obese person or a woman in advanced pregnancy. The maneuver can be done with the victim sitting or standing. The rescuer places the fist against the middle of the sternum.

**FIGURE 5.12**

The abdominal thrust can be performed by kneeling astride a supine choking victim. The proper hand position is shown in the inset (fingers point toward the victim's head). The first-aider presses inward and upward with four quick thrusts.

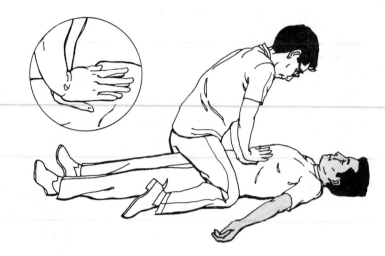

If a chest thrust must be performed on a supine person, the first-aider begins by kneeling close beside the chest and placing the heel of the hand on the lower half of the sternum about one and one-half inches from the end. The fingers of the hand are elevated and the long axis of the heel of the hand is parallel to the breast bone (Figure 5.13). The other hand is then placed directly on top of the first. The first-aider administers chest thrusts by placing his or her shoulders directly over the hands and exerting a downward thrust with the arms and shoulders. Six to ten thrusts are administered.

*FINGER SWEEPS*    Whether the manual thrusts have dislodged the object is determined by viewing or, when the person is unconscious, sweeping the mouth with the fingers. First, the lower jaw is grasped with the fingers and the tongue with the thumb and the tongue is lifted away from the back of the throat. This may open the airway or permit the object to be seen and reached. The first-aider does not reach directly into the

**FIGURE 5.13**

Chest thrust for the supine choking victim is done from the side. The first-aider exerts a downward thrust with the arms and shoulders.

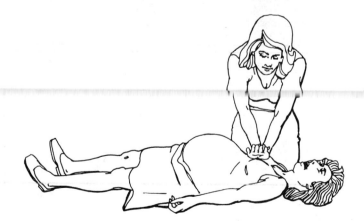

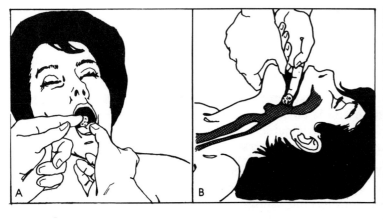

**FIGURE 5.14**

Finger sweep to remove a foreign body in an unconscious person. To see if manual thrusts have dislodged an obstructive object, the first-aider grasps the victim's lower jaw with the fingers and the tongue with the thumb to bring the object into view (*A*). The index finger of the free hand is then slid down one side of the victim's mouth to the base of the tongue, and a hooking motion is used to remove the object (*B*).

victim's mouth—he or she slides the index finger of the free hand down one side of the mouth to the base of the tongue. A hooking motion is used to dislodge the object or push it against the opposite side of the throat, forcing it to move upward in the throat (Figure 5.14). If the object is freed, it is removed from the victim's mouth.

If the mouth must be forced open, a cross-finger technique can be used (Figure 5.15). The thumb and index finger are crossed, placed against the victim's upper and lower teeth, and pushed forcefully to open the mouth. The free hand then removes foreign material.

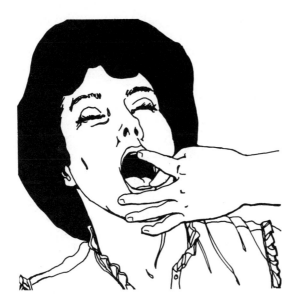

**FIGURE 5.15**

Cross-finger technique to force the mouth open.

### Choking: The Proper Order of Response

Manual thrusts and finger sweeps may both be used in attempts to rescue a choking victim. It is important that they be used properly, that is, executed correctly and in the proper sequence. The sequence differs for the conscious and the unconscious victim. *As soon as the victim can cough or breathe, all emergency choking first aid procedures stop.*

**The Conscious Victim**     If choking is suspected, the victim is asked, "Can you speak?" If the victim cannot speak, he or she is positioned properly and given six to ten manual thrusts immediately. The thrusts are repeated continuously until the victim can either breathe on his or her own, becomes unconscious, or medical help arrives.

**The Unconscious Victim**     When a conscious choking victim becomes unconscious, the immediate concern is for an open airway and adequate breathing. Often the lapse into unconsciousness will relax the choking victim's muscles, lessening the grip on the object. This may allow the victim to resume breathing spontaneously. Again, *the first-aider should not try to remove the object if breathing is only partially obstructed.* He or she should keep the victim calm and have someone seek medical help.

When the choking victim becomes unconscious, the first-aider must call for help (if possible) and open the airway, check for breathing, and attempt to ventilate the non-breathing victim. If ventilation is not possible, a finger sweep and six to ten manual thrusts are done. This sequence—open airway, check for breathing, attempt to ventilate (if the victim is not breathing), manual thrusts (if the airway is obstructed), and finger sweeps—must be carried out in rapid succession.

In some situations the first-aider may come upon an unconscious person who for some unknown reason is not breathing. The procedure then is as follows: The first-aider makes sure the victim is really unconscious. Then he or she calls for help, tries to open the airway, attempts to ventilate, and retilts the head if needed. If ventilation is impossible, the first-aider proceeds as in dealing with a choking victim who becomes unconscious. Manual thrusts and finger sweeps are performed, and (if breathing is not restored) ventilation is attempted. If the victim fails to resume breathing once the obstruction to the airway has been removed, artificial respiration may be required. Restoring breathing must remain as the key goal.

**Infants**     As with artificial respiration, special procedures exist for an obstructed airway in infants less than 1 year of age. If the airway is only partially blocked, someone should call for help while the first-aider tries to keep the victim calm and in a comfortable position. If the infant is actively choking, he or she is positioned face down on the first-aider's forearm with the head lower than the body and four back slaps are delivered. To facilitate this, the infant should be held against the first-aider's thigh or another firm object (Figure 5.16A). After giving four back blows, the first-aider places his or her free forearm on the infant's back while supporting the head and neck. With the free hand, he or she then turns the infant over for delivery of chest thrusts (compressions). The first-aider now places the index finger (of the hand that will be used to apply the compressions) just below an imaginary line drawn between the nipples. The finger is centered on the sternum. The area for compression is one finger width below this

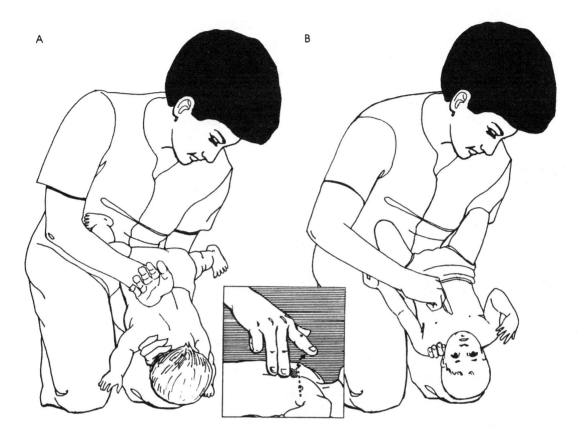

**FIGURE 5.16**

Back blows and chest thrusts for a choking infant. The first-aider holds the infant on his or her forearm and administers four back blows with the heel of the hand (*A*). The first-aider then turns the infant and performs four chest thrusts (*B*) followed by more back blows and chest thrusts.

imaginary line, where the ring and middle finger rest when placed beside the index finger (Figure 5.16*B*). This is the same finger positioning used for CPR with infants (see Chapter 6). Four chest thrusts are given in this position, using two or three fingers, followed by more back blows and then chest thrusts.

Controversy exists between Dr. Heimlich and both the American Heart Association and the American National Red Cross. These two organizations believe the method described here is the most effective. The June 6, 1986, issue of the *Journal of the American Medical Association* presents the recommendations from the National Conference on Cardiopulmonary Resuscitation and Emergency Cardiac Care. These recommendations call for the use of abdominal thrusts in children over 1 year of age. For infants under 1 year of age, however, back blows and chest thrusts continue to be recommended.

Dr. Heimlich proposes an immediate abdominal thrust for both infants and children. For infants he recommends an abdominal thrust performed by placing the index and middle fingers of each hand on the infant's abdomen, slightly above the navel and well below the abdomen. Using Dr. Heimlich's techniques, the first-aider performs repeated upward thrusts. The infant can be lying flat or held in the lap.

*Finger sweeps are not recommended for young children or infants.* Dr. Heimlich, the American National Red Cross, and the American Heart Association all agree. Finger sweeps should be used only when the object can be seen and the sweep is not likely to lodge it more securely. The mouths of infants and children are small; the fingers of an adult may easily force an object further into the throat because space prohibits a strong grasp or hooking motion.

---

## SUMMARY

Breathing interruption or cessation is a high-priority injury that demands immediate attention in an emergency situation. All rescue methods begin by ascertaining if the victim, whether unconscious or conscious, is breathing and opening the airway, if necessary. The skills required to open an obstructed airway and provide artificial respiration are not difficult. Caution is needed in the case of possible spinal cord injury.

The first-aider removes obstructions in the airway if necessary. If the victim is not breathing, two full ventilations are given and then artificial respiration begins. The rate of breathing in artificial respiration differs with the size of the victim. The usual first aid procedure for choking is manual thrusts. If the victim is unconscious, the thrusts should be followed by finger sweeps. The victim may need artificial respiration once the airway is cleared.

---

## CHAPTER MASTERY: TEST ITEMS

### True and False

Circle One

1. The best way to find out if someone has stopped breathing is to check the carotid pulse.  T  F
2. Cessation of breathing for four minutes can result in brain damage.  T  F
3. It should take the first-aider about 45 seconds to determine the consciousness of a stricken person, open the airway, and establish breathing.  T  F
4. A chest thrust is never used with obese individuals.  T  F
5. A finger sweep is used immediately after airway obstruction is verified  T  F

in a conscious victim.

6. The proper artificial respiration rate for an adult is one breath every     **T**     **F**
five seconds.

7. Contact with a household electrical current of 110 volts is sufficient to     **T**     **F**
cause cessation of breathing in some situations.

8. The head-tilt/chin-lift method is used for artificial respiration if a     **T**     **F**
spinal cord injury is suspected.

9. Mouth-to-stoma respiration is used with all laryngectomees.     **T**     **F**

## Multiple Choice (Circle the Best Answer)

1. What is the correct order in which to perform the following artificial respiration
procedures on an unconscious victim? (1) Give two full breaths. (2) Position head
back with jaw jutting up. (3) Check for breathing.

    a. 2, 3, 1
    b. 3, 1, 2
    c. 1, 2, 3
    d. 1, 3, 2

2. Initial inability to perform mouth-to-mouth artificial respiration may be due to
all of the following except

    a. a stomach bulging with excess air.
    b. an obstructed airway.
    c. a poor mouth seal.
    d. an incorrect head and jaw position.

3. Which of the following is **not** a sign or symptom of a completely obstructed
airway?

    a. The victim cannot cough or speak.
    b. The victim grasps his or her chest.
    c. The victim grasps his or her throat.
    d. None of the above.

4. The recommended rate of ventilation for a 1-year-old infant is

    a. one breath every three seconds.
    b. one breath every four seconds.
    c. one breath every five seconds.
    d. one breath every six seconds.

5. The ventilation rate for an adult laryngectomee is

    a. one breath every three seconds.
    b. one breath every five seconds.
    c. one breath every seven seconds.
    d. one breath every nine seconds.

**Discussion Questions**

1. List and explain four types of respiratory emergencies.
2. List the signs and symptoms of an obstructed airway in a conscious and an unconscious person.
3. Describe the proper response by the first-aider to a conscious victim with a partial airway obstruction.
4. Compare and contrast the proper response by the first-aider to a choking infant and a choking adult.
5. Characterize the typical adult choking victim.
6. A neighbor just opened the door to her garage and discovered her husband slumped over in the front seat of his car. The car is still running. On the basis of the material presented in this chapter, what actions should the first-aider take to revive him if he is not breathing but has a pulse and the airway is not obstructed?
7. Someone at a hotel just found an infant lying face down in the wading pool. The infant is not breathing but has a pulse. How should artificial respiration be performed on this infant?

—————————————————— **BIBLIOGRAPHY** ——————————————————

American National Red Cross. *Advanced First Aid and Emergency Care.* Garden City, N.Y.: Doubleday, 1979.

Hafen, B. Q., and K. J. Karren. *First Aid and Emergency Skills Manual.* Englewood, Colo.: Morton Publishing, 1982.

Hafen, B. Q., and K. J. Karren. *First Aid and Emergency Care Workbook.* Englewood, Colo.: Morton Publishing, 1984.

National Conference on Cardiopulmonary Resuscitation and Emergency Cardiac Care. "Standards and Guidelines for Cardiopulmonary Resuscitation (CPR) and Emergency Cardiac Care (ECC)." *Journal of the American Medical Association* 255 (6 June 1986): 2905-2960.

Thygerson, A. L. *The First Aid Book.* Englewood Cliffs, N.J.: Prentice-Hall, 1982.

Winkleman, J. L. *Essentials of Basic Life Support.* Minneapolis: Burgess Publishing, 1981.

# 6

# Cardiac Emergencies and Cardiopulmonary Resuscitation

SANDRA J. LEVI, M.S.

After completing this chapter the student will be able to
- • Explain the basic elements in the circulatory system.
- • Describe the signs and symptoms of cardiac emergencies.
- • Assess the need for cardiopulmonary resuscitation (CPR).
- • Describe and demonstrate the CPR procedures for
  - •an adult with one first-aider.
  - •an adult with two first-aiders.
  - •a child or infant.
- • Describe the circumstances under which CPR should be discontinued.

## ——INTRODUCTION

The respiratory and the circulatory systems work together to provide oxygen to the brain and the body as a whole. When the brain is denied oxygen for as little as four to six minutes, permanent and irreversible brain damage usually occurs. If the supply of oxygen is interrupted for six to ten minutes, death usually follows.

The importance of the circulatory and respiratory systems to life cannot be overemphasized. An understanding of the circulatory system provides the foundation of knowledge that the first-aider needs to handle cardiac emergencies.

## ——THE CIRCULATORY SYSTEM

The circulatory system serves several important functions in the human body. This system is responsible for the distribution of oxygenated blood to tissues. It is also responsible for returning deoxygenated blood to the heart to be reoxygenated. Central to efficient blood circulation is the heart.

The heart is a four-chambered pump (Figure 6.1). Each of the chambers has an essential role in heart function. The right atrium receives deoxygenated blood from the body and holds it until it is allowed to flow into the right ventricle. After filling of this ventricle is complete, the right ventricle squeezes the deoxygenated blood through the pulmonary arteries to the right and left lungs. There the blood is oxygenated. It then travels to the left atrium, where it remains until it is allowed to flow into the left ventricle. When filling of this ventricle is complete, the left ventricle contracts, forcing

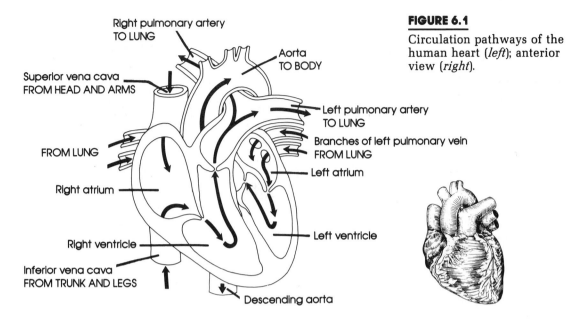

**FIGURE 6.1**

Circulation pathways of the human heart (*left*); anterior view (*right*).

Right pulmonary artery
TO LUNG

Aorta
TO BODY

Superior vena cava
FROM HEAD AND ARMS

Left pulmonary artery
TO LUNG

Branches of left pulmonary vein
FROM LUNG

FROM LUNG

Left atrium

Right atrium

Right ventricle

Left ventricle

Inferior vena cava
FROM TRUNK AND LEGS

Descending aorta

oxygenated blood through the major arteries and subsequently to the body's tissues. All of these events are carefully timed so that the heart pumps or beats 60 to 100 times per minute in the healthy adult.

Circulatory function is closely associated with respiratory function. Human cells cannot exist for long without oxygen. The respiratory system and lungs supply oxygen to the blood, which is distributed to the body tissues via the circulatory system. The circulatory system is also responsible for returning waste products such as carbon dioxide to the lungs, from which the carbon dioxide is expelled into the environment. Both the respiratory and circulatory systems must be functional for human tissue, and especially the brain, to remain alive.

## ___CARDIAC EMERGENCIES

Over 900,000 people die annually in the United States from cardiovascular disease and its complications. This number makes such disease the nation's number one health problem in mortality ranking. Many people are alive today because of the prompt emergency first aid given them for heart attack, including myocardial infarction and cardiac arrest, cardiac injury, or both. Early recognition of a cardiac emergency is essential to effective first aid care. Heart attacks and cardiac injuries are two types of emergency to which the first-aider should be prepared to respond.

**FIGURE 6.2**

Signals of a heart attack. The pain is intense and may radiate to one or all of the areas shown on the left. Other manifestations include dizziness, sweating, nausea, faintness, and trouble breathing. Collapse may be sudden.

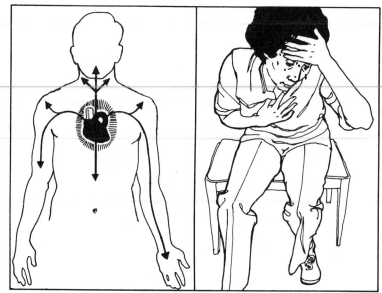

## ⎯ Heart Attack

Acute heart attack occurs when an individual experiences a disruption of the blood supply to the heart muscle. The most common sign of a heart attack is a sensation of squeezing, pain, fullness, or pressure in the center of the chest. Cardiac arrest involves the cessation of effective heart action. The heart may stop beating completely or may beat rapidly and chaotically (fibrillation), failing to pump any blood. Cardiac arrest can result from many causes, though myocardial infarction (death and subsequent scarring of previously healthy heart tissue) is one of the most common. A coronary thrombosis (blood clot in a coronary artery) causes a myocardial infarction. The pain of coronary thrombosis is intense; it can but does not always extend through the center of the chest to the jaw, neck, and back, radiating down the left arm and the fingers of the left hand (Figure 6.2). The pain may be located in the upper abdomen, in which case it may be perceived as indigestion. Pain may be followed by sudden collapse, unconsciousness, cyanosis, defecation, and urination.

The greatest risk of death from a heart attack occurs during the first two hours after onset. Anyone with the symptoms described requires prompt medical attention. A heart attack victim's condition should be closely monitored during transport.

## ⎯ Cardiac Injury

Cardiac injury results from direct trauma to the heart. Most commonly, injury is caused by a weapon, but it could be the result of chest trauma, as incurred in an automobile accident. The most common signs of cardiac injury include external evidence of injury to the area and obvious signs of shock. (Shock and its related first aid care are discussed in Chapter 4.) When cardiac injury is due to a blunt trauma, shock out of proportion to the apparent injury is common. **An object penetrating the chest should not be removed.** Prompt medical attention should be obtained. Other than providing transportation and treating for shock, the first-aider has limited ability to provide assistance to a victim of a cardiac injury.

# ____ASSESSING THE VICTIM

A first-aider who either sees someone collapse or encounters an apparently unconscious person must consider the possibility of a cardiac emergency. Before taking any corrective action, the first-aider assesses the victim's condition as follows:

1 *Check for consciousness.* Kneel, touch the victim on the shoulder and face, and shout, "Are you OK?" If the person does not respond, check for breathing.
2 *Check for breathing.* Tip the person's head back to open the airway. (If spinal cord injury is suspected, use the jaw thrust technique discussed in Chapter 5.) Then perform the LOOK, LISTEN, and FEEL technique, also described in Chapter 5.
3 *Give initial ventilations* (if person is not breathing). If the victim is not breathing, give two full breaths, each 1 to 1½ seconds in length, to inflate the lungs. (See initial ventilations for adults and infants in Chapter 5.)
4 *Check for a carotid pulse and breathing.* After inflating the lungs, feel for a carotid pulse for five to ten seconds. The carotid pulse is found in the grooves beside the adam's apple. Palpate the pulse on the nearest side of the victim, rather than reaching across the victim's neck. While feeling for a carotid pulse, reassess the victim's breathing status. (Review again the procedures for palpating the carotid, radial, femoral, and brachial pulse described in Chapter 2.) Once the victim's status has been assessed, obtain help and initiate first aid care.

# ____OBTAINING HELP

When a respiratory or cardiac emergency occurs, the first-aider tries to obtain help. The first-aider should point to a bystander (if there is one), tell him or her to obtain emergency medical assistance, and briefly state what to say, for example, "Call 911 and report a cardiac arrest at 110 Smith Street." A lone first-aider who comes upon a cardiac emergency scene should quickly assess the victim's condition, telephone for help if possible, and administer CPR if required. If there is little likelihood of obtaining assistance, however, the first-aider should not delay initiating artificial respiration or CPR in order to obtain assistance.

**TABLE 6.1**

Resuscitation action guide

| Assessment Findings | | First Aider Action Guide |
| --- | --- | --- |
| Breathing | Pulse | Action |
| Yes | Yes | Monitor victim<br>Transport to life support unit |
| No | Yes | Give artificial respiration<br>Obtain emergency medical care |
| No | No | Give CPR<br>Obtain emergency medical care |

## ___INITIATING CARE

The first-aider must then initiate first aid care appropriate to the victim's condition (Table 6.1):
- If the victim is breathing and has a pulse, monitor the victim's status and transport him or her to a life support unit.
- If the victim has a pulse but is not breathing, initiate artificial respiration.
- If the victim has no pulse and is not breathing, initiate CPR.

Artificial respiration and patient transportation are discussed in other chapters. This chapter emphasizes CPR.

## ___RESTORING CIRCULATION

Both respiration and circulation must continue for the brain and other body tissues to remain alive. Normally these functions take place without conscious control. When a situation arises in which these functions cannot continue automatically, the first-aider's job is to maintain them artificially.

Chest compressions can be used to restore circulation when the heart is not beating. In chest compressions, the heart is squeezed between the sternum (the breastbone) and the vertebrae (the bones making up the back bone). Blood is circulated through the lungs to the body. *Chest compressions serve no useful purpose in circulation unless the blood is first oxygenated by adequate respiration. Therefore, cardiac compression must always be accompanied by artificial respiration.*

## ___CARDIOPULMONARY RESUSCITATION

Before the CPR sequence is described, it is important for the first-aider to understand the techniques involved in hand placement (Figure 6.3) and giving compressions during a cardiac emergency.

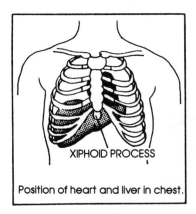

Position of heart and liver in chest.

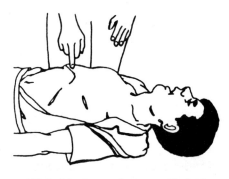

**1** First-aider traces rib cage with right middle finger to notch.

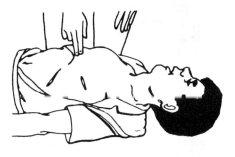

**2** Middle and index fingers are placed along bottom of sternum.

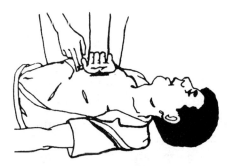

**3** Heel of left hand is placed on sternum just above index finger.

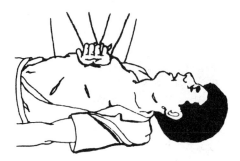

**4** Heel of right hand is placed on top of left hand, keeping fingers of both hands raised.

## FIGURE 6.3

Determining the proper hand placement for cardiopulmonary resuscitation when the first-aider is kneeling to the victim's right. Compression over the xiphoid process (inset) may lacerate the liver and must be avoided.

## __Hand Placement

1 If kneeling to the victim's right, trace up the right side of the victim's rib cage with the right middle finger to the top of the notch.
2 Keeping the middle finger in place, lay the index finger next to it on the sternum (breastbone).
3 Without lifting the right index and middle fingers, place the heel of the left hand on the sternum just above the right index finger.
4 After the heel of the left hand is placed, place the heel of the right hand on top of the left hand.
5 Keep the fingers of both hands in a raised position off the victim's chest, leaving the heels of the hands on the victim's chest. If desired, lock the fingers of the left hand around those of the right.
6 **If chest compressions are done over the xiphoid process, serious liver damage may result.** The xiphoid process is a small piece of bone extending from the sternum just beyond the point where the last of the rib cage curves upward to attach to the sternum.
7 If kneeling to the victim's left, follow the foregoing procedure but reverse the right and left references.

## __Giving Compressions

The object of giving compressions is to squeeze the heart between the sternum and the spine. Compression should depress the adult sternum from 1½ to 2 inches. The first-aider should keep the following principles in mind.

1 The victim must be in a supine position on a firm surface for compressions to be effective.
2 Maintain hand contact with the victim's chest throughout each series of compressions. Let the hands lose contact with the victim's chest only when giving breaths.
3 Before beginning every set of compressions, replace the hands carefully, using the "rib cage trace" procedures outlined in Figure 6.3.
4 Bend at the hips and keep the elbows straight when giving compressions. In this way body weight is used to mechanical advantage in applying the force necessary to depress the sternum.
5 To ensure that pressure is applied in the proper direction, keep the arms perpendicular to the victim's chest. Compressions must be applied perpendicular to, and not at an angle to, the chest (Figure 6.4).
6 Keep the fingers up when giving compressions. Pressure is only applied to the lower half of the sternum; it is incorrect to also apply pressure to the ribs.

## __One-First-Aider CPR

When only one first-aider is present at the scene of a cardiac emergency, he or she has many tasks to fulfill alone. The needs of the victim are assessed first. If the adult victim is not breathing and does not have a pulse, the first-aider telephones for help (if possible)

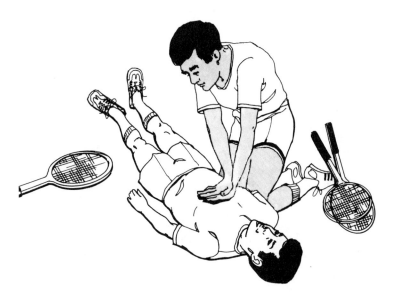

**FIGURE 6.4**

When giving compressions, the first-aider keeps the arms perpendicular to the victim's chest

and then initiates CPR. Shouting for help might be appropriate in the hope that a passerby might hear and respond.

The first-aider begins by giving fifteen compressions at the rate of 80 to 100 compressions per minute. The first-aider says "one and, two and, three and, ... fifteen and" to help pace the compressions correctly. The depth of compression is 1½ to 2 inches. Following the series of fifteen compressions, the first-aider gives the victim two breaths.

The first-aider completes four cycles of fifteen compressions and two breaths in approximately one minute. Following the two breaths of the fourth cycle, he or she stops a maximum of seven seconds to recheck the pulse and breathing status. A carotid pulse is palpated for five seconds. If the pulse is present, breathing is assessed for three seconds. If neither is present, CPR is begun. Once the first-aider begins CPR, he or she must not interrupt the cycles for more than seven seconds at a time until the victim recovers.

If during the check the first-aider finds a pulse and breathing, he or she monitors the victim while obtaining professional medical help. If a pulse is found but no breathing, artificial respiration is administered. If no pulse is found (and therefore no breathing), the first-aider gives the victim two breaths before resuming the fifteen compression–two breath cycles. After resuming CPR, the first-aider performs a simultaneous pulse and breathing check every few minutes (using no more than five seconds to accomplish this task). The sequence of steps in one-first-aider CPR are presented in Table 6.2.

## __Two·First·Aider CPR

The administration of CPR by two first-aiders is usually more effective than its administration by one first-aider. The victim receives more breaths per minute, and the first-aider becomes less fatigued.

**TABLE 6.2**

Action sequence in one-first-aider CPR

Tap victim (e.g., on shoulder) and shout, "Are you OK?"
Tip head and check for breathing.
Give two full breaths.
Check carotid pulse and breathing.
Obtain emergency medical care.
Give four cycles of fifteen compressions and two breaths.
Check pulse for five seconds.
Give two breaths.
Resume fifteen compression–two breath cycles.

First-aider A assesses the victim and initiates CPR, while first-aider B notifies emergency medical personnel. When first-aider B returns, he or she begins to assist in CPR. A special procedure is followed, so that CPR is not interrupted during the transition from one first-aider to the other. First-aider B observes the activities of first-aider A while taking a position near the victim's head on the opposite side from first-aider A. He or she waits until first-aider A begins compressions one through ten and then states, "I know CPR, may I help?" First-aider A says, "Yes, check the pulse." If first-aider B has not waited and has asked to help at an inappropriate time, first-aider A says, "Check the pulse when I return to compressions." After this minimal amount of conversation, the two first-aiders know how they will work together to provide appropriate care for the victim.

In the next step, first-aider B kneels beside the victim's head and feels for a pulse. If a pulse is found, he or she says, "Stop compressions." If a pulse is not found, first-aider B attempts to ascertain whether the pulse-finding technique or the compression technique is inadequate. If either is, he or she takes corrective action, before saying, "Stop compressions." While first-aider A stops compressions, first-aider B continues to check for breathing and a pulse. The procedure at this point depends on first-aider B's findings.

- If the victim has a pulse and is breathing, the first-aiders continuously monitor the victim until professional medical care arrives.
- If the victim has a pulse but is not breathing, first-aider B says, "Pulse present, no breathing, I'll give artificial respiration." First-aider B begins artificial respiration. He or she periodically rechecks the carotid pulse.
- If the victim has no pulse (and is therefore not breathing), first-aider B gives a breath, then says "No pulse, continue CPR."

When CPR is to be continued, first-aider A resumes compressions. *Two-first-aider CPR is given in a five compression–one breath cycle.* The rate of compressions remains 80 to 100 compressions per minute. First-aider B gives a breath between compression five and compression one. First-aider A pauses for 1 to 1½ seconds after the fifth compression to allow adequate time for ventilation. The two first-aiders work together applying CPR in this manner until first-aider A tires or wishes to switch places for other reasons.

A set of procedures is followed for changing positions. First-aider A initiates a switch by saying "Switch one thousand, two one thousand, ... five one thousand," as he or she completes a series of compressions. He or she then goes to the victim's neck area to conduct a check lasting no more than five seconds. Meanwhile, first-aider B gives a breath before placing the hands appropriately for doing compressions. If there is no pulse and no breathing, first-aider A gives a breath and then says, "No pulse, continue CPR." The five compression–one breath CPR cycle is resumed.

## __CPR for Infants and Children

The needs of infants and children during a cardiac emergency differ somewhat from the needs of adults. The CPR technique has to be modified to accommodate the smaller physical size of the victim. The similarities and differences are discussed here in terms of assessment, obtaining help, initiating care, and giving CPR.

The assessment of the infant or child is similar in sequence to the assessment of an adult. For an infant under 1 year of age, the first-aider may tap the infant's foot and say, "Baby, baby, are you OK?" If there is no response the first-aider opens the airway and checks for breathing for five to ten seconds. In the infant the head is tipped slightly to open the airway, whereas in the adult the head is tipped significantly. If breathing is absent, the first-aider gives the baby two slow breaths (1 to 1½ seconds in duration) sufficient in pressure to make the infant's chest rise. These breaths are delivered by the first-aider placing his or her mouth over the infant's mouth AND nose. The first-aider then rechecks breathing status while taking the infant's brachial pulse for five to ten seconds. The brachial pulse is found on the inner side of the baby's upper arm (Figure 6.5A). The first-aider then obtains assistance and initiates care according to the victim's needs.

If the infant requires artificial respiration, the puffs of air are given at the rate of one breath every three seconds (Chapter 5). If CPR is required, the infant is given five compressions to every one breath. Compressions are given with the tips of two fingers placed on the sternum midway between and one finger width below the nipples (Figure 6.5B). The depth of each compression is ½ to 1 inch. Compressions are given at the rate of 100 per minute. The first-aider does a five-second (maximum) pulse and breathing check after one minute of CPR. If there is a pulse and breathing, the first-aider closely monitors the infant while waiting for medical assistance. If there is a pulse but no breathing, the first-aider gives artificial respiration. If there is no pulse (and therefore no breathing), CPR is resumed starting with a breath. *The pulse check must always begin and end with a breath.*

CPR for a child 1 to 8 years of age is similar to CPR for an infant in that the compression-to-breath ratio is five to one. It differs, however, in the following ways: Compressions are given at the rate of 80 to 100 per minute. They are given with three fingers or the heel of one hand (Figure 6.5C). Hand/finger placement is determined by using the rib cage trace method (Figure 6.3, steps 1-3, page 99). The depth of each compression is 1 to 1½ inches. The breaths are slightly fuller.

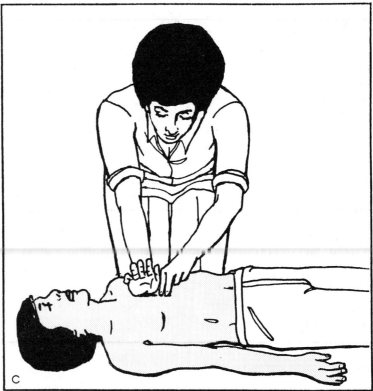

**FIGURE 6.5**

Cardiopulmonary resuscitation in infants and children. (*A*) The infant's head is tipped slightly to open the airway, and the brachial pulse is checked in the inner upper arm.
(*B*) Compressions are given to a depth of ½ to 1 inch with two fingers on the sternum midway between and one finger width below the nipples. (*C*) In children 1 to 8 years of age, compressions are given with three fingers or the heel of one hand to a depth of 1 to 1¼ inches.

**TABLE 6.3**

Compression characteristics by type of CPR and victim needing it

| Type of CPR and/or Victim | Rate of Compressions per Minute | Compression Depth (in.) | Ratio of Compressions to Breaths | Part of Hand(s) Used for Compressions |
|---|---|---|---|---|
| One-first-aider | | | | |
| Adult | 80–100 | 1½–2 | 15:2 | Heels of both hands |
| Two-first-aiders | | | | |
| Adult | 80–100 | 1½–2 | 5:1 | Heels of both hands |
| Children | 80–100 | 1–1½ | 5:1 | Heel of one hand |
| Infants | 100 | ½–1 | 5:1 | Tips of two fingers |

The sequence of activities for giving CPR is the same for infants and children. Table 6.3 presents compression characteristics for adults, children, and infants. Adult CPR techniques are used for children over 8 years of age.

# WHEN TO DISCONTINUE CPR

CPR should be discontinued when
- The victim is able to breathe unaided.
- Medical personnel with more advanced training than the first-aider arrive on the scene and are ready to take over.
- The first-aider is physically unable to continue.

## SUMMARY

Circulation of oxygenated blood is a life-sustaining function of the heart. Recognition of the signs of a cardiac emergency and calling or sending for professional medical care are essential aspects of first aid. Cardiopulmonary resuscitation (CPR) is a first aid technique for a person who is not breathing and has no pulse. The techniques for CPR differ somewhat according to the physical size of the person requiring it (i.e., adult, child, or infant).

## CHAPTER MASTERY: TEST ITEMS

**True and False**                                                                 Circle One

1. If the supply of oxygen to the brain is interrupted for six to ten minutes, death usually results.                                      T        F
2. CPR involves artificial respiration plus compressions for circulation of blood.                                      T        F

3. Obtaining professional medical assistance is an important aspect of CPR.   **T**   **F**
4. In infant CPR, the rate of compressions is sixty per minute.   **T**   **F**
5. In adult CPR, the heels of the first-aider's hands are placed over the victim's xiphoid process.   **T**   **F**
6. In infant CPR, the first-aider's fingers are placed between the nipples.   **T**   **F**
7. A pulse and breathing check is done one minute after initiating CPR.   **T**   **F**
8. Once initiated, CPR may be interrupted if necessary for periods up to a maximum of ten seconds.   **T**   **F**
9. A second first-aider should begin to assist only during the first ten compressions of a CPR cycle.   **T**   **F**
10. CPR should not be discontinued for any reason.   **T**   **F**

## Fill in the Missing Word(s)

1. The four steps involved in assessing the possibility of a cardiac emergency are _____, _____, _____, and _____.
2. The following first aid action is needed when the victim (a) is breathing and has a pulse: _____ and _____, (b) is not breathing and has a pulse: _____ and _____, (c) does not have a pulse (and is therefore not breathing): _____ and _____.

## Multiple Choice (Circle the Best Answer)

1. In one-first-aider CPR, the ratio of compressions to breaths is
   a. 3 to 1.
   b. 5 to 1.
   c. 5 to 2.
   d. 15 to 1.
   e. 15 to 2.

2. In one-first-aider CPR, compressions are given to an adult at the rate of
   a. 40–60 per minute.
   b. 60–80 per minute.
   c. 80–100 per minute.
   d. 100–120 per minute.
   e. 120–140 per minute.

3. In two first aider CPR, compressions are given to an adult at the rate of
   a. 40–60 per minute.
   b. 60–80 per minute.
   c. 80–100 per minute.
   d. 100–120 per minute.
   e. 120–140 per minute.

4. In infant CPR, the depth of the compressions should be
   a. ¼ to ½ in.
   b. ½ to 1 in.
   c. 1 to 1½ in.
   d. 1½ to 2 in.
   e. 2 to 2½ in.
5. In the child, CPR compressions are given with
   a. one finger.
   b. the heels of two hands.
   c. the heel of one hand.
   d. two fingers.
   e. the palm and fingers of one hand.

## Discussion Questions

1. Describe the steps the first-aider must complete to properly place the hands for administering chest compressions to an adult.
2. Explain the advantages of two-first-aider CPR over one-first-aider CPR.
3. Identify the most common signs of a heart attack.

## BIBLIOGRAPHY

American National Red Cross, *Respiratory and Circulatory Emergencies.* Garden City, N.Y.: Doubleday, 1980.

National Conference on Cardiopulmonary Resuscitation and Emergency Cardiac Care. "Standards and Guidelines for Cardiopulmonary Resuscitation (CPR) and Emergency Cardiac Care (ECC)." *Journal of the American Medical Association* 255 (June 6, 1986): 2905-2960.

Parcel, G. S. *Basic Emergency Care.* St. Louis: C. V. Mosby, 1982.

# 7

# Bleeding and Wounds

DAVID M. WHITE, ED.D.

After completing this chapter the student will be able to

- Describe the body's circulatory system.
- Explain the effect of blood loss on body functions.
- Identify the various types of bleeding from open wounds, specifically, arterial, venous, and capillary bleeding.
- Demonstrate techniques for control of external bleeding.
- Explain why the tourniquet is generally considered a last resort to stop bleeding.
- Cite the signs and symptoms of internal bleeding.
- Describe the distinguishing characteristics of various open wounds.
- List and explain first aid measures for open wounds.
- Describe important first aid measures for special wounds, such as bites, crushing injuries, and amputations.
- Explain recommended methods for dealing with foreign objects embedded in wounds.
- Describe infection and basic first aid measures for infection control.

## ___INTRODUCTION

The circulatory system is a complex arrangement of vessels by means of which blood is circulated throughout the body. Circulation is powered by pressure created by the heart. The four chambers of the heart function as two paired pumps. The right-side pump circulates blood from the body to the lungs. The left-side pump circulates blood from the lungs to the body.

There are three basic types of blood vessels: arteries, veins, and capillaries. Arteries carry blood away from the heart; veins bring blood back to the heart. Capillaries provide the connections between the arteries and the veins. Figure 7.1 illustrates the networking of the heart and the blood vessels.

Of the three types of blood vessels, the *arteries* are strongest because of their thick, muscular walls. These walls allow the arteries to withstand large internal pressures. In fact, some arteries have such thick walls that the walls have their own system of capillaries to provide sufficient nutrients and oxygen to the muscular tissue. An extensive network of nerves controls the dilation and constriction of the arteries and the amount of blood passing through.

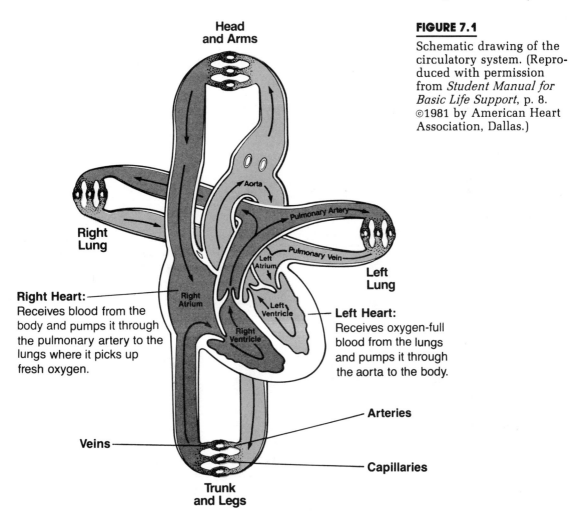

**Head and Arms**

**Right Lung**

Aorta

Pulmonary Artery

Pulmonary Vein

**Left Lung**

Left Atrium

Right Atrium

**Right Heart:**
Receives blood from the body and pumps it through the pulmonary artery to the lungs where it picks up fresh oxygen.

Left Ventricle

Right Ventricle

**Left Heart:**
Receives oxygen-full blood from the lungs and pumps it through the aorta to the body.

**Arteries**

**Veins**

**Capillaries**

**Trunk and Legs**

**FIGURE 7.1**

Schematic drawing of the circulatory system. (Reproduced with permission from *Student Manual for Basic Life Support*, p. 8. ©1981 by American Heart Association, Dallas.)

The arteries gradually decrease in size, turning into arterioles, which in turn become the smallest vessels, the hairlike capillaries. *Capillaries* have very thin walls which allow two-way passsage of nutrients and waste products between the blood and body cells. Blood moves slowly through the capillaries, which permits this exchange to occur. The capillaries join together to form small *veins* (venules), which in turn join to form larger veins. The walls of the veins have a layer of muscle that is not nearly as thick as that of the arterial walls. Veins do not have to withstand the high pressure to which arteries are subjected. One major difference between veins and other blood vessels is the presence in veins of valves, which help to direct the flow of blood back to the heart. When blood is flowing toward the heart, the valves allow free passage. If back pressure develops, the valves close, preventing blood from flowing back into the capillaries. Veins increase in size as they approach the heart.

Oxygenated blood flows from the left ventricle of the heart through the aorta and then through other large arteries to all parts of the body (except the lungs). As just described, the blood returns to the heart in veins and empties from either the superior or inferior vena cava into the heart. The blood then enters the right ventricle and is pumped into the lungs. Gases are exchanged in the lungs and oxygenated blood flows into the left atrium. The left atrium then fills the left ventricle and the cycle begins again. Each cycle takes approximately one minute.

## ——EFFECT OF BLOOD LOSS ON BODY FUNCTIONS

The average adult body contains five to six liters of blood. Content varies with the size and age of the individual. A newborn infant may have only 300 milliliters (ten to twelve ounces) of blood. As a general rule, the loss of one liter (approximately one quart) of blood in an adult, 500 milliliters (approximately one pint) in a child, or 25 milliliters (approximately two ounces) in an infant is very dangerous (Table 7.1).

Normally, the circulatory system adapts constantly to the body's changing needs and conditions, so that the blood vessels are filled to capacity. This helps to ensure that blood is circulated efficiently to all parts of the body and also creates pressure on the vessel walls, called *blood pressure*. The diameter of the arteries and veins varies and is controlled by the autonomic nervous system. When blood is lost, the body reacts by reducing the size of the blood vessels (vasoconstriction). Also, the heart pumps more rapidly to circulate the smaller volume of blood. If the amount of blood lost is not great, these actions maintain normal blood pressure, and all parts of the body receive an adequate supply of blood. However, if the blood loss is great, blood pressure may fall below normal, so that blood is not efficiently circulated.

The amount of blood being circulated may decrease for reasons other than severe bleeding. First, the arteries and veins may become larger in diameter (vasodilation) because of failure of the autonomic nervous system to adjust efficiently in an accident or emergency situation. Massive dilation creates a circulatory capacity far too large for the volume of blood available. The blood pressure is ineffective in forcing the blood through the increased area, and the blood tends to pool in the extremities. Second, the heart may not function effectively, as during a heart attack.

**TABLE 7.1**

Critical circulating blood volumes for adults, children, and infants

|  | **Normal Circulating Volume** | **Loss That May Cause Death** |
|---|---|---|
| Adult* | 5 to 6 liters (5 to 6 quarts) | 1 liter (1 quart) |
| Child (1 to 8 years) | 2 to 3 liters (2 to 3 quarts) | 500 milliliters (1 pint) |
| Infant (0 to 1 year) | 300 milliliters (10 to 12 ounces) | 25 milliliters (2 ounces) |

*Includes persons over 8 years of age.

As the volume of blood in the circulatory system diminishes, blood pressure lowers. The heart reacts to the lowered blood pressure by pumping more rapidly. If the lowering of blood volume is significant and the body cannot adapt adequately, the result is shock. The state of shock worsens as blood volume lessens, and death may result (see Chapter 4).

Therefore, it is extremely important that severe bleeding be controlled and measures taken to improve blood flow throughout the body. A person may bleed to death in a matter of minutes (or less if a major artery is severed), and shock may reach a critical stage in a very short time. This explains why severe bleeding is an immediate life-threatening emergency. Control of severe bleeding is often the responsibility of the first person on the scene, because the time required for medical or paramedical personnel to arrive may be too great for survival of the victim.

## ___TYPES OF BLEEDING

Bleeding may be either internal or external and is caused by blood escaping from arteries, veins, capillaries, or any combination of these. Generally, blood clots in three to ten minutes. However, in some cases bleeding may be so severe that clots cannot form or the person may bleed to death before clotting starts.

The volume of blood loss is very important. The faster blood loss occurs, the more dangerous the situation. Generally speaking, blood loss from an artery is greater than that from either veins or capillaries. Because arteries are under greater pressure than veins or capillaries, blood from severed arteries spurts. Arteries carry oxygenated blood, and thus **arterial blood is bright red.** Arterial bleeding is often profuse. Venous bleeding is usually more slow and steady and **venous blood is dark red.** Venous bleeding may also be profuse, however.

Capillary bleeding is never profuse, but is associated with other problems, such as the likelihood of infection. Figure 7.2 illustrates the principal characteristics of arterial, venous, and capillary bleeding.

External bleeding is relatively easy to spot, but internal bleeding is usually not visible and thus is difficult to detect. Bleeding from any body opening, except for menstrual bleeding, may indicate internal bleeding. For example, bleeding from the ears or nose may indicate a severe head injury. Blood in the urine or feces can result from internal organ damage, such as injury to a kidney. Coughed up blood may indicate a severely bleeding stomach ulcer. A bone fracture may cause internal bleeding by damaging tissue around the break. Thus, even though little or no blood is apparent, the victim may be bleeding to death internally, and it is important for the first-aider to recognize the presence of such bleeding and to administer appropriate first aid measures.

The signs and symptoms of internal bleeding are very similar to those of shock (see Chapter 4). The pulse is weak or rapid and the blood pressure is low. The skin is cool and clammy; the eyes are often vacant and dull. There may be nausea and vomiting. The victim is often thirsty and very anxious. Other signs may give clues to the location or source of the bleeding. For example, internal chest wounds caused by broken ribs may

**FIGURE 7.2**

Characteristics of venous, arterial, and capillary bleeding

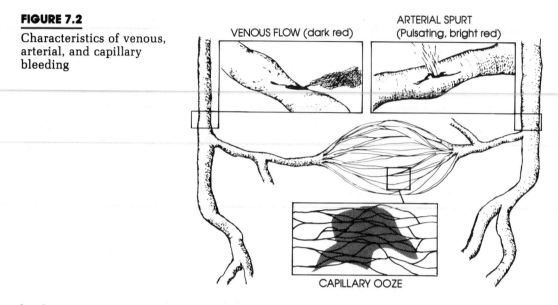

VENOUS FLOW (dark red)

ARTERIAL SPURT (Pulsating, bright red)

CAPILLARY OOZE

lead to coughing up of bright red blood. There may be blood in vomitus. Dark-colored blood, the color and consistency of coffee grounds, usually indicates an older injury, whereas bright red blood generally indicates a recent problem. A victim of abdominal trauma may lose a significant amount of blood into the abdominal cavity. Besides showing signs similar to those just mentioned, this person will also typically have a very tender abdomen. Figure 7.3 illustrates the most common signs and symptoms of internal bleeding.

Evaluating the extent of internal blood loss is often difficult. However, the first-aider should be aware that injuries to specific areas (e.g., penetration of the chest cavity near the heart) or certain types of injuries (e.g., ruptured spleen or liver, broken pelvis,

**FIGURE 7.3**

Common signs and symptoms of internal bleeding

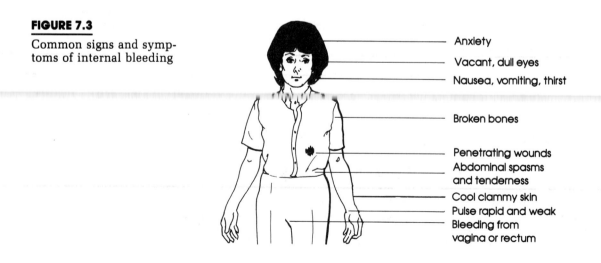

Anxiety

Vacant, dull eyes

Nausea, vomiting, thirst

Broken bones

Penetrating wounds
Abdominal spasms and tenderness

Cool clammy skin

Pulse rapid and weak

Bleeding from vagina or rectum

fracture of the long bones of the arm or leg) may be associated with significant internal blood loss. Any badly bruised area indicates blood loss; the larger and more severe the bruise, the greater the loss of blood.

## ____TECHNIQUES FOR CONTROL OF BLEEDING

Because of the life-threatening effects of severe bleeding, it is essential that the first-aider be familiar with the techniques for control of bleeding. These include, in order of preference, direct pressure, elevation, use of pressure points, and as a last resort, use of a tourniquet (Figure 7.4).

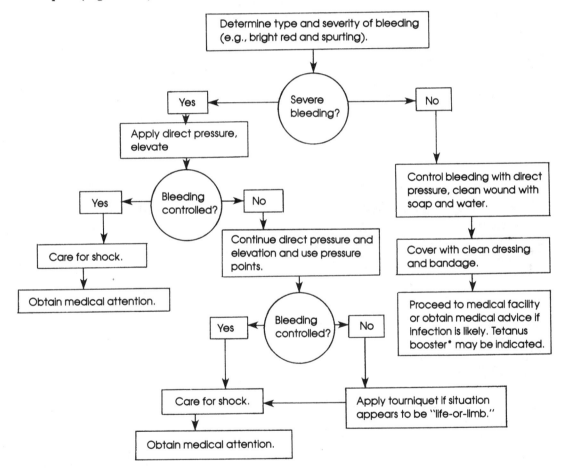

*Tetanus is characterized by sore, spastic muscles, particularly in the head and neck. It usually occurs five to ten days after initial infection. Tetanus boosters are needed once every ten years.

### FIGURE 7.4
Steps in caring for victims with bleeding from open wounds

## ___Direct pressure

Almost all external bleeding is controlled by direct pressure. Pressure applied directly over the injured area usually slows blood flow to the extent that clotting can occur. Direct pressure may be applied with only a bare hand, if necessary. A cloth compress should be applied as soon as possible, with pressure applied directly by the hand or by a pressure bandage (see Chapter 17). Ideally, the compress is sterile gauze. However, a search for sterile gauze or even a freshly laundered handkerchief may require too much time if the bleeding is severe. Even unclean material can be used if nothing else is immediately available. The flow of blood from a severely bleeding wound tends to clean the wound, so that the chance of contamination is lessened. If the compress becomes blood soaked, additional layers of cloth should be added along with additional direct pressure. *The original compress should not be removed, so that any clots formed will not be disturbed.*

A pressure bandage can be applied over the dressing if the first-aider needs to be free for other duties. A bandage or strip of cloth should be centered directly over the wound and dressing. The first-aider maintains a steady pull as he or she wraps the bandage around the injured body part. The bandage is tied over the dressing with a square knot (Figure 7.5) for additional pressure. If the wound is on an extremity, the pulse should be monitored below the wound site to be sure the bandage is not cutting off arterial circulation.

## ___Elevation

Direct pressure should be accompanied by elevation of the injured area above the heart level (Figure 7.6). The force of gravity can slow the bleeding by reducing the blood pressure at the wound site. However, elevation should not be used if it causes additional pain, such as may be the case with an open fracture. In this case, elevation could actually increase the volume of blood lost because the movement of broken bones can damage

**FIGURE 7.5**

Application of a pressure bandage. (*A*) Bleeding wound. (*B*) Pressure bandage is centered directly over the wound and dressing. (*C*) A steady pull is maintained as the bandage is wrapped around the injured part. (*D*) A square knot tied over the dressing provides additional pressure.

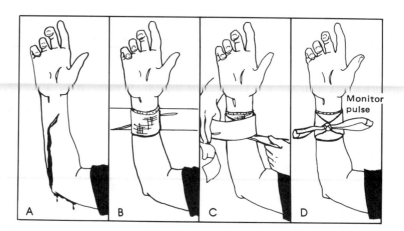

Monitor pulse

A    B    C    D

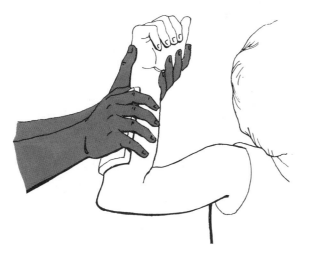

**FIGURE 7.6**
Direct pressure on a bleeding wound and elevation of
the part above heart level
slows blood pressure at the
wound site.

tissue and cause internal bleeding. If elevation causes additional pain, the degree of
shock may also increase.

If elevation is indicated, *direct pressure must be continued.* Elevation alone is not
effective for controlling hemorrhage.

## __Pressure Points

Some instances of severe bleeding cannot be controlled by direct pressure and elevation.
In these cases the first-aider may apply pressure on the major artery supplying blood to
the injured part. The sites where pressure can be applied are called pressure points.
Direct pressure and elevation should be maintained while pressure is applied also to the
supplying artery (pressure point).

Using pressure points to control bleeding is analogous to stepping on the garden hose
to reduce or cut off the flow of water. The supplying artery is pressed against a bony area
with the fingers or heel of the hand, just as the garden hose is pressed against the ground
with the foot. Using a pressure point to control bleeding is generally not as satisfactory as
using direct pressure and elevation, because seldom do all of the injured blood vessels
originate from the same supplying artery. However, its use may slow the flow of blood so
that direct pressure and elevation are effective. **Pressure points should be used to control
bleeding only when absolutely necessary, because circulation within the entire body
part is affected.**

There are several points in the human body where an artery lies close to the skin or
over bony areas (Figure 7.7), and these are appropriate as pressure points. The most
practical and effective pressure points are the brachial artery in the upper arm (found on
the inside of the arm between the biceps and the triceps muscles, about midway between
the elbow and the shoulder) and the femoral artery in the groin. Proper hand positions
for applying pressure to the brachial and femoral arteries are illustrated in Figure 7.8.
*The flat inside surface of the fingers, rather than the fingertip, should be used to press the*

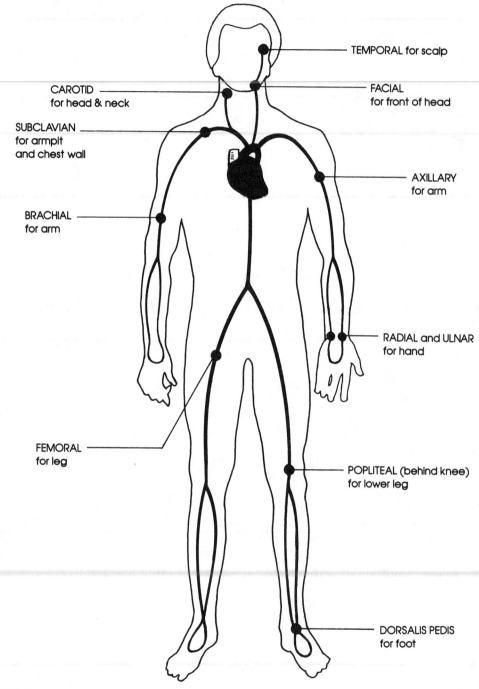

**FIGURE 7.7**

Pressure points help control bleeding in areas supplied by various arteries.

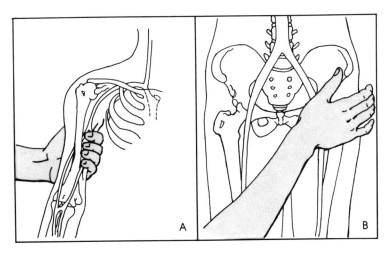

**FIGURE 7.8**

Proper hand positions for applying pressure to the brachial (*A*) and femoral (*B*) arteries

*brachial artery against the humerus (bone in the upper arm).* A pulse will be felt when the artery is located. The femoral artery should be compressed against the pelvic bone in the area just below the crease of the groin. In this case the victim should be lying down and the first-aider should use the heel of the hand to provide pressure. To do this effectively, the victim's clothing will probably have to be disturbed. The victim (if conscious) and witnesses (if available) are informed of the reason for such action, and the privacy of the victim is protected as much as possible. The arm supplying pressure should be kept straight; the weight of the first-aider's body can help provide additional pressure if the first-aider simply leans forward on the straightened arm. Elevation can be maintained by positioning the injured leg on a chair, on a box, or on the first-aider's own leg or shoulder. More intense pressure can be applied to the femoral artery by compressing it with the flat of the fingertips of one hand and using the heel of the other hand over the fingertips for additional pressure. This technique requires the aid of a second first-aider or of a pressure bandage, because *direct pressure should always accompany use of pressure points.*

Other pressure points that may be helpful in controlling severe bleeding are as follows:

1 *Temporal artery.* This artery is located in front of the ear (the "temple"). Bleeding from the head and forehead may be controlled by pressing on this artery.
2 *Facial artery.* This artery is located by pressing behind the notch in the lower jaw. When bleeding from the chin, lips, or lower face is difficult to control, pressure on the facial artery will help.
3 *Carotid artery.* These large arteries are on either side of the neck. **Pressure should be applied to a carotid artery only as a last resort and both arteries should never be compressed simultaneously.** The carotid arteries supply the

brain with oxygenated blood, and brain damage can occur if the flow of blood from both arteries is stopped or significantly hindered.

4 *Subclavian artery.* This artery is located under the clavicle (collarbone). Severe bleeding in the shoulder area can be controlled by pressing the subclavian artery against the collarbone and the first rib.

5 *Ulnar artery.* This artery is located in the wrist area. Pressure on it will assist in controlling severe bleeding from the hand.

The first-aider should be familiar with all of these pressure points, especially the brachial and femoral artery points. Locating these points can be practiced by checking each area until a pulse is detected.

## — Tourniquet

**A tourniquet should be used to control bleeding only as a last resort, when all other methods have failed.** There are few occasions when a tourniquet is required. The most likely is when partial or complete accidental amputation has occurred or when a major artery has been severed or torn.

The "last resort" status of the tourniquet has several reasons. A correctly applied tourniquet cuts off all blood flow to the injured limb; tissue death (gangrene) occurs after any appreciable length of time. The decision whether to apply a tourniquet is thus often called a "life-or-limb" decision: If the tourniquet is applied, the limb may be lost. Application of a tourniquet too tightly, or of one that is too narrow (less than two inches wide), will likely result in permanent damage to blood vessels, nerves, and other tissues. If the tourniquet is too loose it will actually increase blood loss, because blood flow back to the heart will be slowed but blood flow away from the heart will not be affected appreciably. Also, if the tourniquet is released after being applied, blood clots will dislodge, toxins will be introduced into the circulatory system, and the state of shock will worsen. Thus, **a tourniquet once applied should not be loosened until qualified medical personnel evaluate the victim.** Finally, tourniquets are used only for wounds of the extremities, never for use around the trunk, the neck, or the head.

Several commercially made tourniquets are available. Individuals who work around heavy machinery, such as farmers and construction workers, should have one of these tourniquets accessible in a nearby first aid kit. If a commercially prepared tourniquet is not available, a substitute can be improvised from a band of material at least two to four inches wide. A wire, rope, or string should NOT be used. Belts, neckties, stockings, large handkerchiefs, and cravat bandages can be fashioned into tourniquets.

A tourniquet is applied as follows (Figure 7.9):

1 Position the tourniquet between the heart and the wound, near the wound but not touching the wound edges. If the wound is in a joint or just below a joint, place the tourniquet just above the joint.

2 Place a small pad over the supplying artery so that the pressure focuses on that critical area.

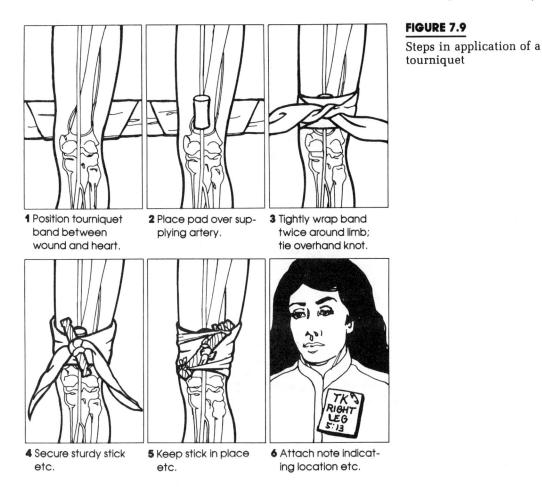

**FIGURE 7.9**

Steps in application of a tourniquet

**1** Position tourniquet band between wound and heart.

**2** Place pad over supplying artery.

**3** Tightly wrap band twice around limb; tie overhand knot.

**4** Secure sturdy stick etc.

**5** Keep stick in place etc.

**6** Attach note indicating location etc.

**3** Center the tourniquet so that it crosses over the main supplying artery to the injured area, and wrap the material twice tightly around the limb, tying in a flat, overhand knot.

**4** Place a short sturdy piece of wood, metal, or other material that will not break over the knot and then tie two overhand knots so as to tightly secure the stick; twist the stick until the bleeding stops.

**5** Secure the stick in place with the loose ends of the tourniquet, another strap of cloth, or other suitable material.

**6** Indicate in a note the location of the tourniquet and the time it was applied, and attach the note to the victim's clothing in plain view. A "T" or "TK" may be written on the victim's forehead with lipstick, or even blood, if it is not possible to write a note.

**7** Do not cover the tourniquet with clothing or blankets or hide it in any way.

**8** Do not loosen the tourniquet unless a physician advises doing so.

## __Internal Bleeding Control

There are definite limits to the extent to which the first-aider can control internal bleeding. Massive injury to soft tissues creates a very serious situation, and permanent disability may result. The first-aider can, however, take several important actions to maintain and possibly improve the condition of the victim of internal bleeding.

Initially, care should be given for shock (see Chapter 4) and the victim should be carefully examined for fractures and other injuries. Areas where fractures are suspected should be immobilized, because the broken bone ends can cause tissue damage and bleeding, especially if the break is within one of the long bones of the arm or leg. The victim with internal bleeding will usually be nauseated and may likely vomit. The first-aider should anticipate this by keeping the victim lying down, preferably on the side. Nothing is administered by mouth, especially if surgery may follow (which is very likely in the case of fractures, abdominal injuries, or diseases that cause internal bleeding). The victim is made as comfortable as possible. Above all, the victim's breathing and pulse are monitored throughout the rescue and the first-aider should be alert to airway blockage that may be caused by vomitus or blood.

## _____TYPES OF WOUNDS AND FIRST AID CARE

According to the American National Red Cross, "a wound is a break in the continuity of the tissues of the body, either internal or extenal" (1979, p. 24). Wounds are classified as either closed or open. A closed wound is damage to underlying tissues without a break in the skin or mucous membrane. An open wound is a break in the skin surface or in the mucous membrane lining the body's natural openings (such as the inside of the mouth). Both closed and open wounds present special problems for the first-aider. For example, open wounds are prone to infection and cause problems from blood loss. Closed wounds are less likely to become infected, but often the damage is difficult to estimate and the amount of blood loss may be as extensive as with an open wound.

## __Closed Wounds

Closed wounds are usually caused by a blunt force striking the body, such as the force created by a car accident or a fall. Closed wounds can also result from situations such as the improper handling of a closed fracture. A broken bone that is mishandled or improperly splinted can cause extensive internal injury. In a closed injury, subsurface damage exists, and this damage may extend to an internal organ. For example, a sharp blow to the lower back may not only create a bruised area just beneath the skin but also bruise the kidneys. The extent of this internal damage is difficult to estimate. If a closed wound appears minor, the first-aider should be cautious, because serious internal injury may have occurred. Further medical care must be sought.

### Signs and Symptoms
Small blood vessels in the tissues are usually crushed or torn, causing a closed wound to exhibit several signs and result in a number of symptoms. The blood that leaks out into

the tissues causes immediate swelling and pain, the extent of which is directly related to the factors causing the injury. Any leaking blood will move toward the skin and cause the familiar bruise (black-and-blue mark). In more serious injuries, such as when large blood vessels are involved, a pool of blood may develop very rapidly, creating a "lump" of blood (a hematoma). The amount of blood lost is often enough to worsen the victim's condition significantly, especially in terms of shock. A closed wound will, therefore, generally produce the following signs and symptoms: redness at the site of the injury, which later changes to a black-and-blue mark; swelling and tenderness at the injury site; a lump, depending on the extent of the injury and the tissue involved; and, if blood loss from the circulatory system is significant, signs and symptoms of shock (see Chapter 4).

### First Aid Care

Small bruises are usually no cause for alarm and require no special first aid care. If swelling and discoloration are evident, indicating internal bleeding, the use of cold compresses is recommended. A bandage, such as roller gauze, may be applied to provide pressure to help control the bleeding (see Chapter 17). First aid care for shock should be administered if any of the symptoms of shock are present or if the first-aider thinks the victim may have incurred extensive soft-tissue damage. Further medical care must be sought.

Anytime that soft-tissue damage is extensive, underlying fractures are likely. Correct handling and splinting of fractures may significantly reduce the amount of internal blood loss, while improper handling may seriously worsen the victim's condition because of additional blood loss.

## —Open Wounds

As mentioned previously, an open wound is a break in the skin or mucous membrane. Open wounds bleed obviously and are subject to infection. Shock, nerve damage, and tissue damage are also concerns. There are several types of open wounds (Figure 7.10). Each type has specific problems, such as bleeding or infection, with which the first-aider should be familiar.

### Abrasion

An abrasion is an open wound caused by scraping or rubbing away of an outer layer of skin. A skinned knee caused by falling on the pavement is an example of abrasion. Abrasions are sometimes called floor burns, rope burns, or strawberries. Generally they are painful, and blood oozes from the damaged capillaries and small veins. The danger of complications resulting from a loss of blood is minimal. However, because the wound bleeds little and in many cases the injured area is large, the danger of infection from contamination is significant.

### Incision

An incision is a smooth cut. Incised wounds are commonly caused by knives, razor blades, glass, or other sharp objects. Incisions tend to bleed freely, with the amount of bleeding depending on the depth and location of the cut. Extensive tissue damage, including damage to nerves, muscles, tendons, and blood vessels, may result from an incision.

**FIGURE 7.10**

Types of open wounds

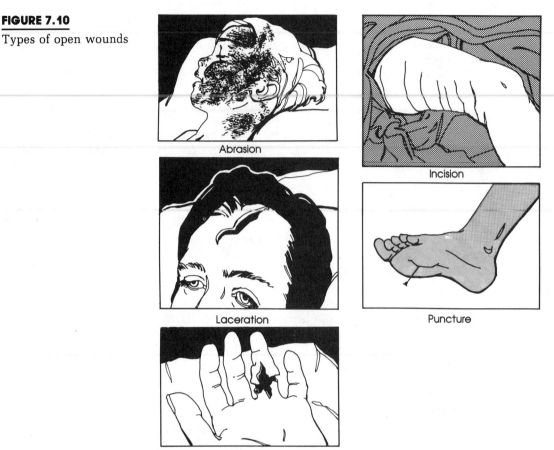

Abrasion

Incision

Laceration

Puncture

Avulsion

## Laceration

A laceration is a jagged, irregular cut or tear in the skin and soft tissues. Bleeding may be severe, especially if a large blood vessel is torn. Because a laceration is often caused by such objects as moving machinery, and because it may involve underlying tissue, the chance of infection is generally greater with a laceration than with an incision. Further, since a laceration is an irregular cut or tear in the tissue, the bleeding is generally more difficult to control than with an incision.

## Puncture

A puncture is a penetrating open wound caused by a pointed object such as a splinter, a nail, a needle, a knife, or a bullet. Generally the opening is small and external bleeding is minimal. However, because the object may have penetrated deeply into the body, with a puncture there is risk of internal damage and bleeding. The nature of a puncture wound makes it highly susceptible to infection. Most infectious organisms, like the tetanus bacterium, thrive in warm, moist environments with little air exposure.

**Avulsion**

An avulsion is an open wound in which tissue is torn completely off or left hanging as a flap. Avulsions may be caused by shooting, machinery accidents, animal bites that tear skin, or other incidents that involve forceful separation of tissue from the body. Any tissue, whether it be a finger, toe, ear, or an entire limb, may potentially be successfully reattached if the part is transported with the victim to the hospital.

**First Aid Care**

As a general rule, the first-aider handles open wounds with three primary considerations in mind. First and foremost, the bleeding must be stopped. Excessive blood loss results in shock, which if not controlled leads to death. Second, additional contamination must be prevented. Third, the injured area should be immobilized. These steps are followed by keeping the victim quiet and caring for shock, if necessary. The severity of the injury will dictate whether additional measures are required. The first-aider should always be aware that with a wound involving more than the superficial layers of the skin, such as a deep puncture wound, there may be associated internal damage. The severity of an open wound cannot be estimated simply by the extent of external bleeding.

The techniques recommended for controlling bleeding have been discussed earlier in this chapter (direct pressure, elevation, use of pressure points, and use of a tourniquet). Often, however, an open wound is partially covered with clothing and may be complicated by foreign matter (e.g., glass or metal) around and in the wound. This compounds the situation for the first-aider. General rules regarding these problems are as follows:

1 Uncover the wound. Clothing over and around a wound can limit assessment of the extent of the injury and should be removed. It is best not to try to remove clothing by pulling it over the arms, legs, or head. The recommended procedure is to carefully cut, tear, or lift it aside. Avoid excessive movement of the injured area. This may aggravate the injury and increase pain for the victim. An increase in pain usually promotes shock. To the extent possible, continue to protect the victim's privacy.

2 Clear foreign matter from around the surface of the wound. Carefully remove any gross matter. *Do not try to clear the wound of any embedded material.* No matter how dirty a wound may seem, the time spent attempting to clean it out, especially a serious wound such as a deep abrasion, is usually wasted and may actually promote, rather than decrease, the chance of infection. Removal of foreign matter embedded in a wound is considered the job of a physician.

When these two tasks have been accomplished, the first-aider proceeds to control bleeding, prevent contamination, treat for shock, and immobilize the injured area. Certainly the extent of bleeding will dictate the amount of time spent uncovering and clearing the surface around the wound. If bleeding is severe, as with arterial bleeding, the time should be minimal. The first-aider must exercise good judgment and avoid misusing time in cases of severe bleeding.

Measures should be taken to reduce the likelihood of infection. As a general rule, the more a wound bleeds, the less prone it is to infection. The blood flushes out contamination. *When a bandage has been applied to control bleeding, it should not be removed even to clean the wound or to apply clean dressings.* Not only may removal disturb clots and lead to additional bleeding, but it will also increase the likelihood of infection.

If bleeding is minor and only the outer layer of skin has been injured, as with most abrasions, it is generally recommended that the wound be cleaned. This is best accomplished with soap and water. If necessary, the area may be soaked in clean water for several minutes or held under water flowing from a tap for several minutes. The area is then blotted dry with a sterile dressing (preferably) or a freshly laundered towel. Absorbent cotton should not be used because it will tend to adhere to, and thus contaminate, the wound. Antiseptics should generally be used only under the direction of a physician, because they may destroy tissue or, in some cases (e.g., through improper application), their use may promote infection by introducing foreign substances into the wound. After cleaning the wound, the first-aider places a sterile dressing over the entire wound area and bandages it into place (see Chapter 17).

## __Bites

Bites, either animal or human, may cause lacerations, abrasions, punctures, or avulsions. They are handled as other open wounds with special consideration given to the fact that they are infection prone. Bacterial infections, such as tetanus, and virus infections, such as rabies, can result from a bite.

### Animal Bites

The incidence of animal bites is fairly high. Every year at least one million Americans are biten by dogs (Thygerson 1982), and many others are bitten by cats, squirrels, and other animals. The injury may range from a seemingly minor puncture wound to an extensive laceration.

When bleeding has been well controlled, the bite wound is thoroughly washed with soap and water for at least ten minutes. Thorough cleansing helps to reduce the risk of rabies, as well as infection from other agents. Application of sterile dressing and a bandage prevents further contamination. *The victim should seek medical attention as soon as possible.*

An animal that inflicts a bite should be observed for at least ten days to determine if it has *rabies.* The animal need not be killed, as is commonly thought. If the animal appears rabid and cannot be safely captured, however, it may have to be destroyed. In such a case the head should be saved for inspection by the proper authorities.

Skunks, raccoons, and bats are the animals that carry rabies most often in the United States and Canada. Rabies is almost always fatal; in fact, only three people are known to have survived this disease. Only about two human cases of rabies a year are reported in the United States; however, of the million Americans bitten by animals each year, about 35,000 will receive rabies vaccinations.

Rabies is primarily transmitted via the virus-laden saliva of a rabid animal. Transmission usually occurs through a bite because rabies makes the animal uncharacteristically aggressive. However, the virus may be transmitted through an open wound such as a scratch. The first symptoms of rabies include fatigue, headache, and irritability. These are followed by a fever and sore throat. Soon the stage from which rabies gets it nickname, "hydrophobia," occurs and the victim chokes and gags when trying to drink. The victim gradually deteriorates and death usually results as a complication of coma.

This sequence can be prevented if immunization is begun after the bite. The first step in dealing with the disease **is to wash the wound thoroughly with soap and water.** Next, rabies immune globulin is administered. Despite its frightening reputation, the currently used vaccine is quite painless and highly effective. The typical treatment is five doses over a four-week period. Adverse reactions are uncommon.

The Harvard Medical School Health Letter (1984, p. 5) indicated that the following factors should be considered when making a decision about immunization:

1 *Species of the biting animal.* Skunks, raccoons, and bats, for example, are more likely to transmit rabies than are squirrels or chipmunks. Statistically, wild animals are much more likely than domestic animals to be rabid.

2 *Presence of rabies in the region.* Local health or wildlife departments may be able to provide this information.

3 *Circumstances of the bite.* An animal that bites without provocation is most likely to be rabid. Bites incurred during feeding or handling are usually regarded as provoked.

4 *Type of exposure.* Bites are more dangerous than scratches or abrasions, unless the animal has drooled or licked broken skin.

5 *Condition of the animal.* A recently vaccinated animal is less dangerous than an obviously sick one.

### Human Bites

The risk of infection is great when a human bite breaks the skin, because the mouth is teeming with potentially harmful bacteria. If bleeding is not excessive and is well controlled, the wound is washed thoroughly with soap and water, covered with a sterile dressing, and bandaged. The wound is then carefully monitored for signs of infection. As with any open wound, if tissue damage is significant medical attention should be sought, because sutures may be required. Self-inflicted bites of the tongue, lip, and inside of the mouth generally present no problem as far as infection is concerned. If the tissue is significantly damaged, however, as when the tongue is cut badly, medical attention may be required.

## __Nonpoisonous Snakebites

Approximately 37,000 nonpoisonous snakebite incidents are reported yearly in the United States. Although the bulk of attention dealing with first aid care for snakebite centers around dealing with the toxic reaction from poisonous snakes, it is also important for the first-aider to know how to care for the puncture wound created by a nonpoisonous snakebite.

The bite pattern of a nonpoisonous snake is distinctly different from that of most poisonous snakes. Nonpoisonous snakes have teeth instead of fangs, and they thus leave a series of small puncture wounds instead of one or two distinct punctures. If there is doubt regarding whether the bite is from a poisonous snake, the first-aider follows directions for caring for the victim of a poisonous snakebite. (See Chapter 10 for a discussion of poisonous snakebite and Figure 10.4 for an illustration of the puncture pattern associated with nonpoisonous snakes.) If the bite is identified as that of a nonpoisonous snake, the following first aid procedures should be followed:

**1** Calm and reassure the victim.
**2** Clean the wound with soap and water.
**3** Consult a physician about antibiotic therapy and prevention of tetanus.

## __Crushing Injuries

Crushing injuries are serious because both external damage, such as open wounds and bleeding, and internal damage, such as broken bones, are often sustained. Bleeding may be severe, and fractures usually complicate the situation. The first-aider controls bleeding in a crushing wound by using the same techniques recommended for other open and closed wounds. However, direct pressure on this type of wound may case more harm than good. Thus, direct pressure must be carefully applied and done only to the extent that is absolutely necessary to control bleeding. Pressure on the supplying artery (see the discussion of pressure points in this chapter and Figure 7.7), elevation, and application of cold compresses are useful for external as well as internal hemorrhage control. Cold compresses and elevation are generally the best way to handle minor crushing injuries, such as a finger closed in a car door. In more serious injuries, a carefully applied splint is recommended, because it will not only immobilize the area, but also help to control internal and external hemorrhage (see Chapter 8 for more information on splinting).

## __Amputations

An amputation occurs when a body part, usually all or part of an extremity, is cut or torn completely from the body. Bleeding associated with an amputation is usually profuse and difficult to control. The first-aider attempts to control bleeding by using the techniques recommended for other open wounds. However, because the tissue damage is usually great and numerous blood vessels are damaged, he or she may need to apply a tourniquet. The victim needs medical care immediately.

The amputated body part should always be saved, if possible, for reattachment. Reattachment attempts have achieved much success in recent years. In fact, a well-preserved body part may be reattached up to twenty-four hours after the amputation. The success of reattachment is somewhat dependent on the first-aider's handling of the transportation of the severed part. The first-aider first wraps the part in dry, sterile gauze or a clean towel or cloth. Even though the part may be dirty, no attempt is made to clean it, because this may reduce the viability of the tissue. The part should NOT be packed directly in ice or immersed in ice water. After the part has been wrapped in gauze or clean material, it should ideally be placed in a plastic bag (like a sandwich bag) and the bag sealed shut. This bag containing the body part should then be placed in another plastic bag that contains ice, and this bag also be sealed. The body part is taken to the hospital along with the victim. Time should not be wasted, however, searching for plastic bags. The most important factor is that the severed part be handled carefully, kept

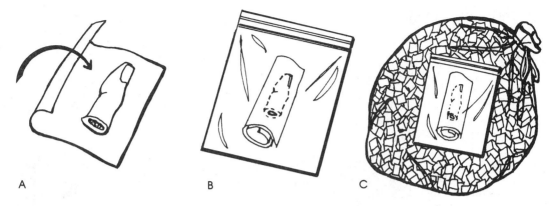

A    B    C

**FIGURE 7.11**

First aid care for an amputated part. (*A*) The part is wrapped completely in clean material. (*B*) The wrapped part is sealed in a plastic bag. (*C*) The plastic bag is placed in another plastic bag filled with ice.

clean and cool, protected from additional damage, and taken as soon as possible to the hospital. Figure 7.11 illustrates the steps that should be taken in caring for an amputated part.

## GENITAL INJURY

The external genitalia are not a common site of injury. When injury does occur, it is usually either from blunt trauma, as with a kick or fall, or from a cut. Such an injury is usually very painful, but unless bleeding is severe, it is generally not considered life threatening. The pain from blunt trauma injury is reduced if the victim lies quietly with a cold compress over the injured area. Bleeding is controlled with direct pressure. If tissue has been severed, it is saved and sent with victim to a medical facility.

The first-aider should respect the victim's privacy and avoid embarrassment as much as possible. The victim is reassured and appropriate first aid measures are briefly explained. The victim is protected from onlookers, if possible.

## FOREIGN OBJECTS IN A WOUND

The removal of foreign objects from a wound is sometimes recommended, as with small splinters and thorns, but there are situations when removal of a foreign object may do much more harm than good (e.g., objects penetrating the eye). The first-aider must exercise extreme caution when determining whether an embedded object should be removed. Removal of a deeply embedded object or a large penetrating object may cause additonal tissue damage and promote bleeding.

## __Thorns and Splinters

Small objects such as thorns, splinters, and wood or metal fragments should be removed from a wound only if they are visible and near the surface of the skin. The wound is flushed with water initially if there is a possibility that the object can be removed by irrigation. Sterile tweezers or the tip of a sterilized needle may be needed. Sterilization can be accomplished by holding the tweezers or needle over a flame for several seconds.

## __Impaled Objects

A knife, a rod, a piece of glass, or other object may be embedded in the body in such a way as to impale it. **The first-aider must not remove such an object.** Trained medical personnel are needed for the task of removal. Similarly, the body should not be removed from a fixed object, such as a fencepost.

If the object is protruding from the skin, the object should be immobilized. This is best accomplished by first carefully cutting or breaking it off near the surface of the skin. The object is then stabilized by covering it with a bulky dressing, such as several layers of cloth or towels. If available, a thick, donut-shaped dressing that fits securely around the object and over the wound is effective. The dressing is then bandaged firmly in place, and medical attention is sought immediately.

If the impaled object is sharp, such as glass or a knife, the first-aider must avoid further injury to the victim and also self-injury during efforts to control bleeding. No pressure should be applied directly on the object or against the tissues touching the edge of it. The best way to apply pressure is to spread the fingers around the object and press the hand flat against the wound site. Figure 7.12 illustrates appropriate care for an impaled object.

## __Fishhooks

It is not uncommon for a fishhook to become embedded in the skin. If only the point of the hook penetrates the skin, it is easily removed by backing the hook out. If the barb of the hook is embedded, however, withdrawing it the way it went in will damage a large

**FIGURE 7.12**

Management of impaled object (A). Pressure is applied to wound site (B). Bulky dressings held in place with bandages immobilize the object (C).

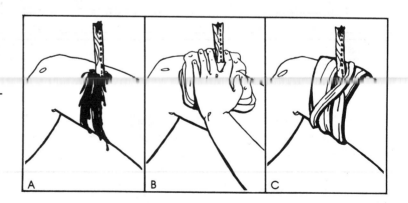

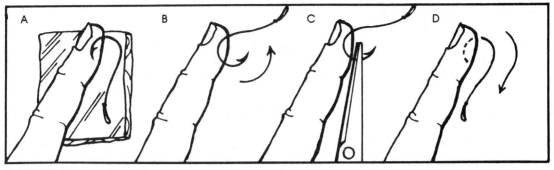

**FIGURE 7.13**

Removal of an embedded fishhook. After the area is anesthetized with ice (*A*), the hook is pushed through until the barb protrudes from the skin (*B*). The barb is then clipped off (*C*) and the hook withdrawn (*D*).

chunk of tissue. If medical care is near, it is best to transport the victim and have a physician remove the hook. If medical care is distant, the hook may be removed in the following manner (Figure 7.13):

1 Apply ice (if available) to the area for several minutes to provide temporary anesthesia.
2 Advance the fishhook in the wound in a curve until the barbed point penetrates the skin and comes out.
3 Clip off the barbed end with pliers or clippers.
4 Withdraw the shank of the hook through the original hole.
5 Cleanse the area with soap and water and cover it with a dressing.
6 Consult a physician.

## ___WOUND INFECTION

Any open wound can become infected, because bacteria are present in all open wounds. Wounds that have had extensive contamination, such as a crushing injury in a machine-related accident, wounds that do not bleed freely, and wounds that prevent entrance of air (especially punctures) are most prone to infection. Normally the body destroys large numbers of bacteria, and with proper care most open wounds can be spared infection. However, if the body cannot resist the bacteria or if the wound is not properly cleaned and maintained, infection can develop. First aid measures for wound infection generally involve simply recognizing the signs and symptoms of infection and referring the victim to appropriate medical attention.

Infection is usually characterized by redness, heat, pain, swelling, and pus accumulation at the site of the injury. Pain and swelling usually accompany a wound and disappear within two or three days. If they continue beyond this time, infection may have set in. As an infection develops it spreads through the lymph system, and red streaks may be noticed radiating from the wound site. The lymph glands of the neck, armpit, or groin may become swollen and tender. Infection that spreads beyond the wound site is serious, and medical attention should be sought. If such attention will be long delayed, the following temporary procedures may be followed:

1 Immobilize the infected area and have the victim avoid excess movement.
2 Elevate the affected part.
3 Apply warm, moist heat (hot water bottle or warm, moist cloths or towels) to the wound dressing. Change the heat source often enough to maintain its warmth.
4 Alternate thirty-minute periods of heat application with thirty-minute periods of no heat. Do this repeatedly until medical help is available.
5 Monitor the victim's temperature and give this and other related information to medical help when available.

*These procedures do not replace medical care.* They are utilized only when medical help will be long delayed.

─────────────────────── **SUMMARY** ───────────────────────

The circulatory system is a complex arrangement of blood vessels—arteries, veins, and capillaries—and the heart. If a breakdown related to the circulatory system occurs (for example, a damaged vessel or ineffective heart muscle), the entire body reacts. This generalized reaction is called shock.

The average adult body contains about five to six liters of blood, and the loss of one liter is very dangerous. Loss may be either internal or external. Because an individual can lose a significant amount of blood in a short period, it is essential that appropriate first aid measures be taken to control severe bleeding.

Arterial bleeding is usually the most difficult type to control because the arterial blood is under pressure and tends to spurt from a wound. Arterial blood is bright red. Venous bleeding is characterized by steady flow and dark red color.

Both arterial and venous bleeding may be profuse. Bleeding from an injured capillary is never profuse, rather the blood tends to ooze slowly from the wound.

Internal bleeding is difficult to assess. The signs and symptoms of internal bleeding are very similar to those of shock. Injury to certain areas of the body tends to be associated with significant internal blood loss.

Bleeding from a open wound is controlled in order of preference, by direct pressure, elevation, use of pressure points, and as a last resort, use of a tourniquet. Direct pressure successfully controls almost all external bleeding. Direct pressure should be accompanied by elevation of the injured part above the heart level in the absence of fracture and if elevation does not increase pain. Pressure applied to pressure points (points where supplying arteries lie close to the skin surface) may be useful if the bleeding cannot be controlled with direct pressure and elevation. **As a last resort,** a tourniquet may be applied. This is generally considered a "life-or-limb" situation, that is, the threat to life posed by excessive bleeding transcends the threat to the limb posed by the tourniquet.

Internal bleeding may be controlled by administering first aid care for shock and immobilizing any injured areas. The victim should receive medical attention as soon as possible.

Wounds may be classified as either closed or open. Closed wounds are usually caused by some external force; there is no break in the skin. Swelling, tenderness, and the signs of shock may be evident. A cold compress held in place with a bandage may be applied over a closed wound. Correct handling is important—many closed wounds are associated with fractures.

Open wounds, wounds associated with a break in the skin or mucous membrane, may be classified as abrasions, incisions, lacerations, punctures, or avulsions. First aid care for these wounds involves controlling bleeding, caring for shock (if indicated), preventing contamination, and immobilizing the injured part.

Other wounds that present first aid problems are bites, both animal and human; crushing injuries; and amputations. Anytime a body part is torn away completely it should be delivered to medical personnel for possible reattachment.

Small foreign objects may be carefully removed from a wound by the first-aider, but large penetrating objects or objects deeply embedded in the wound should not be. An impaled object should be immobilized near the body's surface

Infection is a possibility with any open wound. It is characterized by redness, heat, pain, swelling, and pus accumulation at the site of the injury. An infection that spreads though the lymph system can be very dangerous. If red streaks radiate from the wound or if the lymph glands are swollen and sensitive, medical advice should be obtained as soon as possible.

_____ **CHAPTER MASTERY: TEST ITEMS** _____

**True and False**                                                          **Circle One**

1. Blood coming from a severed artery is usually bright red and spurting.   T   F
2. The average adult body has about ten liters of blood.                    T   F
3. For an adult, the loss of one liter of blood can be very dangerous.      T   F
4. Capillaries provide the connection between arteries and veins.           T   F
5. A tourniquet should be loosened for a few seconds about every twenty     T   F
   minutes.
6. An incision is generally more prone to infection than is a puncture.     T   F
7. A finger that has been torn from the hand should NOT be cleaned          T   F
   before being transported to the hospital with the victim.
8. Severe bleeding is an immediate, life-threatening emergency.             T   F

9. The signs and symptoms of internal bleeding are distinctly different     **T**     **F**
from the signs and symptoms of shock.

10. Red streaks radiating from an open wound site are a phase of the     **T**     **F**
healing process.

### Multiple Choice (Circle the Best Answer)

1. Bleeding that is usually limited to oozing and some danger of infection best
describe a(n)
   a. abrasion.
   b. amputation.
   c. avulsion.
   d. incision.
   e. laceration.

2. When applying a tourniquet, the first-aider should
   a. tighten the tourniquet just enough to control bleeding.
   b. cover the tourniquet with the shirt sleeve or pants leg that was covering the
   injured area.
   c. be sure that the tourniquet touches the wound edge.
   d. release the tourniquet every twenty minutes.
   e. both a and c

3. The first-aider should *initially* try to control severe bleeding from a laceration on
the lower leg by applying
   a. a tourniquet just above the wound site.
   b. direct pressure and pressure on the femoral artery.
   c. pressure on the femoral artery.
   d. direct pressure and elevation of the leg.
   e. elevation only.

4. Which of the following may indicate internal bleeding?
   a. bleeding from the ears
   b. blood in the urine or feces
   c. a fractured femur (thighbone)
   d. coughing up of blood
   e. all of the above

5. The tourniquet is generally recognized as the last resort for stopping bleeding
because
   a. its application is likely to result in tissue death in the wound area.
   b. a great deal of time and effort are required to procure the materials needed to
   make a tourniquet.
   c. its application generally causes intense pain and dangerously increases the
   victim's level of shock.
   d. its correct application is very difficult and usually only medically trained
   personnel use it efficiently.
   e. once it has been applied, constant monitoring of the victim is required, which
   limits the first-aider if other victims need help.

6. Approximately one week after incurring a puncture wound while building a new fence, a neighbor begins to experience stiffness in the neck muscles and painful muscle spasms, especially in the jaw muscles. These signs may indicate
   a. damage to the spinal column.
   b. internal nerve injury.
   c. tetanus infection.
   d. a general secondary infection.

## Discussion Questions

1. Compare and contrast arteries, veins, and capillaries in terms of their function, their size and thickness, and the relative dangers to the victim when they are cut or torn.
2. List and briefly describe the types of open wounds. Indicate a problem associated with each, for example, bleeding, infection.
3. Describe what the first-aider should do for a person with a knife embedded in the abdomen.
4. List the steps recommended if someone has a severely infected foot and medical help is delayed for several days.
5. List several prominent signs and symptoms of internal bleeding.

_____ **BIBLIOGRAPHY** _____

American National Red Cross. *Advanced First Aid and Emergency Care.* 2d ed. Garden City, N.Y.: Doubleday, 1979.
Goldfinger, S., ed. *The Harvard Medical School Health Letter.* 10 (December 1984).
Thygerson, A. L. *The First Aid Book.* Englewood Cliffs, N.J.: Prentice-Hall. 1982.

# 8

# Musculoskeletal Emergencies

JOHN L. ECHTERNACH, ED.D., P.T.

After completing this chapter the student will be able to
- Describe the steps in the assessment of musculoskeletal injury and the purpose of each step.
- Describe the important principles of first aid that relate to care of a musculoskeletal injury.
- Define simple terms clearly, such as open and closed fracture, dislocation, sprain, and strain.
- Explain first aid care including proper immobilization techniques for possible fractures of bones of the shoulder girdle, arms, hands, chest, pelvis, legs, and feet.
- Describe first aid care for dislocations, sprains, and strains.

## INTRODUCTION

*The musculoskeletal system* is made up of the bones of the skeleton, muscles, ligaments (that attach bone to bone, providing stability at joints), and tendons (extensions of muscle tissue that attach muscle to bone). The musculoskeletal system performs two important functions. First, it provides the bony framework (Figure 8.1) to or within which the rest of the body systems and tissues are either attached or enclosed. For example, it provides the basic framework and shape of the body, protects vital organs such as the lungs and heart, and protects the brain and spinal cord. Second, the muscles of the musculoskeletal system fill out the shape of the body and provide the ability to control movement (i.e., to move with deliberateness from one place to another).

Any structure in the system can be injured in major or minor accidents. Musculoskeletal system injuries occur most frequently from automobile accidents, athletic and recreational activities, and falls. Two groups of individuals are most likely to be injured in accidents and falls, young children (up to 4 or 5 years of age) and older adults (over 65 years of age.) Both groups often incur injury to the skeletal system. Among older individuals, fractures occur readily because of the brittleness of bones due to the aging process.

## SPECIAL NOTE: THE FACE, SKULL, AND SPINAL COLUMN

The bones of the face, skull, and spinal column play a major role in protecting the central nervous system (i.e., the brain and spinal cord) from injury. The discussion of musculo-

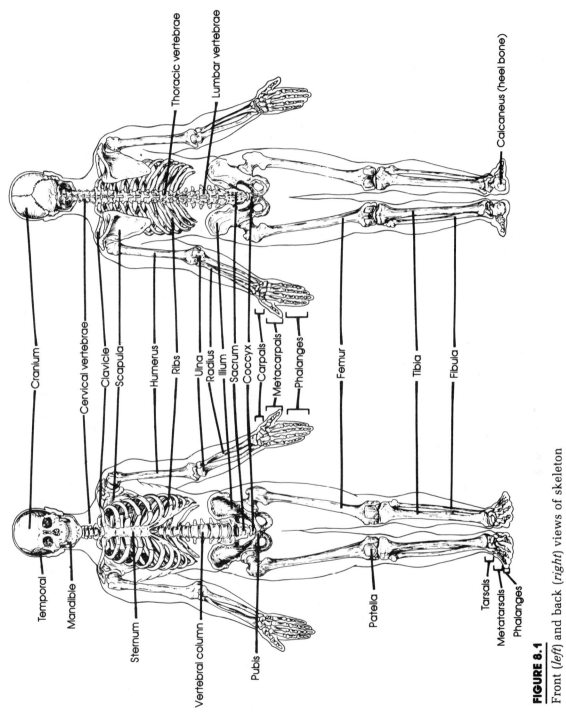

**FIGURE 8.1**

Front (*left*) and back (*right*) views of skeleton

skeletal injuries that follows excludes information pertaining to these particular parts of the skeletal system. Injuries of the face, skull, and spinal cord (and related first aid) are discussed in conjunction with emergencies involving the central nervous system in Chapter 9.

## ____ASSESSING THE EXTENT OF MUSCULOSKELETAL INJURIES

In assessing an individual for any type of problem, the first-aider must first take care of those emergencies that pose the greatest potential threat to the victim. The concept of triage has been dealt with previously (see Chapter 2). Assessment is generally followed by action-oriented decisions based on interpretation of the data by the observer. In an emergency situation, all of this transpires relatively quickly.

The most important source of information about musculoskeletal injury is the victim, if conscious. Information is gathered as part of the subjective interview (Chapter 2). The victim should be able to tell the first-aider how the injury occurred. Did the person fall and strike an object, hear or feel a bone snap? Is any area of the body particularly painful or tender? Is difficulty experienced in moving any part of the body? The victim may report a sensation of grating. This is called *crepitus,* and occurs when broken bones rub together.

Simple observation as a part of the objective (head-to-toe) examination provides a great deal of information. The first-aider compares one side of the body with the other, noting any differences in shape and length of corresponding parts. Obvious deformities such as angulation (crookedness of a bone), shortening, or rotation of a limb may be apparent. The victim is examined for evidence of bleeding, or an open wound over a bony area. Gentle point pressure (palpation) is used to detect swelling. Pain and tenderness in response to this gentle pressure at any site of suspected injury or fracture are noted. The finding of any of these conditions may signal the presence of a musculoskeletal injury. As indicated in Chapter 2, special care must be taken in assessing a person with suspected spinal cord injury. Likewise, caution must be exercised in assessing the musculoskeletal injuries of an individual who has experienced head or facial trauma (Chapter 9).

In all cases of trauma, regardless of the victim's readily observable injuries, the first-aider should conduct the full assessment procedures detailed in Chapter 2. These include the subjective interview (with witnesses, if available, in the case of the unconscious victim) and the objective examination. Additionally, it is prudent to care for all unconscious victims of trauma as if they have experienced spinal cord injury. First aid care for spinal cord injuries is presented in Chapter 9.

## ____TYPES OF FRACTURES

Two types of fractures are of primary importance to the first-aider, closed and open (Figure 8.2). With a *closed fracture,* no wounds are seen on the surface of the body

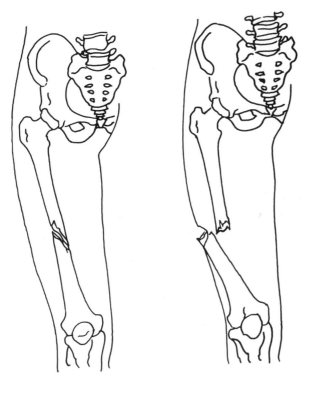

**FIGURE 8.2**

Closed (*left*) and open (*right*) fractures

adjacent to the fracture site, and a definite diagnosis often is not possible until an x-ray film is made. If a fracture is suspected, preventive first aid care reduces the risk of aggravating the injury.

An *open fracture* is much more severe and involved than a closed one. Injuries may be such that the fractured bone protrudes through the skin. In other instances, severe tearing (avulsion) of soft tissues exposes the injured bone.

Other classifications of fractures, such as spiral, oblique, comminuted, or impacted, refer primarily to the relationship of the bone ends to each other. Although important for understanding fractures, they are not of primary importance to the first-aider.

## SIGNS AND SYMPTOMS OF FRACTURE

Signs and symptoms of a fracture are basically those just described in the discussion of assessment. They typically include pain or deformity or both in the area of the fracture (e.g., angulation of the mid lower leg), discrepancy in the lengths of the extremities, crookedness or rotation of the limb, open wounds over the bone, or dislocation of the area, and crepitus with only minor mobility in the area. The first-aider should suspect a broken bone when one or more of these is observed.

## _____BASIC FIRST AID PROCEDURES FOR FRACTURES

In all fractures, the primary objectives of care are to keep the broken bone ends from moving (this includes keeping the adjacent joints from moving) and to prevent shock. Critical life-saving first aid care should always be carried out first. Additionally, care may be needed for shock before the fracture is addressed. After an assessment of critical needs and an appropriate response, the broken bone ends of a fracture can be immobilized to prevent further injury.

Sometimes immobilization can be accomplished by splinting. The first-aider should make no attempt to reduce (restore to normal position) a fracture, to straighten a crooked limb, or to push a protruding bone back through the skin. If competent help is known to be on the way and the injured person does not have to be moved, splinting may not be necessary. Under these circumstances, rolled-up clothing, blankets, or other materials can be placed on either side of the injury to limit movement. With open fractures there is the possibility of hemorrhage. The victim's clothing is moved aside or cut away and bleeding is controlled by digital pressure and a large clean dressing placed over the wound. (Pressure points—sites where digital pressure can be applied to major arteries to control the blood supply to various parts of the body—are identified in Figure 7.7.) It is important that the first-aider not contaminate the wound while controlling hemorrhage.

If ambulance service is readily available, the first-aider should not move the person suspected of having a fracture unless a life-threatening circumstance exists at the emergency scene (e.g., fire or noxious fumes). This holds true even if the injured person is in an automobile involved in an accident or is under the wreckage. If a life-threatening situation does exist, however, the victim must be quickly and safely moved to a protected area. (Chapter 18 discusses extrication and transportation techniques).

## _____PRINCIPLES OF SPLINTING

Before specific first aid procedures for specific fractures are discussed, a review of the principles of splinting is appropriate. The purpose of splinting is to immobilize the fracture area. The purpose of immobilizing the fracture area is to ensure that broken bone ends do not move. Preventing movement reduces the chance of complication of the injury and further damage to the soft tissues around the fracture site. _A splint used to immobilize bone ends of a fracture should extend beyond the joint above the fracture and the joint below the fracture._ This protects against movement at either bone end of the fracture.

A variety of commercial splints are available (e.g., the air splint, Figure 8.3). Ambulance companies, emergency medical technicians, and often even Boy Scout troops have some of these prepared splints in their emergency kits. The first-aider, however, seldom has access to these when dealing with a fracture injury. It is important, therefore, that the first-aider learn to utilize not only prepared splints but a wide variety of materials from which splints may be improvised. One way of doing this is to plan ahead and practice the use of commercially prepared and improvised splinting materials and techniques.

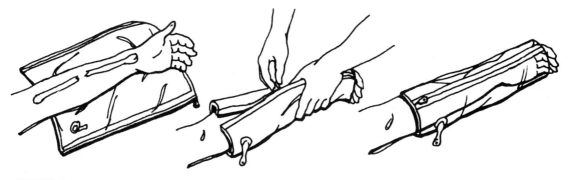

**FIGURE 8.3**

Example of an air splint. The splint must be free of wrinkles before it is zipped shut. It is inflated until the first-aider's thumb makes only a slight indentation. Overinflation reduces blood circulation and must be avoided.

A great number of objects can be used for splinting. Even a pillow can be utilized in certain instances. For example, a pillow can be tied to or pinned around a fracture of the forearm (Figure 8.4). A pillow splint can also be used for a fractured ankle. Cardboard boxes can be used by shaping or cutting them in such a way as to conform to the appendage and then appropriately securing them in place. Rolled-up blankets or newspapers, wooden boards, and sticks all have potential for use as splints.

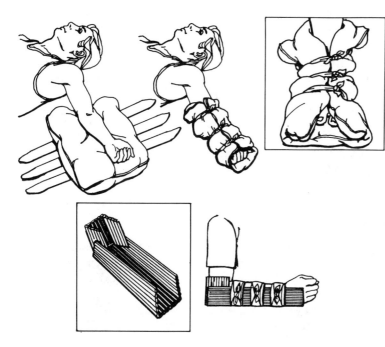

**FIGURE 8.4**

Examples of splinting materials. *Top row:* A pillow can be tied or pinned around a fractured forearm or ankle (*inset*). *Bottom row:* A corrugated box (*inset*) is cut, shaped, and secured to fractured forearm.

**FIGURE 8.5**

Use of intact leg for splinting a broken leg. A blanket
between the legs protects
the break from pressure.
Bandages are tied at the
side of the uninjured leg.

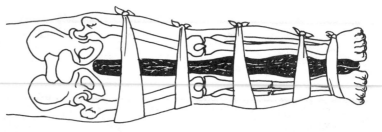

One of the simplest splinting techniques involves the use of a parallel body part. This is helpful in the absence of prepared splints or materials for improvising splints. For example, with fractures of the long bones of one leg, the intact leg can be used as the splinting device. The legs are tied together with anything that is available (Figure 8.5). A fractured arm can be tied, after padding, against the victim's chest if the elbow is bent, or to the side if the elbow is straight.

When tying a splint in place on either the arm or leg, *the first-aider must not cut off the pulse.* Therefore, after the splint is applied and tied in place, the pulse is palpated below each point on the appendage where the splint is secured, to verify continued blood flow to the area. Additionally, the first-aider observes the involved hand or foot for evidence of discoloration (e.g., bluish color), indicating a decrease in blood supply. If the victim complains of numbness or tingling below the site where the splint was applied, the ties should be loosened to prevent damage to the blood vessels, nerves, or both. Indeed, damage to blood vessels and nerves is one of the most common complications of upper extremity fractures. Often this damage can be prevented through careful rendering of assistance and subsequent monitoring of the splints and bandages that have been applied.

Usually it is necessary to place padding (which can be paper, clothing, or other soft materials) between the splint and the victim's skin, particularly if a board splint is used. Neckties, handkerchiefs, or strips of cloth can be used to tie the splint to the body part. Tying can also be accomplished with belts or with prepared or improvised cravat band-ages (see Chapter 17).

## ___FIRST AID CARE FOR SPECIFIC FRACTURES

### ___Fractures of the Clavicle

The clavicle, also known as the collarbone, is broken relatively frequently, especially in children. First aid care for a fracture of the clavicle entails the use of a sling to elevate the arm and the scapula (shoulder blade), thereby reducing their downward pull on the clavicle. The sling consists of a triangular piece of cloth large enough to fit around the person's neck, support the entire forearm and hand, and enclose the elbow. The hand is suspended in the sling slightly higher than the elbow. To prevent the fractured bone

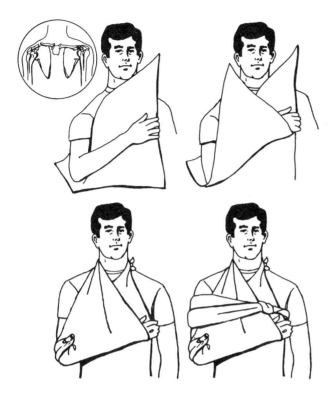

**FIGURE 8.6**

Sling for a fractured clavicle. Elevating the arm and scapula reduces downward pull on the fracture. The hand is suspended higher than the elbow. The bandage around the arm and chest prevents the fractured bone ends from moving.

ends of the clavicle from moving, a second piece of material is placed over the sling and around the victim's chest and upper back. This bandage passes under the arm just below the armpit on the uninjured side. When fastened, this support should effectively hold the arm or the injured side in place (Figure 8.6). The first-aider is careful to monitor the hand on the injured side for the possibility of a restriction in blood supply, taking corrective action as needed.

## Fractures of the Scapula

Fractures of the scapula are not nearly as common as fractures of the clavicle and generally result from a direct blow. They often occur in automobile accidents and athletic contests. Direct blows are associated with other related problems, such as shoulder dislocation or severe contusions around the shoulder blade. First aid care for a fracture of the scapula is similar to that for the clavicle. The first-aider applies a sling with the arm bent and the hand suspended slightly above the elbow. The downward pull of the arm is compensated for by the sling. The injured arm is stabilized against the side of the body (thus preventing horizontal movement) by passing a second bandage over the sling and around the victim's chest and upper back. Again, this bandage passes under the arm just below the armpit on the uninjured side (Figure 8.7).

**FIGURE 8.7**

Sling for a fractured scapula. The sling can be smaller than that used for clavicle fracture. Again, the hand is suspended above the elbow and the arm is stabilized against the body with a second bandage.

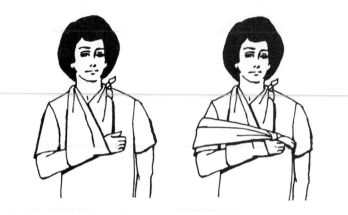

## __Fractures of the Humerus

Closed fractures of the humerus, or upper arm bone, normally call for splinting. A small amount of padding is placed on the outside of the arm and is secured above and below the fracture. Once a splint and padding are applied, the arm is placed in a sling. Again, the sling should cradle the arm and be additionally secured around the upper body (Figure 8.8).

An open fracture of the humerus is cared for in essentially the same way, with one exception and a few precautions. First, a splint is not used until after a large sterile or clean dressing has been applied to the open wound. No attempt is made to clean the wound. Second, the splint is applied in such a way that it does not exert pressure against the area of the break. If a splint cannot be applied, the arm can be supported with a sling, its horizontal movement restricted by encircling the chest with a bandage as previously described.

Sometimes a fracture of the humerus occurring very close to the shoulder is not recognized. Such a fracture is a particular possibility when the victim has fallen on an outstretched hand. This kind of fall can push the shaft of the humerus into its head.

**FIGURE 8.8**

Splinting for an upper arm fracture. Padding on the outside of the arm (*A*) is secured with bandages above and below break. (*B*) Sling supports the arm and shoulder girdle and is held by a second bandage (*C*).

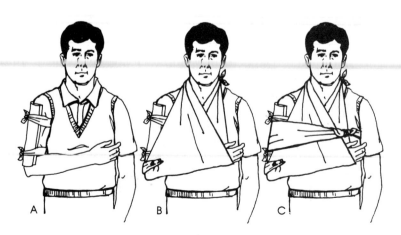

Initially the amount of disability may not seem as severe as with other fractures. Nonetheless, it is very important for a person with this type of injury to be seen by a physician for evaluation of the damage.

## ___Fractures of the Elbow

In assessing fractures involving the elbow, the first determination is whether the fracture is in the lower end of the humerus or in the upper end of the bones of the forearm. If the fracture occurred when the elbow was bent, no attempt should be made to straighten the arm. Instead the forearm is placed in a sling and bound to the body. If, on the other hand, the fracture occurred when the elbow was straight, no attempt is made to bend the arm to put it into a sling. Instead a protective pad or folded cloth is placed in the armpit and well-padded splints are applied along both sides of the forearm and are tied above and below the elbow.

## ___Fractures of the Forearm

The two bones of the forearm (radius and ulna) may fracture individually or together. The best way to handle fractures in the mid shaft of the bones is to splint the forearm with an air splint (if available) or something like newspapers or a padded board. The newspapers or padded board are secured above and below the fracture site (Figure 8.9). After the splint has been applied, the arm is placed in a sling for support. Placement in the sling is such that the thumb is up and the palm of the hand is against the body.

## ___Fractures of the Wrist

Typically, a wrist fracture is the result of falling on an outstretched hand. The victim usually has extended the wrist further than it normally goes, and the result is fracture

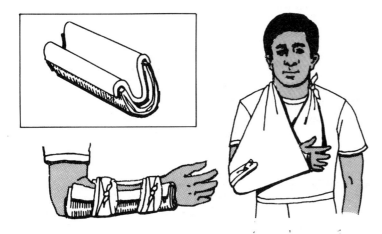

**FIGURE 8.9**

Splinting for forearm fracture. A padded rolled magazine (*inset*) may be applied with bandages above and below the break. A sling supports the arm. An air splint, if available, can also be used to immobilize this fracture.

and angulation of the bones in the lower portion of the forearm. First aid care consists of placing the arm in a comfortable position, generally with the person lying down, and then splinting it. The splint can be improvised from newspapers or magazines, and should be padded. It should extend below the wrist to support the hand and above the wrist to the middle of the forearm.

A fracture of the wrist involving the carpal bones is often difficult to detect. Frequently both the victim and the first-aider assume the injury is a sprain. *Any severe injury to the wrist area should be evaluated medically, particularly if pain and swelling persist.*

## ▬Fractures of the Hands and Fingers

Fractures of the hands and fingers are relatively common. First aid for a fracture of a single finger consists of splinting with a small padded board and placing of the finger in a comfortable, protected position. If two or more fingers are involved, plus crushing of soft tissues, the first-aider should not try to clean the wounds. A large ball of gauze or a bound-up cloth is placed in the palm of the injured hand, and then the entire hand is covered with a large and bulky dressing. These two steps allow the mass of material in the hand to act as a splint and the covering to secure it. The person is made as comfortable as possible until more sophisticated care is available. *The injured hand must be kept raised to reduce swelling.* The arm should not be allowed to hang down at the side. The first-aider may assist the victim to lie with the hand elevated on a pillow until transportation arrives. If it is necessary for the victim to walk some distance for subsequent transportation, he or she should rest the forearm on the head, thus keeping the hand elevated.

## ▬Fractures of the Hip and Shaft of the Femur

Fractures around the hip joint involving the upper portion of the femur (thigh bone) commonly result from falls or from automobile accidents. Because the musculature of the thigh and the buttock region is massive, an open fracture in this area is rare. However, bleeding into the muscle after trauma to this area is NOT uncommon. It is therefore important for the first-aider to be on guard for shock. Bearing of weight on this type of fracture should be discouraged, even if the person does not seem to have much pain and discomfort.

Fractures of the shaft of the femur typically result from falls or athletic or traffic injuries. The fracture is usually easily detected because the victim's foot is characteristically turned outward and the limb appears to be shortened. Shortening is due to overlapping of the bone ends as the muscular spasm associated with the trauma pulls the broken end of the lower portion of the bone up and over the upper portion. Fracture of the shaft of the femur frequently causes severe pain, and the victim typically has to be treated for shock.

The choice of splinting procedure for this type of fracture depends on whether the person will have to be transported some distance and on who is to do the splinting. Fractures of the shaft of the femur respond best to traction splints. Putting a leg in traction is best accomplished by emergency crews who are well trained in the use of the

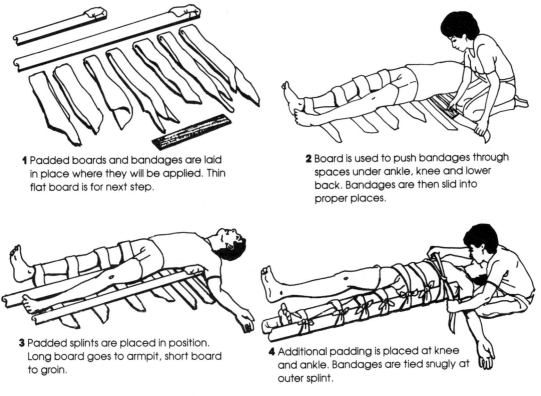

1 Padded boards and bandages are laid in place where they will be applied. Thin flat board is for next step.

2 Board is used to push bandages through spaces under ankle, knee and lower back. Bandages are then slid into proper places.

3 Padded splints are placed in position. Long board goes to armpit, short board to groin.

4 Additional padding is placed at knee and ankle. Bandages are tied snugly at outer splint.

**FIGURE 8.10**

Fracture of the femur managed with board splints

traction splints. Untrained persons should not attempt to use this kind of splint. If the victim is to be transported a short distance on a stretcher, the first-aider may place a blanket between the victim's legs and bind the legs together (see again Figure 8.5). If the victim is to be transported a greater distance, the first-aider may improvise a more rigid splint (Figure 8.10). This splint should stretch from well above the pelvic region to well below the heel on the outside of the leg. On the inside of the leg it should stretch from the groin to below the heel. The entire splint (both boards) should be well padded. The splints can be pulled together by strips of cloth at the ankle, knee, and lower back.

## Fractures of the Patella

The patella (kneecap) is most often fractured by a direct blow. First aid care for this kind of fracture calls for splinting with a pillow, blanket, or other type of padded support, applied from behind the leg. The splints should preferably extend from the buttocks to below the heel, and should be held in place with four bandages or strips of cloth secured at the upper and mid thigh, the upper calf, and the ankle (Figure 8.11).

**FIGURE 8.11**

Splinting for a fractured
patella. A padded splint is
applied under the leg from
the buttocks to below the
heel, with extra padding in
the space under the knee.
Bandages secure the splint
at the upper thigh, above
and below the knee, and at
the ankle.

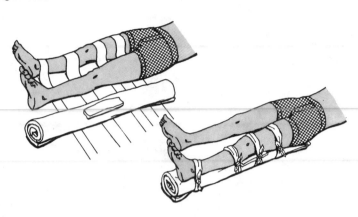

## ___Fractures of the Lower Leg

The tibia and fibula are the two bones that make up the lower leg. The tibia, also known as the shinbone, supports the weight of the body and can be palpated directly beneath the skin along the front of the leg. The fibula forms a strut and also forms the outer portion of the ankle joint. Fractures of the tibia and fibula occur fairly frequently, especially in automobile accidents involving pedestrians, injuries during athletic contests, and certain falls (particularly those in which the ankle is also twisted or sprained).

First aid care for fractures of the tibia and fibula typically involves application of well-padded splints on each side of the leg and foot (Figure 8.12). The foot should point straight up, however, do not turn the foot if it is not in this position. If a rigid splint is not available, blankets, towels, or anything else that might provide a firm support may be used. It is sometimes possible to insert a folded blanket or towel between the victim's legs and tie the legs together for transportation. As in all previous splinting situations, the bandages must not interfere with circulation.

Occasionally a fracture of the fibula, which is not a weight-bearing bone, will go unrecognized. Persistent pain and swelling in the area indicate the need for further medical attention. A person with suspected fracture of the tibia, the fibula, or both, should not try to stand or bear weight.

**FIGURE 8.12**

Splinting for a lower leg
fracture. Well-padded
splints on both sides of the
leg extend well beyond the
foot.

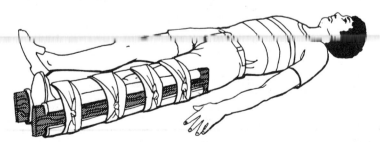

## __Fractures of the Ankle, Foot, and Toes

The ankle joint comprises the lower portion of the tibia and fibula, the tibia forming the inner portion of the joint and the fibula the outer portion. These bones articulate with a bone in the foot called the *talus.* The talus is one of several *tarsal* bones. Immediately beyond the tarsal bones are the *metatarsal* bones, and finally other phalanges (bones that make up the toes of the foot). Fractures of the foot commonly occur from indirect trauma, such as the foot being run over by a car or a heavy object being dropped on the foot. Occasionally heel bones are fractured, for example, by a jump or fall from a height and landing on the heel. Sometimes the small bones of the foot (as well as the metatarsals behind) are broken by crush injuries or by stubbing or twisting the toes.

The person with a fracture of the foot is not permitted to bear weight on the injured appendage. *The leg is kept elevated to help control swelling.* If an open wound is present, the shoe is removed, and sterile (or at least clean), bulky dressings are applied to the wound. The victim must be warned about possible pain when the shoe is removed. The foot may then be splinted with a pillow. Any deformities of the toes or metatarsal bones are not corrected. An adjacent, uninjured toe may be used for support by securing the two toes with bandages or strips of cloth. If medical care is readily available, the shoe can be left on the foot to help control swelling.

## __Fractures of the Pelvis

The pelvis is made up of fused bones and forms a girdle that serves as the junction between the lower extremities and the trunk (see again Figure 8.1). The sacrum, which comprises five fused vertebrae, is the most posterior portion of the pelvic girdle and fits between the two major halves of the pelvis. Each half of the pelvis is made up of three fused bones: the ilium, ischium, and pubis. The head of the femur forms a joint with the pelvis on either side, known as the hip joint.

Housed within the pelvic cavity are a number of important organs, including the bladder, urethra, lower portion of the bowel, and in women, the reproductive organs, as well as large blood vessels. Thus, internal bleeding is often associated with a fracture of the pelvis. When internal organs are injured, the victim usually goes into shock. Pelvic injuries thus can be extremely serious. Many of the procedures associated with first aid care for injuries to the spine apply to fractures of the pelvis. For example, it is important not to handle the victim unless essential; if the person has to be moved, he or she must be supported on a wide broad surface (e.g., a backboard). *A person with a pelvic injury should not be asked to sit up, stand up, or attempt to walk.* Finally, medical treatment should be sought as soon as possible.

## __Fractures of the Ribs and Sternum

The twelve ribs are attached posteriorly to the spinal column by way of articulation with the vertebrae. Ten of these ribs are joined anteriorly to the breast bone of the sternum by way of costal cartilage. The two lowest ribs, those not joined to the sternum, are called

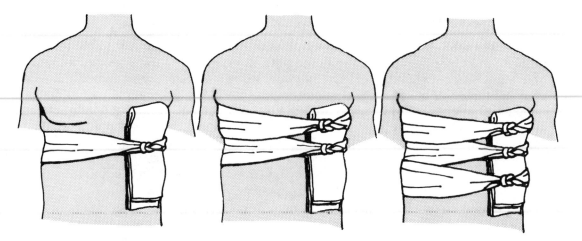

**FIGURE 8.13**

Immobilizing fractured ribs. Bandages are tied over a pad placed on the uninjured side. To support the ribs, the first bandage is placed below the site of pain and the second above it. A third bandage below the first restricts movement.

floating ribs. The ribs and sternum together with the spinal column make up the rib cage, an area known as the thoracic region of the body. The purpose of the rib cage is to protect the heart and lungs as well as their vital supportive arteries. Muscle attachments to the rib cage provide for the muscular movement involved in breathing.

One or more ribs may be fractured by a direct blow or fall. Unless the rib is clearly deformed, the injury is painful but usually not serious. It should, however, be evaluated medically.

Crushing injuries of the chest, in which several ribs are fractured or in which ribs are fractured in several places, may seriously impair breathing. The lungs may be punctured by one or more ribs, allowing air and, perhaps, blood to enter the chest cavity. The intrusion of air or blood into the chest cavity, in turn, compresses the lung tissue and reduces breathing ability. A victim with a punctured lung often coughs up bright red blood. Other internal organs occasionally are damaged, depending on the direction of the blow that caused the injury.

First aid care for simple rib fracture involves wrapping the injured area with an Ace bandage or other bandages to support and immobilize the ribs (Figure 8.13). Wrapping the injured area tends to reduce pain and discomfort, which minimizes interference with breathing. Any open wound, particularly if lung tissue is exposed, is a major emergency. If a puncture has caused a sucking wound in the chest, the victim should be directed to exhale. The wound is then closed with a large pad, which is strapped into place or covered by plastic until a dressing is available. Until help arrives, however, the first-aider may have to seal the wound with his or her open hand or hands if nothing else is available. It is always important to maintain the person in the most comfortable position. A conscious victim can assist in achieving this. If the victim is unconscious, placing him or her on the affected side may be the best procedure, unless the need to care for shock precludes this. The first-aider should watch carefully for signs of respiratory distress.

Injury to the sternum is caused by a blow to the front of the chest. Such an injury can result, for example, from a person hitting the steering wheel during a motor vehicle accident. Many of these injuries can be prevented by wearing of seat belts. Injury to the sternum should be handled in the same way as multiple rib injury, and should be considered serious. Follow-up medical care is needed.

## ___DISLOCATION OF JOINTS

A joint is a point in the skeletal system where two or more bones connect. The connection is formed by fibrous connective tissue or cartilage. Dislocation implies that the end of one of the bones making up the joint has been displaced. Dislocations occur most frequently in joints that are highly mobile but not particularly stable, such as the shoulder joint. Dislocation occurs in the fingers or thumb and less frequently in the elbow. Dislocation of the hip joint is relatively rare. Occasionally the patella becomes dislocated at the knee joint. Dislocations may result from direct blows or from falls, as well as from athletics. With the last, the cause is often attributed to the absence of proper training and protective equipment.

Symptoms of a dislocation typically include pain, swelling, and obvious deformity of the joint (Figure 8.14). A dislocation can be recognized by loss of movement, lengthening or shortening of the limb, loss of normal joint contours, or deformity, or a combination of these. The first-aider should ordinarily NOT try to reduce the joint, particularly if medical care is readily accessible, as this may increase the damage.

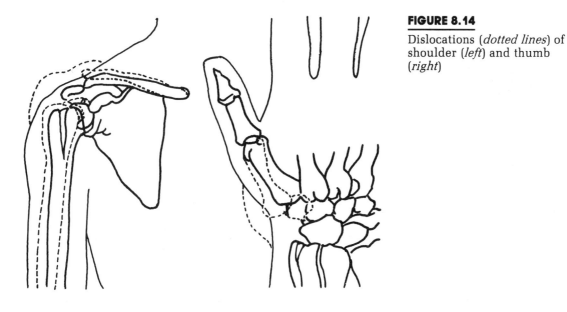

**FIGURE 8.14**

Dislocations (*dotted lines*) of shoulder (*left*) and thumb (*right*)

Finger joint dislocations may be reduced, however, if care cannot be obtained for some time. The application of firm and steady traction to the dislocated joint eliminates a great deal of discomfort. Once medical care is available, radiologic evaluation for completeness of the reduction and for incidental fractures is needed.

Dislocation can damage the soft tissues, ligaments, blood vessels, and nerves that pass close to the joint. The principles for handling closed fractures can be applied to treating dislocated joints, that is, splinting and immobilizing the affected joint in the position in which it is found. A sling is used where appropriate for support, and the victim is urged seek medical attention as quickly as possible.

With a dislocation of the knee joint, the victim often is unable to return the knee to a fully extended position. The knee will feel "locked" into place, because the cartilage displaced in the dislocation becomes a mechanical block to movement. *No attempt should be made to straighten the leg.* The victim should seek professional medical help as soon as possible. If pain is acute and the person needs support, the first-aider can immobilize the leg by splinting it in the position in which it is locked. This action helps prevent further damage to the area.

## ___SPRAINS OF JOINTS

Ligaments are connective tissue structures composed of strong fibrous bands. Ligaments join bone to bone and provide stability for joints. They strengthen the joint capsule, which surrounds the joint completely and contains within it the synovial (lubricating) fluid. By definition, a sprain is an injury to one or more ligaments. Excessive or abnormal joint motion causes the injury. The degree of damage can vary from partial tearing of a few fibers to complete tearing away from the bone of the connecting ligaments. In a sprain, damage is done to the small blood vessels, the joint capsule, and the soft tissues around the joint. Swelling and bleeding generally accompany this damage. The bleeding often leads to accumulation of blood within the tissues (hematoma). Severe sprains may also involve injury to the tendons that attach muscle to bone around the joint.

The most common sites for sprains are the ankle, finger, thumb, and wrist. Sprains of the ligaments of the knee also occur, but less frequently. The victim of an ankle or a knee sprain should not be permitted to place weight on the joint.

*Immediately after injury, the injured area should be elevated and immobilized and cold applied.* The purpose of these three measures (elevation, immobilization, and cold treatment) is control of swelling, which in turn controls pain. Compression also helps control swelling. Severe sprains should always be evaluated medically because of the possibility of concealed fractures and the potential threat to long-term joint stability.

As part of first aid care for a sprain of the knee or ankle, a splint can be applied for immobilization by means of a blanket or towel. Figure 8.15 illustrates a method for immobilizing a severely sprained ankle. An elastic wrap, if one is available, can be placed around the knee or ankle to provide compression and counteract swelling in the respective sprain.

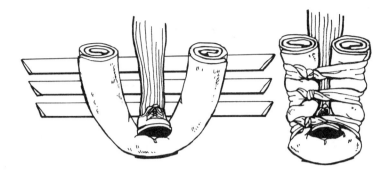

**FIGURE 8.15**
Immobilization of a sprained ankle. A rolled blanket is secured with bandages around the heel, at the ankle, and above the ankle. The shoe provides compression to counteract swelling.

Mild sprains are often cared for successfully at home. Measures include rest, application of cold (ice) compression, and elevation. Cold should be applied for twenty minutes every four to six hours for at least the first forty-eight hours. The victim should perform a mild range of motion activities if this can be tolerated. In general, cold applications should continue until all swelling caused by the sprain has ceased. The use of cold reduces the swelling and sensation of pain and significantly controls the size of hematoma development in the area of the injury.

If home or self-treatment is undertaken for any sprain and the pain and swelling persist more than a week, medical attention should be sought. As previously indicated, all severe sprains should receive prompt medical evaluation.

## ___STRAINS

Strain involves injury to muscle fibers resulting from excessive, forceful stretching of a given muscle. In the absence of definitive medical identification, strains are frequently confused with sprains. With muscle strain, not only is the muscle tissue (and occasionally its associated tendinous tissue) damaged but also adjacent blood vessels. Bleeding from these vessels into the injured area produces swelling and pain.

The goal of first aid care for a strain is to stop the bleeding into the injured area and prevent further tearing of muscle fibers. This is accomplished by using essentially the same measures as used for sprain: rest and immobilization of the injured part, application of cold, application of a compressive bandage, and elevation of the injured part (if an arm or leg). Cold should be applied for approximately twenty minutes five times a day during the first forty-eight hours following the injury. If the strain involves a weight-bearing area, only minimal weight bearing is permitted. Mild strains can often be self-treated or cared for at home. Muscle tears, however, need medical attention for complete management.

Strains of the low back region are relatively common. They typically result from pushing, shoving, or lifting. Because of the many possible complications that can be associated with a back injury, severe back pain should always be evaluated by a medical practitioner. Most of the first aid emphasis for low back strain is on rest (i.e., reduced activity and movement). Cold can be applied, but often this is uncomfortable.

---

## SUMMARY

The musculoskeletal system is often injured in automobile accidents, recreational activities, and falls. Assessment of the musculoskeletal injury requires gathering information from the victim (if conscious) or from witnesses (if available) and conducting a full assessment of the victim's condition regardless of the state of consciousness.

Basic first aid care for fractures is to keep the broken bone ends immobilized, so as to minimize pain and limit further damage. Concurrently the first-aider must be alert for the possibility of shock, and as a precautionary measure, must treat all fracture emergencies as if shock were the expected outcome. Splinting provides a method for immobilizing broken bone ends and is used for care of fractures when immediate medical assistance is not available. Damage to blood vessels and nerves must be prevented by proper splint placement and procedures. In securing a splint, care must also be taken to ensure continued circulation.

Dislocation of a joint includes the symptoms and signs of pain, swelling, deformity, and loss of movement. In general, the first-aider should not try to reduce a dislocation unless there will be considerable delay in obtaining medical care. Immobilization of the dislocated joint is the preferred first aid response.

Sprains of joints are common and vary in severity from mild to severe. First aid care for a sprain involves rest, elevation of the limb, immobilization of the injured part, and application of cold. First aid care for a strain is similar to that for a sprain and includes rest, immobilization, and the application of cold to the injured area.

In dealing with musculoskeletal emergencies, first-aiders must be aware of the potential seriousness of the problem and the possibility of complications involving other body organs and systems. The first-aider must make full use of all his or her complement of skills in assessing the first aid needs of the fracture victim.

---

## CHAPTER MASTERY: TEST ITEMS

**True and False**  Circle One

1. The musculoskeletal system plays a significant role in protecting vital areas of the body.  T  F
2. Assessment of musculoskeletal injuries requires rapid evaluation of a large amount of information in a brief period of time.  T  F
3. A closed fracture produces a break in the skin.  T  F
4. First aid for fractures seldom requires lifesaving procedures, such as caring for shock.  T  F

5. Common items such as pillows, blankets, newspapers, and cardboard     **T**     **F**
boxes can be used for splints.
6. Injuries to nerves or blood vessels are rarely associated with fractures.     **T**     **F**
7. Fractures of the clavicle do not require splinting.     **T**     **F**
8. In dealing with an open fracture, the first-aider should first attempt to     **T**     **F**
clean the wound.

### Fill In the Missing Word(s)

1. The three principal causes of musculoskeletal injury are _____, _____, and
_____.

2. An injury in which ligaments and surrounding soft tissues are damaged is called
a _____.

3. The reasons for preventing motion at the ends of fractured bones are _____.

4. Immediate care for a dislocated shoulder includes _____.

### Multiple Choice (Circle the Best Answer)

1. In an open fracture
   a. the bone is broken in several places.
   b. the bone is exposed.
   c. the bone is not exposed.

2. Pressure from applying a splint may
   a. cause increased swelling.
   b. increase pain.
   c. compress blood vessels.
   d. a, b, and c
   e. b and c

3. When bluish fingers are observed with forearm injury,
   a. elevate the hand.
   b. suspect poor circulation.
   c. take no action.
   d. apply heat to improve circulation.

4. First-aid for sprains
   a. does not include advice to obtain follow-up medical attention.
   b. focuses only on immobilizing the injured part.
   c. includes elevation and heat for swelling and pain control.
   d. includes elevation, cold application, and compression for swelling and pain
      control.

5. First aid for a dislocated joint is essentially
   a. the same as that for a muscle strain.
   b. the same as that for an open fracture.
   c. the same as that for a closed fracture.
   d. simple relocation of the joint.

6. First aid for rib fractures
   a. depends on the seriousness of the injury and the number of ribs damaged.
   b. needs to encompass possible breathing problems.
   c. includes keeping the victim comfortable, and may include bandaging for stability and comfort.
   d. all of the above
7. Muscle strains are
   a. so common as not to require first aid.
   b. are often confused with joint sprains.
   c. are only serious if they involve the low back region.
   d. all of the above

**Discussion Questions**

1. Describe the procedure for applying a splint to a fracture of the forearm.
2. Arriving on the scene, the first-aider finds a young boy lying on the street next to his bicycle. The boy's lower left leg is bent at an unnatural angle. Describe in proper sequence what should be done and why.
3. Hiking in a remote area, the first-aider's partner slips and twists her ankle severely. Describe and justify the first-aider responses that should occur.

# 9

# Central Nervous System and Facial/Head Injuries

DAVID L. BEVER, PH.D.

After completing this chapter the student will be able to
- Describe the various components of the central nervous system.
- Identify injuries most often associated with central nervous system trauma.
- Define cerebral concussion, cerebral contusion, subdural hematoma, epidural hematoma, and depressed skull fracture.
- Perform basic neurologic assessments of patients with head injuries, spinal cord injuries, or both.
- Provide initial management for head and spinal cord injuries.
- Assess soft-tissue injuries of the face and head, then apply basic emergency care for these injuries.

## ____INTRODUCTION

The central nervous system, which includes tissues within the brain and spinal cord, is the most complex of the body's organ systems. Not only is it responsible for control of all conscious body functions, it also closely integrates with the autonomic nervous system to innervate (carry motor impulses to and sensory impulses away from) organs that operate without conscious control, such as the heart, lungs, liver, and kidneys. The following is a brief discussion of the components of the central nervous system and their interrelated functions.

## ____CENTRAL NERVOUS SYSTEM: STRUCTURE AND FUNCTION

### __Brain

The brain, located within and well protected by the bony structure of the skull, is the center of all voluntary and involuntary activity. Each of the brain's three major divisions —cerebrum, cerebellum, and brain stem (Figure 9.1)—plays a specific role in human performance.

The *cerebrum* is the largest part of the brain and is the site of memory, personality, and intelligence (i.e., "what makes us human"). It is composed of two interconnected hemispheres. It is responsible for the interpretation of sensory stimuli, which include sounds, sights, odors, pressure, and temperature. Another major function is initiation of voluntary motor impulses that ultimately result in body movements.

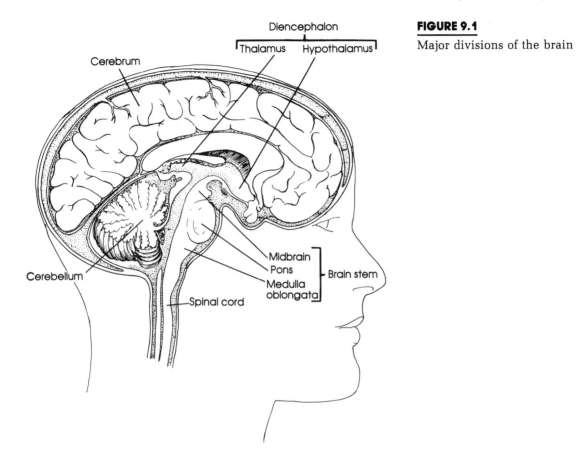

**FIGURE 9.1**

Major divisions of the brain

The *cerebellum,* the second largest part of the brain, lies under the cerebrum in the occipital (back) portion of the skull. Like the cerebrum, the cerebellum is composed of two interconnected hemispheres. Its major functions are coordination of muscle movement, maintenance of balance, and control of muscle tone and posture.

Though nerve impulses for voluntary muscle movement are initiated in the cerebrum, they are refined in the cerebellum so that movement of muscle groups is smooth and coordinated. Likewise, sensory impulses from the inner ear concerning balance and equilibrium are processed by the cerebellum, which in turn sends motor impulses to skeletal muscles so that balance is maintained. Motor impulses from the cerebellum also stimulate muscles that help to maintain posture.

The third major division of the brain is the *brain stem.* It is composed of the diencephalon (thalamus and hypothalamus), the midbrain, the pons, and the medulla oblongata. The most primitive portion of the brain, the brain stem houses the centers of vital activity that control cardiac rhythm, respiration, and size of blood vessels. It is also

involved with control of the visceral organs through the sympathetic and parasympathetic divisions of the autonomic nervous system. Motor impulses originating in the
medulla and hypothalamus are carried to the various organs via the sympathetic and
parasympathetic nerves. The sympathetic nerves generally carry impulses that acceler-
ate organ function, especially during times of stress, while the parasympathetic nerves
carry impulses that slow down organ function and return the body to a state of normal
operation.

A special group of tissues that extends through the brain stem and into the cerebrum
is known as the *reticular activating system* (RAS). These nerve fibers are responsible for
maintaining consciousness. If impulses from the RAS are blocked or the system is
damaged, the individual loses consciousness.

## __ Spinal Cord

Extending downward from the brain stem for a distance of eighteen to twenty-four
inches, the *spinal cord* carries sensory nerve impulses from throughout the body to the
brain and at the same time conducts motor nerve impulses from the brain to the body.
Nerves exiting the spinal cord along its length are responsible for carrying sensory and
motor impulses to and from the cord.

## __ Protective Mechanisms for the Brain and Spinal Cord

Consisting of a series of interconnected immovable bones (eight in number), the skull
provides a significant amount of protection for the highly sensitive brain tissues. At the
base of the skull is an opening in the occipital bone known as the *foramen magnum.*
Through this opening the spinal cord extends downward from the medulla into the
protection of the vertebral column, a series of thirty-three bones (vertebrae) connected to
one another by ligaments, muscles, and fibrous disks (Figure 9.2). This arrangement
allows the vertebrae a considerable amount of movement, while offering maximum
protection to the spinal cord encased within these structures. Not only does the spinal
column protect the nerve tissues of the cord, but it acts as the major means of support for
the skull and upper torso.

Within their protective bony structures, the brain and spinal cord are further protected by three membranous layers, or meninges: the *dura mater,* the *arachnoid,* and the
*pia mater* (Figure 9.3). The dura mater is the toughest and outermost covering. It lines the
skull and the vertebral canal through which passes the spinal cord. The second meninx
is the arachnoid. Between this layer and the third meninx, or pia mater, is an area known
as the *subarachnoid* space. Cerebrospinal fluid, which acts as a shock absorbing agent
for the brain and spinal cord, circulates in this space. The final layer, the pia mater,
attaches directly to the brain and spinal cord; in this delicate layer are the many blood
vessels that supply the underlying nerve tissue.

Though the skull, vertebrae, meninges, and cerebrospinal fluid offer a great deal of
protection for the brain and spinal cord, the extremely sensitive nature of these tissues
makes any injury to the central nervous system a potentially serious one.

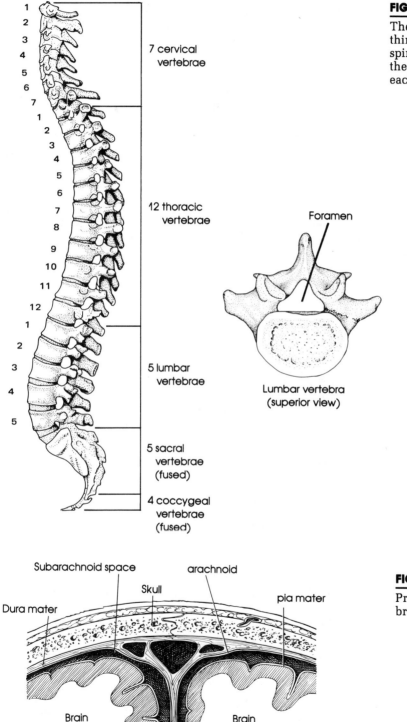

7 cervical
vertebrae

12 thoracic
vertebrae

5 lumbar
vertebrae

5 sacral
vertebrae
(fused)

4 coccygeal
vertebrae
(fused)

**FIGURE 9.2**

The spinal column contains thirty-three vertebrae. The spinal cord passes through the foramen, or opening, in each vertebra.

Foramen

Lumbar vertebra
(superior view)

Subarachnoid space    arachnoid

Skull

pia mater

Dura mater

Brain    Brain

**FIGURE 9.3**

Protective coverings of the brain

# ___INJURIES TO THE CENTRAL NERVOUS SYSTEM

Unlike other tissues, those of the central nervous system have little ability to regenerate. In the case of, for example, a broken bone or a laceration of skin and muscle, the normal healing process replaces the damaged tissues. However, when nerve fibers, especially those comprising the central nervous system, are severed or damaged, return to normal functioning is doubtful, since replacement of these tissues is unlikely. The brain and spinal cord also are damaged more easily by a decrease in the oxygen supply or increased pressure from swelling than are other tissues of the body. A variety of injuries associated with central nervous system trauma are discussed in this chapter.

## ___Head Injuries

Injury to the brain is relatively common. An estimated 30% of all trauma patients entering hospital emergency departments have some type of head injury (Fischer, Carlson, and Perry 1981). Common causes of such injury are motor vehicle accidents, falls, and blows to the head. Head injury occurs in nearly two thirds of motor vehicle accidents, and brain damage is the cause of death in almost 70% of the 50,000 motor vehicle fatalities occurring each year (Rimel, Jane, and Tyson 1981).

### Concussion

Probably the most common and least serious of the brain injuries is *concussion.* It is generally described as temporary loss of consciousness due to disruption of normal neural activity resulting from a sudden blow to the head (Parcel 1982). Loss of consciousness usually lasts no more than a few minutes; however, the victim may have some confusion and loss of memory concerning the accident. Recovery should be complete within twenty-four to forty-eight hours.

### Cerebral Contusion

*Cerebral contusion* is more serious than concussion. It may result from an extremely hard blow or a series of blows to the head. Blood vessels within the brain tear, causing tissues to swell. Since the skull cannot expand as the brain swells, pressure within the cranium reduces the flow of oxygenated blood to these sensitive tissues. Unless the pressure is relieved, the continued compression of brain tissues ultimately leads to respiratory and cardiac failure.

A well-known form of cerebral contusion is the *subdural hematoma.* This condition occurs when blood pools between the brain and its outer layer, the dura mater. Another form of cerebral contusion is the *epidural hematoma* in which blood pools between the skull and the dura mater.

With this injury bleeding tends to be more severe, and rapid intervention by medical personnel is needed. In most cases of subdural or epidural hematomas (Figure 9.4), surgery is required to relieve cranial pressure and correct the damage.

### Skull Fracture

A head injury that may accompany any of the brain injuries discussed thus far is the *skull fracture.* This type of fracture does not necessarily mean that the brain has been seri-

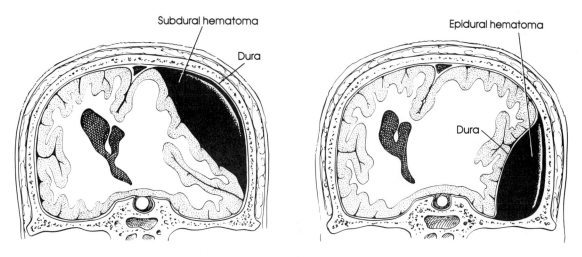

**FIGURE 9.4**

Subdural (*left*) and epidural (*right*) hematomas

ously injured. Serious brain injury is more likely when the skull has not been damaged (Hafen and Karren 1981). The immovable bones of the skull are the primary protection for the brain. These bones are relatively dense and can absorb a significant amount of force. A single high-impact force delivered to a specific area of the skull is likely to result in a fracture. Such a force can be produced in a fall, a motor vehicle accident, or an assault. Depending on how the force is applied, the resulting skull fracture may be linear (a thin-line crack), stellate (fracture lines radiating from the point of contact), or depressed (fragments of bone pushed inward against the brain). Unless the accompanying injuries are quite obvious, the first-aider will probably not detect a skull fracture; most are diagnosed only through x-ray studies.

**Assessment of Head Injuries and First Aid Care**

In the case of a head injury, the first-aider's ability to assess the condition of the victim may be even more important than the ability to provide emergency care. Initial information gathered at the emergency scene by the first-aider can provide medical personnel who subsequently take responsibility for the victim with important information concerning the severity of the injury.

On arrival at the scene, the first-aider's immediate priority is to ensure that the head injury victim has adequate cardiopulmonary function. Is the patient breathing? Is there a pulse? Stabilization of these vital functions (see Chapters 5 and 6) takes precedence over any specific care of the head injury. Once stabilization has been accomplished, patient evaluation can continue.

Since the victim of head injury is likely to be unconscious, witnesses who observed the accident should be questioned thoroughly. (Review again the subjective interview

**FIGURE 9.5**

Manifestations of head
injury

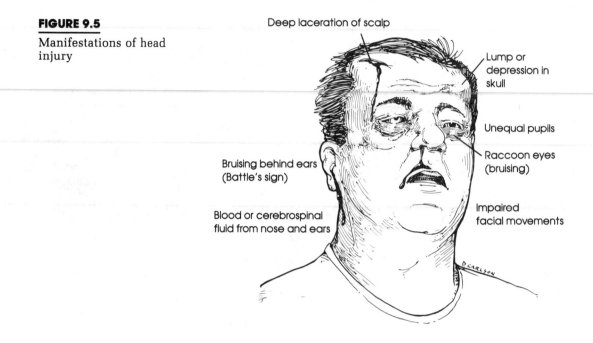

Deep laceration of scalp

Lump or
depression in
skull

Unequal pupils

Raccoon eyes
(bruising)

Bruising behind ears
(Battle's sign)

Impaired
facial movements

Blood or cerebrospinal
fluid from nose and ears

procedures presented in Chapter 2.) If the victim is conscious on the first-aider's arrival,
an important question to ask is, "Do you remember the accident?" Inability to remember
the accident, even if the victim never lost consciousness, is a sign of likely concussion.
Another important observation is how long the memory deficit continues. Continued
inability to recall immediate events (i.e., loss of recent memory) may indicate a more
severe injury. Also, if the level of consciousness of the patient begins to deteriorate,
intracranial bleeding may be occurring. Increasing confusion, lethargy, inability to carry
on a conversation, and agitation are all signs of neurologic deterioration.

Signs of head injury (Figure 9.5) may be observed in both the conscious and unconscious individual. They include the following:

- Deformity of the skull (noticeable lumps and/or depressions)
- Deep lacerations of the scalp
- Bleeding or discharge of cerebrospinal fluid from the ears, nose, or both
- Unequal pupil dilation
- Discoloration around the eyes (commonly called raccoon eyes)
- Bruises and discoloration behind the ears (known as Battle's sign)(often occurs
  with basal skull fracture)
- Rigidity of the limbs (becomes more pronounced with increasing swelling of
  the brain)
- Impairment of facial movements

A person exhibiting a combination of these signs should be considered to have a serious
head injury. Because of the gravity of the situation, the first-aider must act without
delay. As repeatedly emphasized throughout this text, the first priority is to maintain an

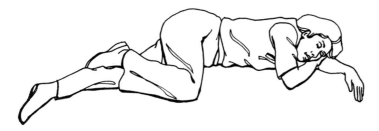

**FIGURE 9.6**

The coma position for a person with head injury

adequate airway and respiration. Care of other injuries has to be delayed until immediate life-threatening conditions are stabilized.

Treatment of external bleeding from a head wound is the second priority after cardiopulmonary functioning. Due to the rich supply of blood vessels in the scalp, even superficial wounds can bleed profusely. Direct pressure over the wound using a clean dressing is usually sufficient to control bleeding (Chapter 7). However, if there is evidence of bony fragmentation of the skull (as in the case of a depressed skull fracture), a dressing should be placed loosely over the wound but direct pressure not applied. The dressing will assist in the clotting process but will not inhibit the flow of cerebrospinal fluid from the wound. If pressure is applied at the wound site, stopping cerebrospinal fluid drainage, pressure will develop inside the cranial cavity. Likewise, pressure from a dressing applied to the skull may lead to laceration of the cerebral cortex by bony fragments, thus creating further intracranial damage.

Though cerebrospinal fluid leaking from the nose and ears is indicative of a serious head injury, the first-aider should not attempt to stop the flow. Attempts to pack the ears or nose may result in infection of brain tissues because of the introduction of bacteria via the ear canals or nasal passages. Forced lessening of the drainage of cerebrospinal fluid may result in increased intracranial pressure.

Another important consideration for the first-aider treating a head-injured patient is the possible presence of spinal cord injury. If the victim is unconscious, especially after an automobile accident or fall, he or she should be cared for as if an injury to the cervical spine has also been sustained.

If a head injury victim is unconscious and additional spinal cord injuries are not evident, the person is placed in the coma position (i.e., on the side with an arm tucked under the head and the face angled downward) (Figure 9.6). This position allows mucus and vomitus to drain from the mouth, thus reducing the chance of airway blockage. The coma position can also be used with a conscious patient who is nauseated or having trouble with mucous secretions draining into the throat. An alternative position for the conscious person is elevation of the head and shoulders to reduce blood flow to the brain and consequently alleviate intracranial pressure.

Any head injury leading to loss of consciousness, even for a short period, should be evaluated by a physician. A conscious victim is transported after initial assessment (described in Chapter 2). In the case of an unconscious person, it is wise to have professional emergency personnel (emergency medical technicians or paramedics) do this. If such assistance is not available or cannot be obtained in a reasonable time, or if the victim was unconscious for a short period of time but thereafter seems fully alert, transport to a medical facility by personal vehicle is an acceptable alternative.

After the initial physician evaluation, a decision will be made whether the victim should be admitted to the hospital for further evaluation and treatment or be released. If the victim seems to have fully recovered and is released, family members should check on him or her every hour for the first twenty-four hours in case any of the signs or symptoms mentioned should recur. If there is recurrence, further medical assistance is indicated.

## ___Spinal Cord Injuries

The most debilitating central nervous system injuries are those to the spinal cord. Though modern technology has greatly improved the chances of survival after a cord injury, it has not improved the chances of a return to normal functioning, since nerve tissues have little ability to regenerate and are very susceptible to swelling and pressure.

Damage to the spinal cord can occur in a variety of ways. The most common involves fracture of one or more of the vertebrae. Bony fragments from the fracture site may be displaced and completely sever the cord, or can shift and compress it. Once the cord has been severed the damage is permanent, and nerve impulse conduction from this point downward and to this point upward ceases. Compression of the spinal cord by displaced vertebral fragments results in the same permanent damage unless the pressure is quickly reduced (Figure 9.7).

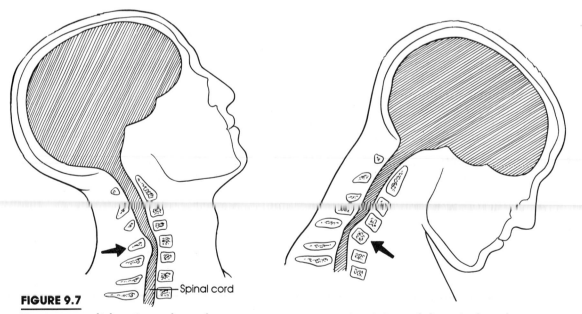

Spinal cord

**FIGURE 9.7**

Fractures or dislocations of vertebrae may cause compression injury of the spinal cord.

In other instances, dislocation of the vertebrae or of the cartilaginous intervertebral disks can occur without fracture. However, this can be just as traumatic, since these unstable structures can also compress the cord.

**Assessment**

As noted previously, the spinal column is a series of small bones separated by cartilaginous disks and bound together by ligaments. This arrangement allows considerable flexibility and, at the same time, protects the spinal cord. In evaluating for possible fractures of the spinal column, the first-aider must keep in mind that a piece or section of bone from a fracture, or displacement of one of the vertebrae making up the spinal column, could compress the spinal cord, causing paralysis or weakness of the body below the injury site. The rib cage tends to stabilize the thoracic portion (Figure 9.2) of the spinal cord. Similarly, the pelvis stabilizes the sacral and coccygeal areas. The neck (cervical) region and the lumbar region (area below the chest wall and above the pelvis), however, have no additional support structures and are more prone to injury. Because people who have fractures of vertebrae, particularly in the cervical region, respond well to treatment if there is no spinal cord injury, *it is mandatory not to create more damage or new damage to the spinal cord when trying to render first aid.*

Circumstances that are most likely to result in spinal cord injury include motor vehicle accidents, falls from heights, and recreational activities requiring physical involvement (e.g., diving and collision sports) (Rimel, Jane, and Edlich 1981). The key to proper management of injuries to the spine involves the recognition of the likely signs and symptoms associated with such injuries.

In a conscious person, local tenderness and pain over a portion of the spine are sufficient reasons to suspect an injury. (Gentle palpation by the rescuer will help pinpoint the areas of damage.) Tenderness and pain over the spine may occur even with a relatively simple soft-tissue injury. Since these symptoms are almost always present with a fracture or dislocation, however, it is best to suspect spinal cord injury and provide appropriate first aid care (Rimel, Jane, and Tyson 1981). Another sign is paralysis or numbness in the extremities. The first-aider can use a number of simple tests to determine the degree of injury. (A review of the assessment measures for injury to the neck, upper and lower back, and the extremities covered in Chapter 2 would be appropriate here. These assessment measures are conducted as a part of the head-to-toe examination of the victim.)

Spinal injury in the neck region is likely to cause loss of sensation in and paralysis of all four extremities (quadriplegia), while fracture in the thoracic or lumbar region will result in paralysis of the lower extremities (paraplegia). A useful technique for the rescuer is to clearly mark with a pen the line on the body where the patient has no feeling, indicating exactly where sensation is lost (Jordan and Calabrese 1980). Weakness of the extremities, tingling sensations, and difficulty in moving the fingers, hands, toes, and feet may indicate spinal cord damage.

A condition that occurs in many cervical spine injuries is known as diaphragmatic breathing. The muscles of the thoracic cavity no longer receive motor impulses. However, the diaphram (separating the chest and abdominal cavity) still functions, thus allowing continued respiratory movements. The first-aider will notice that the victim's abdomen distends with breathing but the chest wall does not move.

Because of the potential for irreversible damage with any spinal cord injury, the first-aider should be overly cautious rather than not cautious enough. Therefore, *all patients with head injuries and those who have lost consciousness at the scene of an accident should be considered to have sustained a spinal cord injury.* With an unconscious individual, the rescuer has to rely on the body's response to painful stimuli. As indicated in the head-to-toe examination (Chapter 2), a pointed object such as a safety pin, car key, or ballpoint pen can be used to stimulate the soles of the feet and the palms of the hands. Movement of the foot or curling of the toes in response to this painful stimulus indicates the likelihood of an intact spinal cord. No response by the hands or feet to painful stimuli indicates cervical spine damage. Hand response but no foot response generally indicates spinal cord damage below the neck. Again, because findings associated with response to painful stimuli can be inaccurate from time to time, *it is recommended that any unconscious accident victim be cared for as if he or she had a spinal cord injury.*

### First Aid Care

As with any injury, the first priority is to establish and maintain respiratory and circulatory function. With suspected spinal cord injury, the rescuer must pay particular attention to the position of the neck. Any flexion or hyperextension of the neck may lead to compression of the spinal cord by fractured or displaced vertebrae. It is imperative to keep the cervical vertebrae in alignment by using gentle traction on the head. The first-aider can slide a rolled-up towel under the victim's neck to help maintain correct positioning and traction. *The head should not be moved to place a support under the neck.* If breathing difficulties occur, the jaw thrust method is used to open the airway (Chapter 5).

A final note of caution: *the victim of suspected spinal cord injury must not be moved unless absolutely necessary.* Patient movement and transport should be handled by trained emergency personnel who have the equipment needed to perform this task safely. When a victim does have to be moved to assure safety, the first-aider should seek the help of at least three other individuals with placing and stabilizing the victim before lifting and carrying (Chapter 18). The importance of keeping the head and trunk as rigid as possible without twisting, bending, or side-to-side movement must be explained to these helpers. If a regular or improvised backboard is to be placed underneath the victim, it is best to practice this beforehand on an uninjured individual at the scene of the accident. Some first aid experts advocate placing a roll of clothing or a blanket around the person's head and anchoring it, as depicted in Figure 9.8, to prevent the victim from turning the head. If the victim is to be placed on a backboard, this procedure for immobilizing the head might be helpful. If a backboard will not be used and the victim will remain lying in place, the head may be immobilized by blocking it into place with whatever is available (e.g., bricks or stones). Techniques for immobilizing a victim for transportation are discussed extensively in Chapter 18.

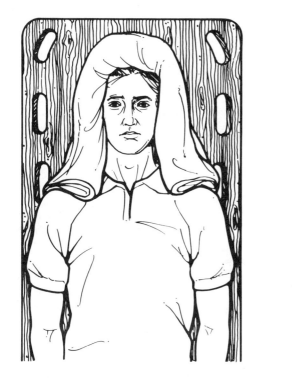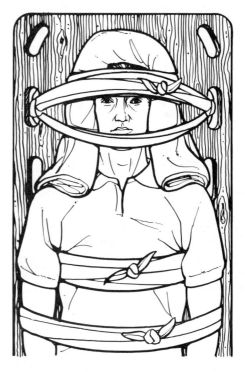

**FIGURE 9.8**

Before a person with suspected spinal cord injury is moved, the head and neck are immobilized with a rolled blanket held with bandages across the forehead and chin. The neck is kept in a straight line with the center of the trunk.

## ____ SPECIFIC HEAD AND FACIAL INJURIES

In addition to causing brain and spinal cord injuries, trauma to the head region can produce a variety of problems involving the eyes, nose, face, oral cavity, and ears. Injuries to these tissues may be minor, requiring little more than direct pressure to control bleeding, or major, requiring surgical intervention. The role of the first-aider in handling these emergencies is discussed in the following sections.

### ___ Facial Trauma

A blow to the face, such as may occur in a motor vehicle accident, can cause a variety of injuries, including lacerations, contusions, and fractures. On initial evaluation these injuries often look worse than they actually are. The majority present no threat to life.

**Signs and Symptoms**

Though the only sure method of identifying a fracture is an x-ray examination, the first-aider must know the signs and symptoms associated with facial fracture. A lack of symmetry in the victim's features is indicative of displacement of underlying bony structures. Damage to the cheekbone (zygoma) may be apparent in a flattening of the face on the injured side. Likewise, fracture of the lower jaw (mandible) on one side results in asymmetry. Damage to the upper jaw (maxilla) along with mandibular fracture produces an elongation of the face. Mandible and maxilla injuries should be suspected when the bite is irregular or the mouth remains open.

Facial trauma is also likely to result in fractures of the bony orbits supporting the eyes. Common complaints of victims include double vision, limited eye movement, and loss of sensation in the cheek and above the eyebrow.

As previously noted, facial injuries are rarely life threatening. It must be remembered, however, that trauma to the face has the potential to create serious associated injuries. For the victim of a motor vehicle accident who has hit the windshield, facial injuries may be the least of his or her problems. In this incident the first-aider would need to consider the possibility of associated brain and cervical injuries. The force of a severe blow to the face is transmitted to both the brain and spine. Incidents that cause massive facial injuries are also likely to damage other regions of the body, such as the chest and extremities.

**First Aid Care**

The first aid approach to facial injuries should consist of (1) establishing an adequate airway, (2) controlling bleeding, (3) identifying and protecting fracture sites from further injury, and (4) recognizing the potential for associated injuries.

Clearing the oral cavity of loose teeth, dentures, clotted blood, or vomitus is usually sufficient to provide an open airway. If the lower jaw (mandible), is damaged, however, the tongue of a supine victim can fall back and block the airway because it is no longer well supported. To avoid this problem the victim is placed in a prone or upright position *if the first-aider has ascertained that spinal cord injury is absent.* This allows the tongue to fall forward and keeps the airway open.

Because of the rich vascular beds underlying the face and scalp, injuries to these tissues tend to bleed profusely. Other than in rare instances, however, facial bleeding can be controlled by direct pressure, because the pressure is applied against a bony underlying surface and closes off blood vessels quickly. Clot formation should occur within five to ten minutes.

Significant swelling will occur with any of the facial injuries discussed, so it is important for the first-aider to apply cold packs to these damaged areas. Control of swelling speeds the healing process, allows medical personnel to perform definitive therapy, and provides psychological benefits to the victim and his or her family.

With facial fracture, surgical intervention is often needed to correct the damage. But the actions of the first-aider can be the key to rapid recovery. A well-padded bandage wrapped around the head and face and placed under the chin supports and protects damaged facial structures from further injury while alleviating discomfort (Figure 9.9).

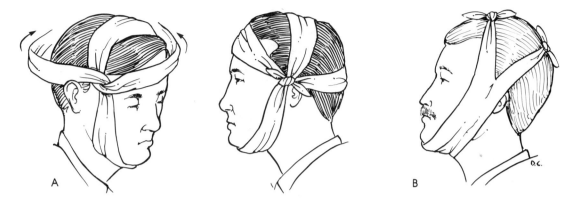

**FIGURE 9.9**

Protection for facial fracture: cravat bandage (*A*) and four-tailed bandage (*B*) well-padded bandages give support and also alleviate discomfort.

The bandage should be tied off at the top of the head to allow for easy removal in case the patient becomes nauseated or vomits. Bandaging is discussed in detail in Chapter 17.

## __Injuries to the Eye

Ophthalmic (ocular) injuries are caused by a variety of mechanisms, which can affect any number of different structures. Injuries include penetration of the globe of the eye, corneal abrasion from foreign bodies, retinal detachment, and damage to structures surrounding the eye.

Stereotypically, penetrating injuries of the eye are most often envisioned as involving an object (such as an arrow or large stick) impaled in the globe of the eye. Certainly this does happen and is a serious injury. More common, however, is penetration or perforation of the eye by small pieces of metal propelled from machinery at a high velocity. Besides causing marked visual loss, these injuries may lead to leakage of vitreous fluid and collapse of the globe. Of utmost importance is protection of the eye from further trauma (Figure 9.10). If the foreign body is sticking out from the eye, it should be covered, for example with a Styrofoam or paper cup (making sure that the cup is big enough to fit over the object). The cup is anchored firmly in place with a roller bandage and the uninjured eye is patched to reduce movement. The eyes move in unison, so that movement of the uninjured eye is likely to create further damage in the injured eye. If the object has completely penetrated the globe or has caused a perforation, care must be taken not to apply pressure to the eye, since this will cause loss of vitreous fluid. The first-aider closes the lid and covers the eye with a patch.

Another extremely serious injury that requires surgical intervention is retinal detachment. The role of the first-aider involves identification of this problem. The retina is the light-sensitive lining covering the back of the eyeball. In susceptible individuals,

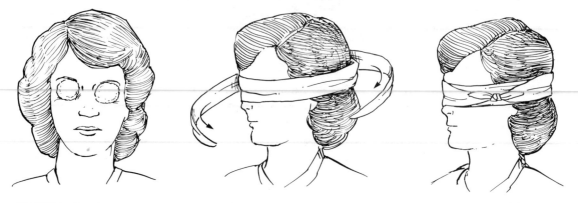

**FIGURE 9.10**

Protective bandaging for eye injury without protruding object. If one eye is injured, both are patched to prevent movement of the eyes in unison causing further trauma.

the lining can be torn away. Repeated blows to the face and head, which occur in some contact sports, can lead to retinal detachment. Symptoms include light flashes or dark spots in front of the eyes or a partial blocking of the field of vision (as if a black curtain were blocking part of the view from the damaged eye). If such an injury is suspected, the person should be transported to an emergency facility immediately. The victim should lie flat and care should be taken not to jar or bump the head, since this may increase the amount of tearing.

As sports such as racquetball, tennis, and squash have increased in popularity in recent years, emergency personnel are seeing a steadily increasing number of injuries to the structures that surround or protect the eye. Injuries to the eye are generally the result of contact with the ball, while damage to the eyelid, brow, and bony orbit occurs from contact with the racquet.

Two common ball-related injuries are corneal abrasion and hyphema. With corneal abrasion, the top layers of this transparent covering of the iris and lens are scraped away. Corneal abrasion is common in wearers of hard contact lenses who exceed the wearing time. Though it is not a serious injury, it is a painful one. The damaged eye should be covered with a patch until the victim can be given medication for pain relief and an antibiotic for the prevention of secondary infection of the abraded area.

Hyphema is a condition in which the anterior chamber of the eye fills with blood after vessels in the globe of the eye have been ruptured. A common symptom, besides bleeding into the sclera (white of the eye), is blurred vision. A person with this injury should be examined by an ophthalmologist to rule out any underlying severe injury.

Surprisingly, racquet-related injuries are often self-inflicted. While attempting to hit the ball, the player will inadvertently hit himself or herself in the forehead or brow, lacerating the skin. Direct pressure applied to the laceration will control the bleeding; however, suturing may be necessary for proper wound closure. A note of caution needs to be sounded at this point concerning laceration of the eyelid. Because of the delicate nature of this tissue, a tear requires special attention in terms of wound closure. Also, a laceration of the lid may be indicative of damage to the eye as well.

---

**Preventing Eye Injury in Racquet Sports**

Because of the confined space in which they are played, racquetball and squash require special precautions to protect the players' eyes. Of primary importance is the use of goggles by all participants. Goggles typically consist of special polycarbonate lenses mounted in a wraparound, impact-resistant plastic frame. Additionally, players, especially novices, should never turn around to view the opponent's return. Players should keep their eyes on the front wall until they are ready to make a shot.

---

## __Injuries to the Nose

*Epistaxis,* or nasal bleeding, is common. Spontaneous bleeding from the nose has numerous causes, most relatively minor. Fracture of the nasal bones and cartilage, often a result of facial trauma, can present two problems: bleeding and displacement of the nasal septum. A serious complication of nasal fracture is the deviated septum. The cartilaginous tissue dividing the nostrils may be dislodged to one side or the other, severely hampering breathing.

### First Aid Care for a Simple Nosebleed
The standard procedure for treating a simple nosebleed is as follows:

1 Have the victim sit up and slightly forward so that blood will not run down the back of the throat (Figure 9.11A). Blood draining into the back of the throat can lead to nausea and vomiting.
2 Pinch together the lower half of the nose between the thumb and forefinger and hold the nose closed for about ten minutes (Figure 9.11B).

This procedure takes care of most nasal bleeding in about ten minutes. If bleeding continues, application of an ice pack to the face and nose helps to constrict arteries, thus slowing blood flow to the damaged area. The pinching action should be maintained. One other possible step is to roll two gauze strips and place one in each nostril. This will assist with clot formation. Approximately one-half inch of each strip should be left outside the nasal cavity to allow for ease of removal once clot formation has occurred.

If these measures do not stop the blood flow within an additional ten to fifteen minutes, the person should be taken to a medical facility for further treatment.

### First Aid Care for Nasal Bone or Cartilage Fracture
Physician intervention is needed to correct a fracture of the nasal bones, cartilage, or both. The application of cold packs to the damaged tissues, however, is an important step

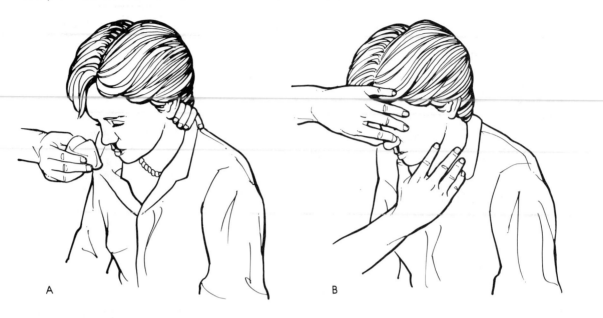

**FIGURE 9.11**

(*A*) A person with a nosebleed should sit up and lean forward to prevent blood from draining into the throat. (*B*) Pressure from pinching the nostrils stops most bleeding within ten minutes.

for the first-aider to take immediately after the injury. If this is not done, swelling and edema of the nose and face will delay and complicate treatment.

## ▬ Injuries to the Ear

A common problem among young children is their tendency to place small objects in the external ear canal. Because attempts to dislodge the foreign body without the appropriate instrument may wedge it more tightly into the ear canal, the first-aider should do no more than transport the child to a medical facility for further treatment.

Sudden changes in air pressure may perforate the tympanic membrane (eardrum). Rapid descent in an airplane, scuba diving at a considerable depth, or slapping of the ear in a water skiing accident can create a rapid pressure buildup, causing the eardrum to rupture. Rupture may also occur if a sharp object is introduced into the ear canal.

Perforation of this thin membrane can cause severe pain and bleeding, tinnitus (ringing in the ears), vertigo (loss of balance), and partial deafness. The activity of the victim at the time of onset of the pain suggests the mechanism of injury. Whatever the cause of injury, the first-aider should not attempt to irrigate the ear canal or to control bleeding from the ear. Before the victim is transported to medical care, the ear should be covered with a clean (preferably sterile) dressing, to prevent possible contamination of the canal and membrane.

## __Orthodontal Injuries

Another injury that often occurs as a result of facial trauma is the evulsion (knocking out) of a tooth. Because of the more flexible structure of the tissues surrounding the teeth of children and adolescents, tooth evulsion in them is more common than in adults.

Recent advances indicate that if an evulsed permanent tooth is replanted within thirty minutes, a 90% success rate may be achieved. If the tooth is replaced after two hours, the success rate drops to 5% (Berkowitz, Ludwig, and Johnson 1980).

The evulsed tooth is washed off under running tap water, **care being taken not to touch the root of the tooth.** The tooth is then gently inserted into its normal position. The victim should hold the tooth in position with a finger while being transported to a dental facility (Berkowitz, Ludwig, and Johnson 1980; deWet 1981; Hafen and Karren 1981).

If the individual cannot tolerate placement of the tooth into its original position, he or she should place it under the tongue during transport. Saliva is the best medium for maintaining tooth viability (Berkowitz, Ludwig, and Johnson 1980). The victim should be cautioned to take care not to swallow the tooth.

---

### SUMMARY

Located within and well protected by the bony structures of the skull and vertebral column, the brain and spinal cord are responsible for control of all conscious body functions, as well as for innervation of organs that operate without conscious control. The central nervous system is protected by a number of body parts, including the skull, vertebrae, meninges, and cerebrospinal fluid. Any injury is potentially serious, owing to the extremely sensitive nature of its tissues.

Since as many as 30% of all trauma victims incur some type of head injury, it is imperative that a first-aider have the ability to assess head injury. Whether the injury is a concussion, cerebral contusion, or possible skull fracture, its assessment at the scene by the first-aider can provide emergency personnel with important information.

A consideration in the first aid care of any person with head injury is the possibility of a concurrent spinal cord injury. Damage to the spinal cord can occur in a variety of ways, the most common being fracture and displacement of vertebrae which in turn sever or compress the cord and interrupt impulse conduction. This is likely to result in permanent damage to the cord.

As with head injuries, the key to proper first aid management of spinal cord injuries is the recognition of the signs that accompany cord trauma. Because of the potential for irreversible damage in any spinal cord injury, it is better for the first-aider to be overly cautious than not cautious enough. Patient movement and transport should, whenever possible, be handled by trained emergency personnel who have the equipment needed to safely perform this task.

Trauma to the head region can produce, in addition to brain injury, a variety of problems involving the face, eyes, nose, ears, and mouth. First aid care for most of these injuries should consist of (1) establishing an adequate airway, (2) controlling bleeding, (3) identifying and protecting fracture sites from further injury, and (4) recognizing the potential for associated injuries.

_____ CHAPTER MASTERY: TEST ITEMS _____

### Fill In the Missing Word(s)

1. Cessation of cardiopulmonary functioning may result from injury to the most primitive portion of the brain, the _____.
2. The brain and spinal cord are covered by three protective layers or meninges: _____, _____, and _____.
3. Unlike other tissues, those of the central nervous system have little ability to _____.
4. Bruises and discoloration behind the ears are often signs of basal skull fracture, known as _____.
5. Circulating through the subarachnoid space, _____ acts as a shock-absorbing agent for the brain and spinal cord.
6. The position in which a head injury victim is placed on the side with the arm tucked under the head and the face angled downward, thereby reducing the chance of airway blockage by allowing mucus and vomitus to drain from the mouth, is known as the _____.
7. Areas of the spine that have no additional support structures and therefore tend to be more susceptible to injury are the _____ and _____.
8. The basic approach to first aid for any facial injury consists of four steps: _____, _____, _____, and _____.
9. An important step to be taken by the first-aider in controlling the swelling and edema associated with facial injuries is the application of _____.
10. The best medium in which to transport a tooth that has been knocked out is _____.

### Multiple Choice (Circle the Best Answer)

1. The three major divisions of the brain are the
   a. cerebrum, medulla, and brain stem.
   b. cerebellum, diencephalon, and cerebrum.
   c. cerebrum, cerebellum, and brain stem.
   d. cerebrum, reticular activating system, and hypothalamus.
2. The special group of tissues that extends through the brain stem into the cerebrum and is responsible for keeping a person conscious is the
   a. autonomic nervous system.
   b. reticular activating system.
   c. peripheral system.
   d. diencephalon.

3. Jerky, uncoordinated movements or problems with balance and posture, or both, are caused by damage to the
   a. medulla.
   b. brain stem.
   c. autonomic nervous system.
   d. cerebellum.

4. Tissues of the brain and spinal cord are damaged most easily by
   a. decreased oxygen level and increased pressure from swelling.
   b. pressure changes.
   c. increase in carbon monoxide level.
   d. heat.

5. The percentage of all trauma patients entering hospital emergency departments with some type of head injury is approximately
   a. 50%.
   b. 75%.
   c. 40%.
   d. 30%.

6. In the case of a head injury, a first-aider's first responsibility is to
   a. control bleeding.
   b. assess the condition of the victim.
   c. locate the mechanism of injury.
   d. immobilize the victim.

7. In a victim of head injury who has not lost consciousness, a likely sign of concussion is
   a. inability to remember the accident.
   b. bleeding from the nose.
   c. a rapid pulse.
   d. pupil dilation.

8. Deterioration in the level of consciousness of a victim of head injury is generally caused by
   a. hyperventilation.
   b. neurogenic shock.
   c. intracranial bleeding.
   d. cardiac arrest.

9. Leakage of cerebrospinal fluid from the nose and ears is indicative of a serious head injury; however, the first-aider should not attempt to stop the flow of this fluid because
   a. this may increase the blood pressure.
   b. this may inhibit blood clotting.
   c. this may increase the intracranial pressure.
   d. this may cause loss of consciousness.

10. All persons with head injuries and those who have lost consciousness at the scene of an accident should be considered to have sustained
    a. a spinal cord injury.
    b. respiratory distress syndrome.
    c. multiple injuries.
    d. internal vascular damage.

11. In a conscious victim, a sign(s) almost always present in a spinal cord fracture or dislocation is (are)
    a. sweating and nausea.
    b. local pain and tenderness at the fracture site.
    c. gross deformity of the vertebral column.
    d. muscle cramping.

12. In the assessment of an unconscious person suspected of having a spinal cord injury, a lack of foot or hand response to painful stimuli suggests damage to the
    a. thoracic spine.
    b. lumbar spine.
    c. sacrum.
    d. cervical spine.

13. For maintenance of an open airway in a victim of lower-jaw trauma, he or she should be placed in a
    a. supine position.
    b. reclining position.
    c. shock-trauma position.
    d. prone or upright position.

14. With an eye injury, covering the undamaged eye with a patch
    a. will reduce movement in the damaged eye, thus reducing the likelihood of further injury.
    b. is unnecessary.
    c. can be dangerous.
    d. will increase movement in the damaged eye.

15. The correct procedure to prevent possible contamination of the ear canal and tympanic membrane after an injury is to
    a. irrigate the canal with water.
    b. lightly cover the ear with a sterile dressing.
    c. pack the ear canal with cotton.
    d. place eardrops into the canal.

## Discussion Questions

1. Describe the tests that a first-aider has available to determine the severity of spinal cord injury in a conscious person.

2. Describe the four-step approach for responding to an unconscious victim of a motor vehicle accident who has severe lacerations around the nose and mouth. (The mechanism of injury was the vehicle's windshield.)
3. In a facial injury involving evulsed permanent teeth, what special measures can be taken by the first-aider?

_____ BIBLIOGRAPHY _____

Baigelman, W., and J. C. O'Brien. "Pulmonary Effects of Head Trauma." *Neurosurgery* 9 (1981): 729–740.

Bell, J. A. "Eye Trauma in Sports: A Preventable Epidemic." *JAMA* 246 (10 July 1981): 156.

Berkowitz, R., S. Ludwig, and R. Johnson. "Dental Trauma in Children and Adolescents." *Clinical Pediatrics*, March 1980, pp. 166–171.

Council on Scientific Affairs. "Brain Injury in Boxing." *JAMA* 249 (14 January 1983): 254–257.

deWet, F. A. "The Prevention of Orofacial Sports Injuries in the Adolescent." *Journal of International Dentistry*, December 1981, pp. 313–319.

Doxanas, J. T., and C. Soderstorm. "Racquetball as an Ocular Hazard." *Archives of Ophthalmology* 98 (November 1980): 1965–1966.

Fischer, R. P., J. Carlson, and J. F. Perry. "Postconcussive Hospital Observation of Alert Patients in a Primary Trauma Center." *Journal of Trauma* 21 (November 1981): 920–924.

Hafen, B. Q., and K. J. Karren. *Prehospital Emergency Care and Crisis Intervention* 1981. Englewood, Colo.: Morton Publishing.

Ingram, N. M. "Trauma to the Ear, Nose, Face, and Neck." *Journal of Emergency Medical Services,* June 1980, pp. 41–43.

Jordan, L., and D. Calabrese. "Treating Spinal Cord Injuries" *Emergency,* June 1980, pp. 41–43.

Kewalramani, L. S., M. S. Orth, and J. F. Krauss. "Cervical Spine Injuries Resulting from Collision Sports." *Paraplegia* 19 (1981): 303–312.

Kiwerski, J., M. Weiss, and T. Chrowstowska. "Analysis of Mortality of Patients after Cervical Spine Trauma," *Paraplegia* 19 (1981): 347–351.

Lankford, T. *Integrated Science for Health Students.* 2d ed. Reston, Va.: Reston Publishing, 1979.

Lindsay, K. W., G. McLatchie, and B. Jennett, "Serious Head Inury in Sport." *British Medical Journal* 281 (20 September 1980): 789–791.

Lowdermilk, T. "Trauma to the Head and Neck." *Journal of Emergency Medical Services,* May 1980, pp. 1–6.

Miller, N. I. "Trauma to the Ear, Nose, Face, and Neck." *Journal of Emergency Nursing,* July/August 1980, pp. 8–12.

Parcel, G. S. *Basic Emergency Care of the Sick and Injured.* 2d ed. St. Louis: C. V. Mosby, 1982.

Rimel, R. W., J. A. Jane, and R. F. Edlich. "An Educational Training Program for the Care of the Site of Injury of Trauma to the Central Nervous System." *Resuscitation* (1981): 23–28.

Rimel, R. W., J. A. Jane, and G. W. Tyson, "Emergency Management of Head Injuries." *Resuscitation* 9 (1981): 75–97.

# 10

# Poisoning and Toxic Reactions

RICHARD S. RIGGS, ED.D.

After completing this chapter the student will be able to

- Define the term "poison."
- Explain the four ways that toxic substances enter the human body.
- Identify clues to look for in attempting to ascertain the kind of poison ingested and the amount.
- Cite the functions of poison control centers.
- List the information a first-aider must have to utilize a poison control center effectively.
- List in proper sequence and explain the first aid procedures for ingested poisons.
- List the instances in which the victim of an ingested poison should not be made to vomit and explain the reasons why not.
- Identify common toxic substances, cite their signs and symptoms, and explain the proper first aid procedures for ingestion of each.
- Identify four types of food intoxications or infections, cite the signs and symptoms of each, and explain the first aid procedures for each.
- Demonstrate the first aid procedures for inhaled poisons.
- Describe the first aid procedures for stings from hymenoptera.
- Describe the first aid procedures for marine life stings.
- Distinguish between pit vipers and coral snakes, compare and contrast the signs and symptoms of their bites, and explain the first aid procedures for bites from each.
- Identify poison ivy, poison oak, and poison sumac.
- Identify common drugs and specify the signs, symptoms, and proper first aid for an overdose of each.

## INTRODUCTION

Poisons are solid, liquid, or gas substances that harm the human body or disturb the function of its structures through chemical action. Poisoning is the condition produced by a poison or toxin when it contacts or enters the human body. Poisoning emergencies may be life threatening and must be dealt with quickly and accurately, to reduce the effect the toxic substance has on the body and, in the most serious instances, to save the victim's life. Poisoning emergencies arise from a variety of circumstances. An individual may misread a medicine label and ingest too much of a substance, or a child may accidentally swallow a cleaning agent that was left accessible. A poisoning emergency also occurs when a suicidal individual takes an overdose of a toxic substance or when someone deliberately gives a toxic substances to another in an attempt to harm that person. The first-aider must respond immediately in such situations to assess the victim's condition, determine the poisoning source, and enact the sequence of first aid procedures that will provide the greatest chance for survival.

Poisons can enter the human body in a number of ways. Accidental poisonings most commonly involve ingestion of the toxic substance through the mouth. Household substances that are frequently ingested and produce poisoning emergencies include medicines, household products, and plants. Poisons can also enter the body through inhalation via the nose or mouth or both. Inhalation of toxic gases and vapors accounts for a significant number of poisoning emergencies each year. Common toxic gases and vapors include carbon monoxide, cooking and heating gas, and an array of volatile substances. Poisons can also enter the body as a result of injection. The sting or bite of an insect, reptile, or animal, or an injected drug can produce a toxic reaction. Finally, toxic substances can enter the body by absorption through the skin. Insecticides, herbicides, plants, and other substances that contact the skin or contaminate clothing can create local allergic reactions, or can be absorbed into the system in large enough quantities to be toxic.

## ____POISON CONTROL CENTERS

Poison control centers, open twenty-four hours a day, have the function of providing information about the toxicity of various substances, the symptoms the substances may produce, and emergency care and first aid procedures. The National Clearinghouse for Poison Control Centers gathers information from the manufacturers and distributors of new products that may be poisonous. It also gathers information regarding modifications made in the composition of existing products. A number of other agencies work with the Clearinghouse. Generally, the manufacturers and distributors of products supply information to the Clearinghouse on the formulation of their products. A few also supply information regarding the toxicity of their products and needed treatment if they are ingested.

---

### ⚕ Locating the Poison Control Center

Many communities have a local poison control center. The first-aider and all other interested persons should check the telephone directory for the availability of such a center and its phone number. If a center is not available in the immediate community, any local hospital or physician should be able to identify the location of a regional center. The telephone number for a poison control center should be on the list with other emergency numbers.

From all of this information, the Clearinghouse has compiled a card-filing system that indexes by trade name a substance's composition, its concentration, and the lethal dose. Also listed are the symptoms and treatment for accidental poisoning by the agent. These card files are supplied to poison control centers throughout the United States Supplements are sent as new products come to market.

When placing a call to a poison control center during an emergency, the first-aider must remain calm and speak clearly, because the center will need certain critical information. The first-aider should be prepared to provide the following:

- Name, age, and weight of the victim
- Address and telephone number of the emergency site
- Name of the ingested substance
- Ingredients listed on the container of the toxic substance
- Amount of the substance ingested
- When the poisoning occurred
- Condition of the victim
- Emergency care that has been provided

The first-aider should then write down and follow exactly the instructions provided. The first-aider should be the last person to hang up the telephone, since this will guarantee the poison control center that the respondent has all the information needed.

## ____POISONING BY INGESTION

Any substance, solid or liquid, has the potential to produce toxic effects when ingested. In an ingested poisoning emergency, symptoms and observable signs will depend on four principal factors: (1) the *toxicity rating* of the poisonous substance, (2) the *amount ingested* (some poisons such as certain pesticides, are so toxic that even minute quantities are lethal), (3) the *kind of substance ingested* (corrosive substances burn sensitive tissues, while barbiturate drugs produce depression of the central nervous system, or sleep), and (4) the *time that has elapsed since the substance was ingested* (certain substances, such as caustic acids and alkalis, show effects almost immediately; others, such as aspirin, have delayed effects).

There is an almost endless number of potentially toxic substances. The following discussion presents general principles for responding to poison ingestion emergencies.

### ____Assessment

To ascertain whether poisoning has occurred, the first-aider must depend on his or her knowledge of the situation and what can be determined from clues provided by the victim and the environment. A conscious victim is asked what happened, what substance was ingested, and how much was taken. Any available witnesses are questioned about the poison. The subjective interview procedures presented in Chapter 2 could be reviewed here). With an unconscious victim, the first-aider must examine clues. What was the victim doing before becoming poisoned? The victim's respiration and pulse are checked. Are there burns or stains around the mouth? Are there odors on the victim's breath or clothing that suggest a specific type of toxic substance? Has the victim been vomiting? Does the victim have convulsions or tremors? An attempt is made to determine whether pain or unconsciousness were sudden. Are the pupils of the eyes responsive to light, or are they fixed and pinpointed? Does the skin feel hot and look flushed? Is the victim in shock? Is the skin cool and clammy? Is the victim perspiring profusely?

Next, the environment is surveyed. In what room was the victim found? The kitchen and bathroom account for a majority of poisoning locations in the home, but the bedroom and garage are other areas where toxic substances are often stored. Is a container for a potentially toxic substance lying near the person? Is the lid missing from such a container sitting nearby? Are the contents of any such containers spilled or missing? Does anything else in the room provide evidence the person has ingested a toxic substance rather than being injured in some other manner?

The first-aider must determine the specific emergency care to be given for the particular type of ingested poison. The first source of information about the poison is the container, if one if found. The label should identify the substance and its ingredients. Many authorities in first aid and emergency care believe that the first aid information found on the labels of many substances is outdated or inaccurate. The first-aider should use the label to identify the substance and then phone a physician or poison control center.

## ___General First Aid Procedures

As previously indicated, a multitude of substances exist that may prove toxic to the human organism when ingested. The first aid procedures that follow are generally appropriate. Greater specificity for a given substance should be sought from an appropriate medical authority or a poison control center.

1 Dilute the poison; give water or other liquids to drink, but **only if the victim is conscious and not convulsing.** Water is usually most readily available; milk is preferable because it coats and protects the gastrointestial tract.
2 Phone the poison control center or a physician.
3 Carefully follow the directions given by the poison control center or the physician.
4 If these directions call for inducement of vomiting, do so with syrup of ipecac. Syrup of ipecac can be purchased in any pharmacy in one-ounce bottles and is inexpensive. Experts recommend that all households have at least one bottle of ipecac for poisoning emergencies. In families with children under the age of 5, one bottle per child should be available.

   Ipecac is given by mouth and the dose varies with age and weight of the person. A normal dose for children under 1 year of age is two teaspoonfuls (10 cc); for children 1 year of age and over one tablespoonful (15 cc); and for adults two tablespoonfuls (30 cc). Follow ipecac administration immediately with at least eight ounces of water. In this instance milk should not be the fluid given, since it delays the desired action of the ipecac. Ipecac usually works in a short time, but may take as long as thirty minutes. The victim will usually vomit three to four times within a fifteen-minute period. If ipecac does not induce vomiting, repeat the dose once. If ipecac is not available, tickle the back of the victim's throat with a finger.

5 During vomiting, keep the victim's head lower than the rest of the body to prevent aspiration or choking on the vomitus. Save the vomitus, container, and other evidence of the poisoning event and send this evidence to the hospital with the victim.

6 If the directions from the physician or poison control center call for it, give activated charcoal in the recommended dose. Activated charcoal can be purchased in any pharmacy. This agent is highly effective in absorbing toxic substances from the gastrointestinal tract and thereby preventing toxicity. (This form of charcoal is the only type effective against toxic substances. Burnt toast and other forms of charcoal are totally worthless in absorbing poisons.) Activated charcoal is mixed with water and administered orally. Ipecac and activated charcoal should not be given together. Ipecac is given first; following vomiting the activated charcoal is administered.

7 Maintain an open airway and monitor vital signs. Administer artifical respiration (Chapter 5) or CPR (Chapter 6) if necessary.

8 Treat the victim for shock (see Chapter 4). Keep the victim lying down and comfortable and maintain a normal body temperature. Place the victim so vomitus will drain from the mouth in case of spontaneous or uncontrolled vomiting.

9 Provide for medical care. Either transport or call for an ambulance to transport the victim. Many of these first aid procedures should be implemented as the victim is being transported to the hospital. Figure 10.1 shows the sequence of first aid procedures for poison ingestion.

A victim of poison ingestion should NOT be made to vomit in the following instances:

1 *When the substance ingested is corrosive (acid or alkali).* Corrosive substances burn and severely damage tissue as they pass through the esophagus into the stomach. Regurgitation of the corrosive substance could cause the damaged esophagus to rupture. Additionally, in vomiting, the substance again comes into contact with the tissue, causing further damage. Aspiration of the corrosive substance into the lungs can also result from vomiting.

2 *When the substance ingested is a petroleum product (e.g., gasoline, kerosene, turpentine).* The most serious danger from a petroleum product is the possibility of aspiration into the lungs. Petroleum products coat as well as destroy airways and capillaries in the respiratory passages. Those who die from ingestion of a petroleum product almost always die from the damage that occurs in the lungs due to aspiration, rather than from absorption of the product from the gastrointestinal tract.

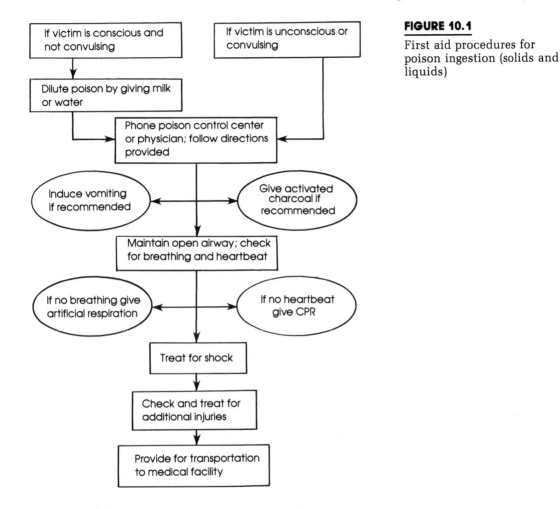

**FIGURE 10.1**

First aid procedures for poison ingestion (solids and liquids)

**3** *When the victim is unconscious, rapidly becoming unconscious, convulsing, has a depressed gag reflex, or a combination of these.* Each of these conditions greatly increases the risk for aspiration of the toxic substance into the lungs, for blockage of the airway, or for both.

## ___Common Ingested Poisons: Types, Signs and Symptoms of Ingestion, and First Aid Care

### Corrosive Substances

**Alkalis**    There is a wide variety of caustic alkalis on the market for use in a number of ways in the typical home. Common household alkalis include liquid and crystalline drain openers, oven cleaners, and dishwasher detergents.

The signs and symptoms of alkali poisoning include burns around the mouth or in the mouth and throat, or both; excessive drooling; if in a child, pulling at the mouth and crying as if in pain; refusal to drink liquids; and respiratory distress.

**Acids**     A large number of substances found around the home and work area are caustic acids. Sulfuric acid is found in automobile batteries. Toilet bowl cleaners contain chemicals that ultimately form sulfuric and hydrochloric acids. Other cleaning agents contain phosphoric or oxalic acids. Many acids are used in hobbies. Most acid poisonings in the United States occur as a result of inhalation of acid fumes or from ingesting acids. Acid poisoning occurs with less frequency than does alkali poisoning.

On ingestion of a strong acid, the victim complains immediately of pain and often does not swallow the acid. In this case burns will be confined to the mouth and lips. If the acid is swallowed, most of the damage will be in the stomach. The victim will experience nausea and vomiting; have intense thirst; and show signs of shock, such as a weak, rapid pulse and clammy skin. Asphyxia due to swelling of the larynx or glottis may occur.

**First Aid Care for Corrosive Substance Poisoning**     Since much of the damage to body tissues will already have occurred by the time the victim of corrosive substance poisoning is found, and since vomiting should not be induced, first aid care is limited. If the victim is conscious and can swallow, the best and safest substance for the first-aider to give is milk. Milk will dilute the poison as well as coat and protect the gastrointestinal tract. If milk is not available, water can be given. The poison control center is then called and the steps shown in Figure 10.1 are followed.

## Petroleum Distillates

These products are commonly found in the home and garage. The most common examples are kerosene, charcoal lighter fluid, liquid pesticides, and mineral spirits. A large number of children under age 5 ingest petroleum distillates each year.

**Signs and Symptoms of Ingestion**     Petroleum distillates produce a burning sensation in the mouth. The victim may spontaneously vomit, greatly increasing the likelihood of the material being aspirated into the lungs. The breath of the victim should have a characteristic petroleum odor. Diarrhea often occurs and may be blood tinged or have a petroleum odor. Respiration and pulse rates increase, hypoxia may occur, and there may be transient cyanosis.

**First Aid Care**     The victim of petroleum distillate poisoning should be transported immediately to a medical facility. The poison control center is called, the victim is treated for shock, and vital signs are monitored. If spontaneous vomiting occurs, the victim's head is kept lower than the rest of the body to prevent aspiration into the lungs. The person is calmed and reassured.

## Salicylates

Salicylates are commonly known as aspirin. Over 200 different consumer products contain salicylates, and these substances are probably the most common cause of poisoning in children. The group primarily affected are children between 1 and 5 years of age. The attractive color and flavor of certain salicylate products, as well as the similarity among bottle labels, are related to the significant number of childhood poisonings by these substances.

**Signs and Symptoms of Ingestion**    The victim of salicylate poisoning manifests the following signs and symptoms: tinnitus (ringing in the ears) and some degree of deafness; profuse sweating and warm, flushed extremities; rapid and bounding pulse; nausea and vomiting (commonly but not always); hyperventilation; and respiratory distress.

First aid care for salicylate poisoning is the same as for acetaminophen poisoning (see below).

## Acetaminophen
Acetaminophen is used alone or in combination with a number of other drugs and has an analgesic effect. Acetaminophen is found in many over-the-counter products, including Tylenol, Datril, Tempra, and a number of cough and cold preparations. Acetaminophen is relatively safe when used in therapeutic doses; however, the incidence of poisonings from an overdose of this substance is increasing in the United States.

**Signs and Symptoms of Ingestion**    Acetaminophen is rapidly absorbed, especially in liquid form. Acute symptoms of overdose include nausea, vomiting, drowsiness, and profuse perspiration. Reduced blood pressure, confusion, and anorexia often occur.

**First Aid Care Salicylate or Acetaminophen Poisoning**    The poison is diluted by giving the victim milk or water. The poison control center is called. Syrup of ipecac is given to induce vomiting; after vomiting, activated charcoal is given for absorption of the salicylate. The first-aider keeps the victim calm and reassured, treats for shock if necessary, and monitors vital signs, remaining alert to the possibility of having to administer artifical respiration or CPR. The victim must be transported to a medical facility.

## Iron
Products containing iron are a common source of poisoning in the United States. Many products containing iron are available in over-the-counter preparations, and they tend to be sugarcoated and bright in color. Many of these are used in homes with small children, increasing the likelihood of accidental ingestion. Since the amount of iron varies with different products, even a small number of tablets may produce a toxic response.

**Signs and Symptoms of Ingestion**    Signs and symptoms of iron toxicity may occur within thirty minutes of ingestion or may take as long as six hours to appear. Iron most commonly affects the liver and gastrointestinal tract. The victim experiences vomiting and diarrhea that is often bloody. Fever; a weak, rapid pulse; and other indicators of shock occur. Coma and seizures are possible, and the victim may appear cyanotic. Even though the victim appears to be recovering, the first-aider should realize that improvement will probably be temporary and that the symptoms will generally grow more severe.

**First Aid Care**    The victim of iron poisoning should be given milk or water to dilute the substance. The poison control center is called. Syrup of ipecac is given to induce vomiting; activated charcoal is of NO value in iron poisoning. The victim is treated for shock and transported to the nearest medical facility.

## Soaps, Detergents, and Household Bleaches

These substances are readily accessible in the home and are often ingested by children. Soaps have a low toxicity level and are responsible for few poisoning emergencies. The symptoms that soaps produce are very mild and are classified mainly as irritants. Detergents are more toxic; they contain a mixture of organic and inorganic ingredients, with some being more toxic than others (and possibly corrosive). Household bleaches are primarily weak solutions of ammonia. Since all of these substances are mixtures of ingredients, their effects on the human organism are not always predictable.

**Signs and Symptoms of Ingestion**     Soap poisoning is recognized primarily by the irritation it produces. When ingested, soaps irritate the oral and gastrointestinal tract. When ingested in large amounts, they cause vomiting or mild diarrhea or both. Detergents also have low toxicity except when they have a high alkaline content. Signs and symptoms of detergent poisoning include irritation of the oral and gastrointestinal passages and adverse effects on the central nervous system. The latter include restlessness, confusion, convulsion, muscle weakness, and cyanosis. Bleaches are mild to moderate irritants but usually do not produce serious tissue destruction. Signs include mild oral and esophageal burns or irritations in the gastrointestinal tract. Solid bleaches are more toxic than liquid bleaches, because the liquids are more diluted. Mixing of cleaners and/or bleaches can produce highly toxic gases that can cause severe irritation to the pulmonary tract (see Poisoning by Inhalation in this chapter).

**First Aid Care**     The first-aider should dilute the poison by giving water or milk. The poison control center is called. In the case of certain household cleaners, the victim should be kept in an upright position, since vomiting may occur spontaneously. Because soaps, detergents, and bleaches may cause skin irritations, burns, or both, any area of the body that is contaminated by such a substance should be thoroughly irrigated with running water.

## Plants

Ingestion of indoor plants is one of the leading causes of childhood poisoning. A formidable array of plants are accessible to children. Plants produce compounds during their growth and development, which concentrate in various parts of the plant or are generally distributed throughout the plant. Examples are alkaloids, coumarins, oxalates, resins, resinoids, flavonoids, and oils. These compounds may be toxic to humans when ingested. These compounds vary in level of concentration depending on stage of growth of the plant. Therefore, a part of or the whole plant may be toxic due to accumulation of the toxic compound.

According to most experts, the majority of plants are relatively harmless, producing mild reactions. However, a number are highly toxic when ingested. A listing of all poisonous plants in the United States would be rather impractical for a first aid text. A variety of factors limit the usefulness of such a list, including the variance in toxicity from plant to plant and the confusing array of common names by which plants are known in different parts of the country. Even if such a listing were given with accompanying illustrations, identification of specific plants would be difficult. It is therefore recommended that all plant ingestions be viewed as potential emergencies requiring immediate first aid care.

**Signs and Symptoms of Ingestion**     The signs and symptoms produced by ingestion of a poisonous plant differ according to the type of plant. The first-aider should examine the victim's mouth for any signs that a plant has been eaten. Accessible plants are examined for missing leaves or berries or for portions of leaves. The victim is observed for sweating, cramping, vomiting, unusual behavior, and unconsciousness.

**First Aid Care**     The first-aider gives the victim water or milk to dilute the poison from the plant. The poison control center is then called and the suspected plant is described as accurately as possible. Vomiting is induced with syrup of ipecac. Activated charcoal is given for absorption of toxic agents from the plant. The victim is treated for shock, if necessary, kept calm and reassured, and transported to a medical facility. To aid with identification of the plant, sufficient remaining portions of the suspected plant should accompany the victim to the medical facility.

## __Food Poisoning and Infection

Most, if not all, food appropriate for human consumption can become contaminated with organisms that produce food infections or food intoxications. Food poisoning and food infections are extremely common and affect nearly everyone at one time or another. They can range in severity from a self-limited inconvenience to a life-threatening emergency. Staphylococcal, *Clostridium perfringens,* and botulism food poisoning, as well as salmonella food infection are discussed here.

**Staphylococcal Food Poisoning**
The most common of all food poisonings is staphylococcal poisoning, a food intoxication rather than a food infection like salmonellosis. Staphylococcal food poisoning results when staphylococci bacteria are introduced into a food. The bacteria produce a toxin (enterotoxin), which is responsible for food poisoning symptoms. Thoroughly cooking a food destroys the bacteria but not the enterotoxin.

---

### Preventing Food Poisoning

Staphylococcal food poisoning is best prevented by promptly serving and consuming food after its preparation or removal from refrigeration. Foods should be kept above 140° F or below 45° F to prevent or at least minimize bacterial growth. Persons with pus-producing skin, eye, or respiratory infections should be prevented from handling, preparing, or serving food. All food handlers should be educated regarding measures necessary to prevent food-borne intoxication and food infection outbreaks.

---

Sources of staphylococcal food poisoning include meats, poultry, eggs and egg products, milk, cheese, ice cream, cream-filled bakery items, and a variety of salads including chicken, potato, egg, tuna, and macaroni. Bacteria usually enter the food during preparation or afterward, when the food is kept warmed or unrefrigerated for a number of hours before being served. This delay allows bacteria time to multiply and produce toxin.

---

**⚕ Prevention of Botulism**

Botulism is prevented by examining food for odor, appearance (cloudy or unclear), gas, or softening. Any food that is foul smelling or in a bulging container (the bulge due to accumulated gas) should not be eaten. Cans that are bulging should not even be opened, to prevent accidental tasting or possible absorption of the toxin through a cut on the hands. If there is ever any doubt about the quality of a food, the food should be thrown away without being opened, tasted, or eaten. Foods containing botulism spores may exhibit no observable changes. Persons who preserve food must be educated in the prevention of food intoxications and infections.

---

**Signs and Symptoms**     Staphylococcal food poisoning manifests itself within two to four hours after ingestion of the contaminated food. Specific signs and symptoms include salivation, nausea, vomiting, retching, abdominal cramping, diarrhea, and prostration. In severe cases the victim may show signs of shock. Most often the condition runs its course in one to two days.

**First Aid Care**     Typically, no first aid measures are called for. Fluids are given to replace those lost through vomiting and diarrhea. If discomfort is severe, medical attention should be sought.

**Salmonellosis**

Salmonella bacteria, of which there are over 1000 varieties, are responsible for the food infection called salmonellosis. Salmonellosis is often referred to as a food poisoning but is in reality a food infection. Salmonellosis results from the infestation of a food by a salmonella bacterium and subsequent multiplication. In a typical year more than 20,000 cases of salmonella infection are reported. Generally, reported cases involve only the most seriously infected individuals. Many thousands of additional, less severe cases go unreported. Foods that are most often the source of salmonella infection include raw meats, poultry, eggs, milk, and fish and various dishes containing these products. Pets such as dogs, cats, turtles, fish, and birds are potential sources of salmonellosis. Food infestation by salmonella cannot be detected by observation, since the foodstuff does not change in appearance, smell, or taste. The bacteria are destroyed by thorough cooking of the food and proper reheating of leftovers. Salmonella infection is prevented by sanitary handling of food and adequate cooling below 45° F or heating above 140° F.

**Signs and Symptoms**     The signs and symptoms of salmonellosis usually manifest themselves within twelve to twenty-four hours. Typically they include fever, nausea, headache, vomiting, muscle weakness, abdominal cramping, and diarrheal stools that may become watery and green.

**First Aid Care**     First aid measures are generally not necessary. Only soft, bland foods and liquids should be given to the victim. If the infection appears severe, medical attention should be sought.

### *Clostridium perfringens* Food Poisoning

The strain of the clostridium bacterium responsible for the food poisoning *Clostridium perfringens* is extremely common and widely distributed through human and animal feces, soil, air, and water. In food the spores of the organism produce an enterotoxin that is responsible for the signs and symptoms of the poisoning episode. *Clostridium perfringens* poisoning occurs most commonly after consumption of inadequately cooked or reheated meats (e.g., stews, meat pies, or gravies made from beef, chicken, or turkey). Inadequate heating allows the spores to survive, germinate, and multiply during cooling or rewarming of the food. Food outlets that are inadequately prepared for large-scale cooking and refrigeration of foods are most often responsible for outbreaks of this type of food poisoning.

**Signs and Symptoms**     The symptoms of *Clostridium perfringens* poisoning manifest themselves within four to twenty-four hours, the average time being ten to twelve hours. Specific signs and symptoms include abdominal pain, diarrhea, vomiting, and vertigo. The typical episode continues for one to two days.

**First Aid Care**     First aid measures are not necessary, since the intoxication is usually mild and the victim recovers in a short time. If the intoxication is severe, medical attention should be sought.

### Botulism

*Clostridium botulinum* is a spore-forming anaerobic (without air) bacterium responsible for the severe form of food intoxication known as botulism. As the spores grow in an anaerobic environment, they produce a highly lethal toxin. At present, types A, B, E, and F toxins are responsible for most human outbreaks of botulism. Growth and toxin release most frequently occur in underprocessed nonacid or low-acid foods, such as home-canned vegetables, particularly spinach, asparagus, beets, corn, and string beans, and fruits. However, meats and fish are potential sources for botulism. Home-canned foods should be baked or boiled for ten to fifteen minutes before they are served as a precaution against botulism.

**Signs and Symptoms**     The manifestations of botulism usually appear within twelve to thirty-six hours but may be delayed for several days. The exotoxin of botulism primarily affects the nervous system. The victim experiences blurred or double vision, dry mouth, and sore throat. The victim may vomit and have diarrhea, or will occasionally have constipation. Lassitude or fatigue with dizziness or headache often accompanies the digestive tract disturbances. The victim generally experiences difficulty in speaking and has progressive paralysis of the respiratory system. Respiratory failure is the most frequent cause of death in botulism poisoning. The fatality rate for botulism has declined in recent years due to better medical treatment and the use of antitoxins.

**First Aid Care**    The victim of botulism food intoxication must receive medical attention immediately. He or she must be monitored for an open airway and respiratory status, artificial respiration or CPR being administered if necessary. The victim is treated for shock and transported to a medical facility.

# ___POISONING BY INHALATION

Inhalation of toxic gases and vapors is responsible for several thousand deaths per year. A number of gases and vapors are potentially toxic if inhaled. These include but are not limited to carbon dioxide, frequently accumulated in wells or sewer systems; carbon tetrachloride, commonly found in industrial settings; methyl bromide, often used as a fumigant; vinyl chloride, used in the manufacture of plastics, solvents, glues, gasoline, and aerosol propellants; and benzene, occasionally encountered by industrial workers who enter storage tanks for cleaning purposes. Many of these gases and vapors may also be encountered in the home.

Most deaths resulting from poison inhalation are attributed to carbon monoxide poisoning. Carbon monoxide is an odorless, colorless, and tasteless gas that results from the incomplete combustion of fossil fuels. When carbon monoxide is released into the environment, it may be inhaled into the respiratory system. The hemoglobin of the red blood cells has an affinity 250 times greater for carbon monoxide than for oxygen. The presence of carbon monoxide in hemoglobin prevents oxygen from bonding with the hemoglobin. It also diminishes the ability of the hemoglobin to release the oxygen it is carrying to the various cells and tissues of the body.

## ___Signs and Symptoms

The victim of inhalation poisoning may experience any or all of the following: headache, dizziness, shortness of breath, chest pain, irritability, fainting, unconsciousness, cessation of breathing, and cardiac arrest. The victim's skin often changes color, tending toward a cherry red, especially the lips and mucous membranes. These signs and symptoms in conjuction with an environment conducive to inhalation poisoning should prompt strong suspicion of an emergency situation.

## ___First Aid Care

The first-aider must recognize that the same substance that has poisoned the victim may rapidly affect himself or herself. The greater the concentration of gases and vapors in an environment, the greater the danger and the shorter period of time the environment can

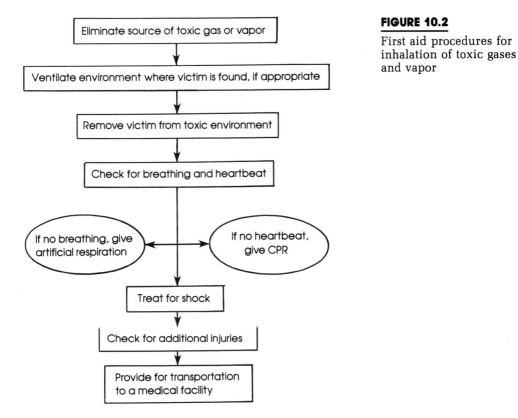

**FIGURE 10.2**

First aid procedures for inhalation of toxic gases and vapor

be entered to effect a rescue. In such an environment, the safety of the victim, first-aider, and bystanders, if any, requires moving the victim.

First aid procedures for all types of inhalation poisonings are essentially the same (Figure 10.2). These procedures are as follows:

1 While holding the breath, quickly open windows or doors to allow fresh air to enter the room or space. If possible, turn off or remove the source of the gas or vapor.

2 Remove the victim to fresh air as quickly as possible. This area should be a safe distance from the site of the initial emergency.

3 Check the victim for breathing and heartbeat. Initiate artificial respiration or CPR if necessary.

4 Administer oxygen, if available. Oxygen hastens the elimination of carbon monoxide from the body.

5 Keep the victim lying down and comfortable. Loosen tight clothing and treat for shock.

6 Check for additional injuries and provide appropriate care for these injuries.

7 Seek medical attention immediately.

## ___POISONING BY INJECTION

This section examines poisoning emergencies that result from the bite or sting of insects, forms of marine life, arthropods, and reptiles.

### ___Hymenoptera

The order *Hymenoptera* includes bees, wasps, hornets, and yellow jackets. More people die each year from the stings of these insects than die from any other group of insect bites. Of greatest concern are persons allergic to the venom and at risk for anaphylactic shock.

**Signs and Symptoms of Sting**
Hypersensitivity to hymenoptera venom manifests itself in a severe systemic reaction characterized by respiratory distress and vascular collapse and often by vomiting and abdominal cramps. This is a true medical emergency and the first-aider must respond quickly.

**First Aid Care**
Commercially prepared kits are available that contain preloaded syringes with two doses of epinephrine, a constricting band, alcohol swabs, and directions for use. The individual with known hypersensitivity to hymenoptera sting should have these kits available in convenient places. The first-aider can administer the epinephrine or get the victim to a medical environment where the epinephrine can be administered.

First aid care for all bee, wasp, hornet, and yellow jacket stings is as follows:

1 Remove the stinger, if one is present. The stinger will have a venom sac attached. When removing the stinger, be careful to not squeeze the sac, because this will inject more toxin or venom into the victim. Use a knife or other sharp instrument to tease the stinger back and forth, as is done in removing a splinter. Honeybees are the only hymenoptera to leave their stinger.

2 Check the victim for a Medic Alert tag that shows hypersensitivity to venom.

3 For a victim not hypersensitive to venom, wash the affected part and apply cold, using either cold water or ice wrapped in a towel. Cold applications should reduce the swelling and also venom absorption. Use a commercial sting/bite preparation to reduce swelling and itching. Nothing more need be done.

4 For a person who is hypersensitive to the venom and shows an allergic response with severe swelling or difficulty in breathing, administer the victim's own medication, if available, and seek medical attention immediately.

   a Apply a constricting band above the sting site. This band is tied firmly but not so that it impedes arterial blood flow. When the band is tied properly, a finger can be wedged between the band and the skin. Monitor the victim's pulse.

**b** Maintain a close watch on respiration and heartbeat. Administer artificial respiration or CPR, if needed.

**c** Treat the victim for shock.

**d** Seek medical attention immediately.

## ___Poisonous Arthropods

### Spiders

Spiders are plentiful and widespread, being found in almost all regions of the world. For the most part, spiders are of little concern to humans. Spiders are responsible for very few deaths, even though spider bites are relatively common. Two genuses of spider are of significance to this discussion on poisons, the black widow and the brown recluse (Figure 10.3). Tarantulas are also briefly reviewed.

**Black Widow Spider**   These spiders are approximately one inch long, are deep black, and carry a unique red mark on the abdomen. This mark is often hourglass in shape, but many variations are seen, as indicated in the figure. They are found in bushes, garages, woodpiles, sheds, and other outside and indoor areas. Black widow spiders inject a venom into their victim through two small fangs (chelicerae). Death rarely occurs from a black widow spider bite; however, children, elderly people, the chronically ill, and those who sustain multiple bites are at risk. An antivenom is available if risk is great.

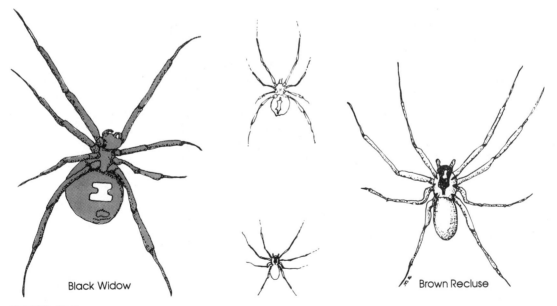

Black Widow

Brown Recluse

**FIGURE 10.3**

The black widow and brown recluse spiders are responsible for most poisonous spider bites in the United States. Center illustrations show the relative size of the two spiders.

Two small red marks indicate the location of injected venom. The victim experiences severe localized pain shortly after being bitten. The pain gradually spreads throughout the body. Cramping may occur in the abdominal muscles and elsewhere. The victim perspires profusely, is nauseous, and may vomit. Respiration and speech may be impaired.

**Brown Recluse Spider**    These spiders, sometimes referred to as "violin" spiders, are very small, usually less than one-half inch in length. They are light brown in color and easily identified by a dark-brown violin-shaped marking on their back. Brown recluse spiders are most often found in dark locations, storage areas, closets, and other places not frequented by human beings.

Usually little or no pain is felt immediately after a bite by a brown recluse spider. A short time later the site is painful, red, and swollen. A generalized body rash may appear. In a few days, tissue at the bite site darkens and necrosis occurs. The dead tissue falls off, leaving an ulcer. The ulcer tends to enlarge, increasing the likelihood of secondary infection. Children or persons who are chronically ill may have more severe symptoms. The victim of a brown recluse spider bite needs medical treatment for the bite to heal properly. No antivenom is available at present for brown recluse spider bites.

**First Aid Care for Black Widow and Brown Recluse Spider Bites**    If the bite is minor and the victim does not show severe symptoms, the bitten area is washed with soap and water, cold is applied, and calamine lotion is used. The bite is monitored for infection and the victim for severe reaction. In the case of severe reaction:

1 Calm the victim and have him or her lie down with the affected part below the level of the heart. Treat for shock.
2 If the bite is on an extremity, apply a constricting band above the level of the bite. Even if the bite occurred some time earlier, the band should be applied as a precautionary measure. The band should not remain on the arm or leg more than thirty minutes. Monitor pulse and insert a finger under the constricting band to determine that it is not too tight.
3 Apply cold, either cold water or ice wrapped in a cloth.
4 Give aspirin if pain relief is needed.
5 Seek prompt medical attention.
6 Administer artificial respiration or CPR if necessary.

**Tarantula**    These large, hairy spiders are present in many areas, particularly in the southwestern part of the United States. The venom of the tarantula is so mild that it rarely presents a medical problem for humans. There is a possibility for an allergic reaction to the venom. If this should occur, medical treatment must be sought immediately.

## Scorpions

Scorpions are arthropods that have elongated, segmented bodies and a long, segmented, active tail. The last segment of the tail contains a stinger that can inject venom. Only two species of scorpions are of concern from a first aid perspective, and both are indigenous

---
**⚕ Beware of Crawlers in the Night**

Scorpions often crawl into the shoes of campers and hikers at night and are found the next morning. Shoes and boots always should be checked before dressing when in areas inhabited by these arthropods.

---

to Arizona. Scorpions live under rocks or bury themselves in sand. They are mainly active at night and prefer cool, damp environments.

**Signs and Symptoms of Sting** The venom of scorpions is locally irritating; often the victim has an allergic response. Convulsions or seizures are possible. Nausea, vomiting, abdominal pain, and shock may also occur.

**First Aid Care** If reaction is severe medical treatment is needed as soon as possible. An antivenom is available. The first-aider maintains an open airway, monitors vital signs, and administers artificial respiration or CPR if necessary. The victim is calmed, reassured, and treated for shock. A constricting band may be of benefit. Cold applications are used to reduce swelling and venom absorption.

## Poisonous Marine Life

Some of the most potent toxins known are found in marine life. The three most common marine organisms causing emergency room visits in the United States are jellyfish, stingrays, and catfish.

### Jellyfish

Jellyfish have long threadlike tentacles that contain nematocysts, stinging structures that contain toxins. These toxins produce symptoms and signs ranging from mild rash, weakness, and intense burning pain to shock, muscular cramping, nausea, vomiting, and respiratory distress.

First aid procedures include removing the tentacles, because they tend to cling where contact was initially made. Removal is accomplished by gently rubbing with a towel or by drying the area with powder or sand. Drying makes removal of the tentacles much easier. Rubbing alcohol can be used to wash the affected area. A commercially prepared meat tenderizer sprinkled on the affected part helps to neutralize the protein toxin. Aspirin may be given for pain relief. If the victim has an allergic reaction, immediate medical treatment is needed. The victim is treated for shock and vital signs are monitored. Artificial respiration or CPR is given, if needed.

### Stingrays

Stingrays are commonly found in coastal waters and may grow quite large. A stingray buries itself in the sand or mud, and when stepped on, lashes out with its tail. Most injuries are thus on the leg or foot. The tail contains bony spines that inject a venom. The signs and symptoms of stingray poisoning include severe pain, nausea, vomiting, and fainting. More serious symptoms include shock, convulsions, irregular breathing, and cardiac distress.

First aid procedures for stingray injection include:

1 Remove all pieces of the spine, if possible, and immerse the wound in saltwater.
2 Soak the wound in hot water for approximately one hour to deactivate the toxin.
3 Control bleeding, as necessary, and dry, dress, and bandage the wound.
4 Obtain medical treatment for further removal of foreign material from the wound and treatment for additional injuries.

### Catfish
Catfish are smooth, scaleless fish with whiskers around their mouth. The dorsal and pectoral spines are venomous and can inflict very painful wounds, usually when the victim is handling the catfish. The wound becomes swollen and infected. Usually the victim finds later that the barb from the catfish spine has remained in the wound.

The victim will probably need a tetanus shot and antibiotics for the infection.

## ▁Snakes

### Pit Vipers
Pit vipers include three species of venomous snakes: rattlesnake, copperhead, and water moccasin (often called a cottonmouth). These three species contain a number of subspecies. Pit vipers as a group can generally be identified by the following characteristics: a triangular-shaped head that is larger than the neck; facial pits that serve as sensors for locating nearby objects that have a higher temperature than the surroundings; elliptical pupils; and at least one or two large fangs (one having possibly been lost)—elongated cone-shaped teeth that are folded against the roof of the mouth and rotated to a biting position when the snake's mouth is opened.

Rattlesnakes have these characteristics plus rattles at the end of the tail. Sometimes, however, the rattles have broken off. The head of copperheads tends to be copper to reddish brown in color and is a distinguishing feature. Water moccasins are usually olive, black, or brown in color; when they open their mouth, the characteristic "white mouth" shows, hence the name cottonmouth. Distinctive features of poisonous and nonpoisonous snakes are shown in Figure 10.4.

At least one, and generally two, puncture wounds occur at the site of a pit viper bite (and in the case of multiple bites, three wounds or more). Swelling occurs at the site of the bite and pain is generalized. The victim experiences weakness, sweating, or chilling, or a combination of these. The pulse is rapid and weak, nausea or vomiting or both are present, and respiration may cease. The likelihood of shock is great.

### Coral Snakes
The coral snake is the only other species of venomous snakes that is found in the United States. There are three subspecies of coral snakes: the Eastern, Texas, and Arizona or Sonoran coral snake. Coral snakes are readily identified by their colorful bright rings of red, white and yellow, and black (Figure 10.5). The red and yellow bands touch one

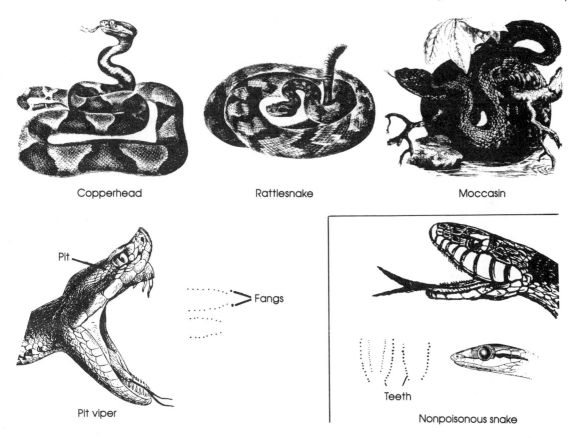

Copperhead        Rattlesnake        Moccasin

Pit

Fangs

Teeth

Pit viper        Nonpoisonous snake

**FIGURE 10.4**

Poisonous and nonpoisonous (*inset*) snakes. The copperhead, rattlesnake, and moccasin are all pit vipers, distinguished by triangular heads, facial pits, elliptical pupils, and one or two large fangs. Bite patterns are shown.

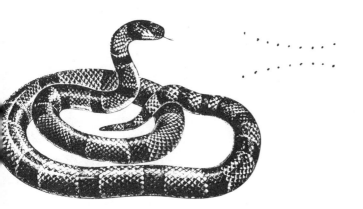

**FIGURE 10.5**

Unlike pit vipers, coral snakes do not have facial pits, fangs (note bite pattern), or elliptical eyes. The mouth area is always black, a feature that distinguishes coral snakes from similarly colored nonpoisonous snakes.

another, hence the admonition, "Red and yellow, kill a fellow." The mouth area is always black. The eyes are round and there are no facial pits, as in pit vipers. Coral snakes burrow, are docile, and are relatively small, generally ranging in length from fifteen to thirty inches. When these snakes bite, they do not strike and release, but hold onto the part and chew, allowing the venom to flow from the fangs over the wounds produced by the chewing and into the bite. Since coral snakes are small, bites tend to be on fingers, hands, toes, and feet. The venom from coral snakes primarily affects the nervous system.

The bite of a coral snake produces one or more toothmarks. Pain is relatively mild and remains localized in the affected part. The degree of pain, however, is associated with the amount of venom injected; the more venom, the greater the pain. After a short period, the victim experiences numbness and weakness in the affected part. Swelling is uncommon. The victim typically begins to feel drowsy, or has a feeling of impeding unconsciousness. The victim also has difficulty in swallowing, becomes nauseous, and may vomit. Convulsions sometimes occur.

### First Aid Care for Snakebite

The victim of a venomous snakebite requires immediate medical treatment. Since the vast majority of such snakebites occur in locations within approximately one hour of medical care, the first-aider must establish as a priority the transportation of the victim to the nearest medical facility. Additionally, the first-aider can take a number of steps that should benefit the victim, and also reduce the chance of additional harm.

**Pit Viper Bite**     First aid care for pit viper snakebite differs from that of coral snakes. Steps are as follows:

1 Have the victim lie down or sit down and remain as quiet as possible.
2 Help the victim relax; provide reassurance; keep the person comfortable; and maintain the body temperature.
3 Immobilize the bitten part in a position such that the victim can use it if necessary. For example, immobilize the foot in a functional position so that, if necessary, the person can walk or use the foot for support in assisting with his or her own transportation. The bitten part should remain at or below the level of the heart.
4 Apply a constricting band just above the bite site, but not on a joint, the neck, or head. The constricting band should be approximately two to three inches wide and only tight enough to restrict venous and lymph flow. Check the tightness of the constricting band by inserting a finger between the band and the skin. If this can be done without much effort, the band is properly applied. Also, monitor the pulse to ensure that arterial blood flow is not impeded. The constricting band may need to be loosened as swelling progresses.
5 *If a physician or a medical facility may be reached within approximately forty-five minutes, do nothing more and immediately transport the victim.*

If a physician or a medical facility *cannot be reached* within approximately forty-five minutes, complete the following additional measures.

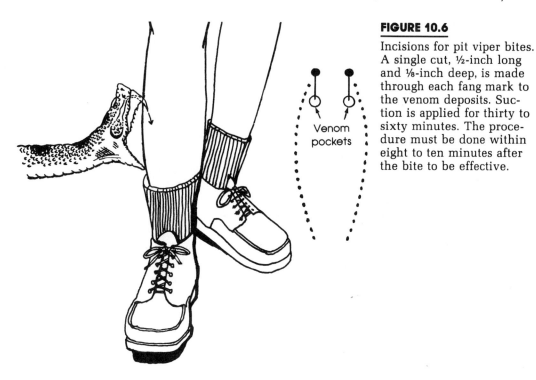

**FIGURE 10.6**

Incisions for pit viper bites. A single cut, ½-inch long and ⅛-inch deep, is made through each fang mark to the venom deposits. Suction is applied for thirty to sixty minutes. The procedure must be done within eight to ten minutes after the bite to be effective.

1 Make a single incision through EACH fang or puncture mark to the believed venom deposit site (see Figure 10.6). Each incision should be approximately one-half inch in length and not more than one-eighth inch deep. Immediately apply suction over the incisions. Suction can be applied with suction cups found in snakebite kits, with the mouth, or with any other means available. When suctioning with the mouth, be certain to spit the suctioned material out and rinse the mouth liberally. Apply suction for approximately thirty to sixty minutes. **This procedure must be done within eight to ten minutes after snakebite.** Beyond that time it may be ineffective.
2 Treat the victim for shock.
3 Monitor respiration and heartbeat. Provide artificial respiration or CPR if necessary.
4 Provide for transportation to a physician or medical facility as quickly as possible.
5 Do NOT apply cold to the affected part.
6 Do NOT give alcohol, aspirin, or stimulants to the victim.
7 Kill the snake if this does not cause additional risk or delay in helping the victim or in seeking medical care. Take the dead snake along with you to help the health care provider determine the specific type of treatment to give the victim.

If the victim is alone, or if no one can assist, he or she should begin walking slowly to the nearest form of transportation or medical care facility. The victim should avoid overexertion and rest frequently.

**Coral Snake Bite**    The first-aider must provide for immediate transportation to the nearest medical facility. Additional steps are:

1 Have the victim sit or lie down and remain as quiet as possible.
2 Keep the victim warm or maintain normal body temperature, make the victim comfortable, and provide reassurance.
3 Monitor respiration and heartbeat. Provide artificial respiration or CPR if needed.
4 Do NOT give any liquids or food.
5 Do NOT use ice, a constricting band, or incision and suction, since these measures have no proven value for coral snake bites.
6 Kill the snake (if this can be done safely and does not delay transporting the victim) and take it to the medical facility to aid the health care provider in implementation of proper medical treatment.

## ____POISONING BY PLANT CONTACT

Poison ivy, poison oak, and poison sumac (Figure 10.7) are plants to which a large number of people are hypersensitive. The hypersensitivity manifests itself as an allergic reaction of the skin on contact with the plant. The responsible toxic substance is

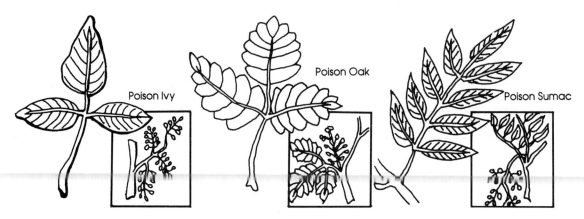

**FIGURE 10.7**
Plants that commonly cause allergic reaction.

urushiol. Urushiol is found in all parts of the plant: roots, stem, leaves, fruits, and sap. Contact may be direct or indirect. Direct contact occurs when the skin touches any part of the plant. Indirect contact occurs when the skin touches an object that has touched the plant and becomes contaminated with urushiol. Pet fur, clothing, shoes, tools, and other objects can serve as a continuous source of urushiol until the object is thoroughly cleaned. Smoke containing urushiol can also produce the allergic response on contact with the skin or the respiratory passages. The latter is a life-threatening event.

Poison ivy can be identified by the cluster of three shiny green leaves that are somewhat oval shaped with pointed tips. The plant may also have green or white flowers and a white, waxy fruit that looks like a cluster of small berries. The plant grows as a vine that attaches itself to other objects (e.g., fences, other plants, trees), as a shrub that grows along the ground, or as an upright shrub that resembles a small tree. Poison ivy is most frequently found in the central and eastern portions of the United States.

Poison oak also has three glossy green leaves that are similar in shape to the leaves of the oak tree. The plant is most commonly found as a low-growing shrub in the western portions of the United States. Other varieties are found in eastern regions.

Poison sumac grows primarily in the eastern part of the United States in marshy, damp areas, either as a shrub or a small tree. Poison sumac can be identified by the number and appearance of its leaves. The leaves are orange in the fall and spring and change to various shades of green during the summer months. The leaves are oval shaped and have pointed tips. There are seven to thirteen leaves on a branch.

## Signs and Symptoms of Contact Poisoning

The signs and symptoms of contact poisoning from poison ivy, poison oak, and poison sumac are the same. They usually appear within a few hours, though they may be delayed one or two days. They typically include redness of the skin, swelling, and itching. Blisters form later with intense itching or burning or both. The blisters or lesions crust over, and itching then usually subsides. Healing commonly occurs in ten days to two weeks.

## First Aid Care

Contaminated skin, clothing, and other objects should be thoroughly washed with soap and water when possible. The affected body parts should be washed immediately; however, this will probably not prevent the allergic reaction. The affected body parts should be kept clean and dry. Calamine lotion may relieve itching and will dry the skin. Warm baths may also be of some benefit in relieving itching.

The first-aider must recognize that hypersensitivity varies among individuals. Severe cases may need medical attention. A physician should also be consulted in the case of inhalation of fumes from a burning poisonous plant or for relief from other symptoms.

## ___DRUG REACTIONS: TYPES OF DRUGS, SIGNS AND SYMPTOMS, AND FIRST AID CARE

### ___Opiates

Opiate drugs are usually referred to as narcotics. This class encompasses all drugs derived from opium—codeine and morphine, semisynthesized drugs such as heroin and Dilaudid, and totally synthetic drugs such as Demerol, Darvon, and Lomotil. Narcotic drugs are mostly prescribed for the relief of severe pain. Opiates produce physical and psychological dependence, tolerance, and withdrawal symptoms when the drug is not present in the body. When more drug is taken into the body than the body is accustomed to, overdose may occur. Overdose usually occurs as a result of intravenous injection of heroin or of oral use of methadone.

Signs and symptoms of an overdose include pinpointed pupils; depression of the central nervous system ranging from stupor to profound coma; difficulty in breathing; convulsions; and shock that includes lowered blood pressure, cool and clammy skin, and pulmonary and cardiac arrest. There may be needle marks (tracks) in the skin from repeated injections.

Withdrawal reactions from opiate drugs begin gradually and increase in severity. They reach a maximum in thirty-six to seventy-two hours and gradually subside over the next seven to ten days. Early withdrawal signs and symptoms include yawning, sweating, and lacrimation (tearing); followed by tremors, restlessness, irritability, and skin flushing; and finally fever, nausea, diarrhea, vomiting, and involuntary muscle spasms.

### ___Amphetamines

Amphetamines are synthesized prescription drugs that have a stimulating effect on the central nervous system. Common amphetamines include Benzedrine, Dexedrine, Methedrine, Desoxyn, and Preludin. Amphetamines serve a number of medical purposes. They are used, for example, to treat obesity or mild depression and to relieve fatigue. The effects are initially exhilarating and described as a "rush" or "flash." Exhilaration is followed by a long period of euphoria, excitement, and the perception of clear thinking and self-confidence. Those who inject amphetamines often engage in a cyclic abuse pattern (a "speed binge"): Amphetamines are injected intravenously as often as ten times a day for three to four days, the abuser neither eating nor sleeping during this time. The binge ends in exhaustion. The abuser then sleeps for twenty-four to forty-eight hours or longer and awakes with a ravenous appetite. Severe depression follows and the person typically begins another speed binge.

The signs and symptoms of amphetamine abuse range from mild to very severe. Mild signs and symptoms include irritability, restlessness, insomnia, tremors, and hyperreflexia. The next level of manifestations include hyperactivity, confusion, mild fever, and sweating. Next are delirium, mania, irregular heartbeat, and marked hypertension. In the most severe instances, signs and symptoms include convulsions, coma, circulatory collapse, and possibly death. The first-aider should check the pupils of the eyes for extreme dilation. Hallucinations, nausea, vomiting, and aggressive behavior may also be exhibited.

## __Alcohol

Ethanol is the type of alcohol contained in widely consumed beverages. Ethyl alcohol is a sedative-hypnotic drug that has acute primary effects on the central nervous system. Alcohol use produces physiologic and psychological dependence, tolerance, and withdrawal symptoms. Alcohol alone can produce serious effects, but when it is consumed in combination with other depressant substances, a synergistic effect occurs. (Synergism is when the combined effect of two drugs is greater than the sum of their effects would be.) Alcohol is used, misused, and abused in most parts of the world.

Other types of alcohol are also consumed, but not widely. Methyl (or wood) alcohol is a highly toxic poison that can produce blindness or death. Rubbing alcohol is also considered toxic.

The signs and symptoms of ethyl alcohol intoxication are generally recognized by most individuals. The greater the concentration of alcohol in the blood, the more marked the symptoms and intoxication. In the early stages, the victim tends to lose inhibitions, and judgment, coordination, and reaction time are adversely affected. As the concentration of alcohol in the blood increases, the sedative and hypnotic effects of the drug increase. Unconsciousness, coma, vomiting, and depression of respiration and other vital organ function are possible with severe alcohol intoxication.

## __Barbiturates and Benzodiazepines

Barbiturate drugs are available by prescription only and are referred to as sedative-hypnotic because they depress the central nervous system and produce sleep. When taken in small doses these drugs reduce anxiety or excitement (the sedative effect). At higher doses they produce sleep, (the hypnotic effect). Barbiturate drugs are often used in suicide attempts. In children and drug abusers, barbiturates are a common source of accidental poisoning. Common barbiturate drugs include secobarbital, butabarbital and phenobarbital. Use of barbiturates produces physical and psychological dependence, tolerance, and withdrawal symptoms. Their effects are synergistic when they are ingested with other depressant substances such as alcohol.

Benzodiazepines are tranquilizers. They include Xanan, Librium, Valium, and Tranxene. These drugs cause few problems if used as prescribed. Rarely they cause significant respiratory or circulatory depression, or both, if abused.

Barbiturate drugs depress the central nervous system and the cardiovascular system. Drowsiness is the most common symptom. With mild to moderate intoxication, the pupils of the eyes are constricted but respond to light. As intoxication progresses, however, the pupils become dilated, breathing slows, and shock develops with its symptoms of sweating, rapid-weak pulse, and cool, clammy skin. Loss of muscle coordination is common and the victim shows confusion.

## __First Aid Care for Emergencies Involving Opiate, Amphetamine, Alcohol, or Barbiturate Abuse or Overdose

First aid for opiate, amphetamine, alcohol, or barbiturate abuse or overdose is as follows:

1 Protect the victim from injury.
2 Maintain an open airway, monitor vital signs, and if needed, administer artificial respiration or CPR.
3 Treat the victim for shock, be supportive and reassuring, and keep the victim calm. For barbiturate abuse or overdose, keep the victim conscious.
4 Seek medical treatment. Withdrawal responses from barbiturates can be most severe, and a medical environment is needed.

## __Hallucinogens

Hallucinogens are drugs that some believe are more appropriately called psychedelic or illusinogenic. Common psychedelic drugs include lysergic acid diethylamide (LSD), psilocybin, mescaline, peyote, and phencyclidine (PCP). These drugs are usually ingested and generally cannot be differentiated. LSD is one of the most widely abused and potent of the hallucinogens. LSD is quickly absorbed from the gastrointestinal tract and its effects begin within thirty to forty minutes. Psilocybin, a mushroom, is similar. Mescaline and peyote come from cactus and are typically ingested as a fresh or dried plant. Sometimes they are injected. These two drugs are rapidly absorbed and their effects are felt within thirty to sixty minutes. PCP, or angel dust, is smoked or ingested; its use has now declined. Mortality from hallucinogens is infrequent.

The hallucinogens as a group produce similar effects: a slight increase in blood pressure, flushing of the skin, increase in saliva flow, trembling, and hyperreflexia. Mydriasis (marked dilation of the pupils) and photophobia (sensitivity to light) are common. With massive ingestion, respiratory and central nervous system depression occurs. Individuals may experience a "bad trip" from any of these drugs. Bad trips are frightening and often produce panic states.

## __Marijuana and Hashish

Marijuana is the name for the tobaccolike preparation of flowers and leaves from the *Cannabis sativa,* or hemp, plant. Hashish is the resin extracted from the tops of the flowering plants. The active ingredient in both marijuana and hashish is delta-9-tetrahydrocannabinol (THC). Hashish has a much higher concentration of THC than does marijuana. These drugs are usually smoked, but some individuals ingest them by mixing them with food. Use rarely presents a serious overdose problem, since THC has a hypnotic effect and puts the user to sleep. A "bad trip" can occur from use of either drug.

Indicators for marijuana or hashish use include an odor of burnt leaves or hemp on the breath or clothes, pink or reddened (often inflamed) eyes, and the usual signs of intoxication.

## __First Aid Care for Users of Hallucinogens, Marijuana, or Hashish

First aid care for users of hallucinogens, marijuana, or hashish primarily consists of counteracting the panic of a bad trip. The first-aider should

1 Place the victim in a safe, quiet, and relaxed environment.
2 Reassure the victim that he or she will be all right and will return to a normal state when the effects of the drug wear off.
3 Monitor vital signs if a large amount of hallucinogen has been used. Administer artificial respiration or CPR if necessary.
5 Seek medical assistance if the adverse reaction is severe or if pulmonary or cardiac distress occurs.

## __Volatile Hydrocarbons

Volatile hydrocarbons include plastic model glues and cements, gasoline, aerosols, spray paint, and nail polish remover. Usually these substances are inhaled, either by being placed in a paper or plastic bag that is held tightly over the mouth and nose or by being sprayed or poured liberally on a cloth that is then rolled up and held against the mouth or nose or both. Inhalation of volatile hydrocarbons can cause serious damage to a number of body organs.

### Signs and Symptoms of Use
Volatile hydrocarbon inhalation depresses body function. It produces intoxication, poor muscle coordination, confusion, and disorientation. The eyes become watery, and nose runs. Odors of the substance are normally found on the user and his or her clothing.

### First Aid Care
First aid procedures include:

1 Remove the source of volatile vapors.
2 Maintain an open airway, check for breathing and pulse, and, if necessary, provide artificial respiration or CPR.
3 Provide fresh air or oxygen.
4 Seek medical care.

_____ **SUMMARY** _____

Poisonous substances can be ingested, inhaled, injected, or absorbed. Regardless of the manner that a poison enters the human body, poisoning presents an emergency that must be dealt with immediately and accurately. For poison ingestion, the first-aider should immediately give water or milk to dilute the poison and then phone a poison control center or a physician. On the basis of the information received, the first-aider implements a prescribed course of action. In most instances the first aid procedure is to induce vomiting, treat for shock, and transport the person to a medical facility. In the case of ingestion of a corrosive substance or a petroleum product, or if the victim is unconscious, the first-aider must not induce vomiting. With an inhaled poison, the first-aider should provide the victim with fresh air and be prepared to administer artificial respiration or CPR. With a poison injected by a bee, spider, form of marine life, or snake, the first-aider has to be alert to the possibility of hypersensitivity reaction. Anaphylactic shock can accompany such a reaction, and the person must be transported immediately to a medical facility.

The potential for adverse reactions from drug misuse or abuse is great. The first-aider should immediately determine if respiration or heartbeat are affected. Victims with a severe reaction must be transported to a medical setting.

## CHAPTER MASTERY: TEST ITEMS

### True and False

**Circle One**

1. The most common poisoning emergencies are those that result from inhalation.    T    F
2. The signs and symptoms produced by ingestion of a toxic substance vary according to the amount and type of substance and the time lapsed since ingestion.    T    F
3. The first-aider can determine much important information regarding a poisoning event by examining the victim, even if unconscious, and the location in which he or she is found.    T    F
4. Poison control centers provide information about emergency procedures only to physicians.    T    F
5. Poison control centers want to know the victim's age and weight in order to determine proper first aid procedures.    T    F
6. The best method of inducing vomiting in a poison victim is to tickle the back of the throat with a finger.    T    F
7. Vomiting should be induced in all poison ingestion emergencies.    T    F
8. The primary age group affected by salicylate poisoning is age 10 to 18.    T    F
9. Carbon monoxide is a toxic gas that is responsible for most gas and vapor poisonings.    T    F
10. First aid for pit viper bites includes packing the bitten part with ice to reduce swelling and venom absorption.    T    F

### Fill in the Missing Word(s)

1. A poison is defined as _____.
2. Of all the stinging hymenoptera, the only one that leaves the stinger embedded in the victim is the _____.

3. The phenomenon in which the combined effects of two drugs are greater than their sum is referred to as _____.
4. The form of marine life that has stinging cells on its tentacles is the _____.
5. In the application of a constricting band in a case of poison injection, the best way to check the band to determine if it is too tight is to _____.

## Multiple Choice (Circle the Best Answer)

1. The recommended amount of syrup of ipecac to give a child over 1 year of age is
   a. 1 teaspoonful.
   b. 2 teaspoonfuls.
   c. 1 tablespoonful.
   d. 2 tablespoonfuls.
2. A substance that produces tinnitus in the human is
   a. carbon dioxide.
   b. salicylate.
   c. kerosene.
   d. acetaminophen.
3. The rooms in a house in which most poisonings occur are the
   a. bedroom and garage.
   b. kitchen and bedroom.
   c. bathroom and bedroom.
   d. kitchen and bathroom.
4. The victim of poison ingestion should be made to vomit when
   a. the poison is an alkali.
   b. he or she is rapidly becoming unconscious.
   c. the poison is kerosene.
   d. the poison is aspirin.
5. When symptoms of snakebite include drowsiness, convulsions, little or no swelling, and difficulty in swallowing, the snake is a
   a. water moccasin.
   b. coral snake.
   c. rattlesnake.
   d. copperhead.

## Discussion Questions

1. Investigating a noise in the bathroom, a first aid-trained father finds his 3-year-old daughter on top of a vanity and next to her a half-empty bottle of adult aspirin. The child tells him that she has taken some of the aspirin. What should he do?

2. Arriving home late one night, a first-aider notices that her next-door neighbor's automobile is running inside the garage and the door is closed. Looking through a window, she sees that someone is slumped over the steering wheel. What should she do?

3. A family is camping in a remote region of a large national park. The father has just been bitten by a rattlesnake. There are three puncture marks on his ankle, the ankle is beginning to swell, and he is in severe pain. The nearest hospital is approximately 1½ hours away. What first aid procedures should be implemented?

4. A neighbor's son has been stung by a honeybee. The stinger is still embedded in his cheek adjacent to his mouth. The boy is known to be hypersensitive to insect bites and stings. What should the first-aider do?

5. A next-door neighbor has rushed into the first-aider's home to tell him that her husband has tried to commit suicide by overdosing on prescription sleeping pills. He is unconscious and cannot be aroused. What first aid care should be given to him?

6. A small girl is found lying on the garage floor. She is not moving, and an empty cola bottle is nearby. Her brother states that their father usually keeps kerosene in the bottle. What should the first-aider do?

--------- **BIBLIOGRAPHY** ---------

American National Red Cross. *Advanced First Aid and Emergency Care.* Garden City, N.Y.: Doubleday, 1979.

Dreisbach, R. H. *Handbook of Poisoning.* Los Altos, Calif.: Lange Medical Publications, 1980.

Haddad, L. M., and J. F. Winchester. *Clinical Management of Poisoning and Drug Overdose.* Philadelphia: W. B. Saunders, 1983.

Hafen, B. Q., and K. J. Karren. *First Aid and Emergency Care Workbook.* Denver: Morton Publishing, 1980.

Parcel, G. S. *First Aid in Emergency Care.* St. Louis: C. V. Mosby, 1977.

Russell, F. E. *Snake Venom Poisoning.* Great Neck, N.Y.: Scholium International, 1983.

# 11

## Burns

IRIS G. BROWN, ED.D.

After completing this chapter the student will be able to
- Explain the structure and function of human skin and its response to various types of burns.
- List and describe burns by degree and by source of injury.
- Identify, describe, and demonstrate appropriate first aid and emergency care for victims of each type of burn.

✢

## ____INTRODUCTION

The seriousness of burn injuries is exemplified by the number of people they and related injuries kill annually. More than 7000 people are estimated to die from burns yearly. Approximately 2000 children under age 14 and more than 1000 under age 5 die as a result of fires. Additional thousands endure great suffering and disfigurements from burns. The most disheartening aspect of the morbidity and mortality count is that *most (75%) accidental burns are preventable.* Nearly all of the pain, damage, hospital and medical cost, time away from employment, and other aspects of burns could be eliminated if people practiced prevention.

## ____FIRST AID OBJECTIVES FOR BURNS

Even though safety behavior is important in reducing the number of burn injuries and the morbidity and mortality rates associated with them, emergency burn situations still can occur at almost anytime and anyplace. It is therefore necessary for the first-aider to understand such crises and to know what to do when they occur. The types of burns (and related first aid care) to be discussed in this chapter are
- First-degree burns
- Second-degree burns
- Third-degree burns
- Fourth-degree (full-thickness) burns
- Chemical burns
- Burns of the eyes
- Electrical burns
- Sunburn
- Radiation burns

---

⚜ **Prevention of Burns in the Home and Out**

Many serious burn injuries, particularly in or near the home, result from poor safety behavior. Thus, perhaps the most significant contribution to prevention of burn injury is the practice of safety behavior in the home.

- Do not smoke in bed. Thoroughly extinguish all cigarettes, pipes, and cigars.
- Use appliances and equipment according to manufacturer's directions.
- Turn pot and skillet handles away from the edge of a stove, table, or counter.
- Keep matches and other flammable materials out of the reach of children.
- Do not overload electrical plugs and outlets.
- Make recommended safety checks on all house and garage wiring.
- Teach children to stop, drop, and roll when clothes are on fire.
- Maintain heating and equipment units properly.
- Provide a home fire escape and practice an escape plan.
- Maintain an appropriate extinguisher in strategic places in the home and car.

- Handle all chemicals as directed.
- Do not expose the skin to hot sunlight for long, uninterrupted periods.
- Do not remove the radiator cap in a vehicle until the vehicle has cooled.
- Wear appropriate clothing and an exposure-sensitive badge if it is necessary to be near radioactive materials.
- Keep flammable fluids away from sparks, fires, and other items capable of starting a fire.
- Do not store explosives or materials that are potentially explosive in improper containers or inside the house.
- If possible, participate in a first aid course. Such courses are sponsored by schools, colleges, and universities; hospitals; community agencies; and other organizations. The courses are usually thorough and very beneficial. They contribute to the secondary level of prevention (minimizing the seriousness of the outcome after a person has been burned) rather than to primary prevention (keeping the burn injury from occurring).

---

The first-aider should keep three general objectives in mind when treating a burn victim regardless of the type or degree of injury:

1 Prevent contamination of the injury.
2 Prevent or treat for shock.
3 Relieve pain.

# ___THE SKIN

The skin, like a cloak, covers the entire body and is its oldest, most sensitive, and largest organ. The skin is crucial for survival and for the protection of body organs. Its size ranges from approximately 2500 to 3000 square inches.

Skin functions are diverse. The skin is largely responsible for regulation of body temperature, protection of all parts of the body, excretion of respiratory waste, retention of body fluids, and maintenance of electrolyte balance within the body. The skin is also

**FIGURE 11.1**

Layers of the skin

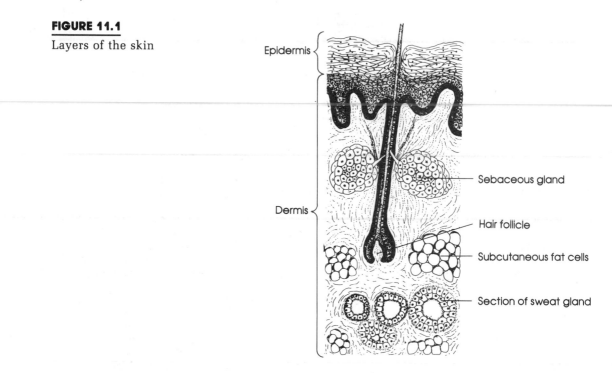

Epidermis

Dermis

Sebaceous gland

Hair follicle

Subcutaneous fat cells

Section of sweat gland

the best natural barrier against insects, pathogens, and other disease sources that attempt to invade the body.

Throughout the discussion of burns and their first aid care, reference will be made to three layers of skin. In reality, however, the skin is composed of only two layers: the epidermis, or outer, thinner layer, and the dermis, or inner, thicker layer (Fig. 11.1). The dermis consists of blood vessels, lymph spaces, nerve endings, sebaceous and sweat glands, and the hair and its follicles. Tissue below the dermis, frequently referred to as the third layer, consists of muscles, tendons, nerves, blood vessels, internal organs, and bone. The severity of damage to the various layers is used to classify burns.

*A burn is an injury to the skin that results from contact with heat, a chemical agent, radiation or a hot liquid, including water.* The severity of a burn injury varies according to depth and size. The ability of the skin to heal spontaneously depends on the depth of the burn.

The first-degree burn heals most quickly, because only the top layer (epidermis) is involved. The second-degree burn is the next fastest to heal; this injury involves the two top layers of skin. Third-degree and fourth-degree burns usually heal slowly, because all three skin layers are burned. Fourth-degree burns generally cause bone damage. In each type of burn the heat involved is detected by antennas in the skin.

First-, second-, and third-degree burns are painful, but the fourth-degree burn may not be, because nerve endings are often wholly destroyed. The presence of pain with a burn may be used to help reassure the victim that the burn is not as serious as a fourth-degree burn.

# ___TYPES OF BURNS BY DEGREE

## ___First·degree Burns

A first-degree burn is a superficial injury usually characterized by reddening of the epidermis. The burn may be very painful, but usually heals without difficulty unless infection occurs. In such a case a physician should be consulted and instructions should be closely followed. Infected first-degree burns can create unnecessary discomfort and unsightly scars.

It is not likely that a first-degree burn over 10 to 20% of the body will pose a life threatening situation. Still, if such a first-degree burn does occur over this much body surface, medical attention is recommended to eliminate the possibility of complications leading to long-term illness and pain. Immediate medical attention is needed if the victim is an infant. Figure 11.2 depicts the "rule of nines" for estimating the seriousness of burns.

Once the first-aider has determined that the burn is a first degree injury, he or she can apply cold water, since this helps to relieve the pain and promote healing. When the affected area can be immersed in cold water with shaved ice, this is advisable. Ice water applied immediately may prevent a first-degree burn from developing into a second-degree injury. A mild local analgesic may be applied on the recommendation of a physician. To reduce the chance of infection or contamination, only those creams, ointments, or other medications recommended by a physician should be used. Whatever medication is used, it should be a type that easily washes off, rather than one that requires painful rubbing for removal. It is important that the victim follow the instructions given by the physician and properly take the medication prescribed. An example of a burn care instruction form is presented in Figure 11.3.

## ___Second·degree Burns

Second-degree burns are painful to touch and are characterized by blisters, deep reddening, sensitivity to cold air, and loss of body fluids (plasma and electrolytes). These characteristics result from extension of the injury into the deep layers of the skin and the capillaries there. The outer epidermal cells are destroyed by heat.

Healing depends on the number of damaged cells and their ability to survive and multiply to the point of resuming normal cell function. Partial skin loss occurs in nearly all cases, but scarring and skin grafting are not associated with this type of burn.

A second-degree burn is not serious if restricted to a small portion of the skin. But like the first-degree burn, the second-degree injury can become life threatening if it is contaminated, if shock occurs, or in this case if the injury covers 30% or more of the victim's body surface (Figure 11.2). A second-degree burn over 25% of an adult's body surface or 20% of a child's body surface is considered a major burn injury. Such an injury

**FIGURE 11.2**

The "rule of nines" is used to determine the amount of a burned area in both adults and infants. Numbers represent percentages.

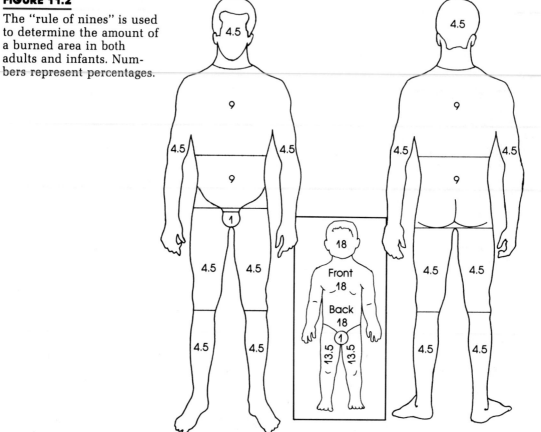

requires the assistance of a physician to reduce the risk of it developing into a life-threatening situation. Figure 11.4 presents guidelines for determining which injuries are major burns.

The second-degree burn is usually very painful, readily complicated by shock, and easily infected when not cared for properly. First aid care for this type of burn is governed by the extent of body involvement (mild or extensive) and by the three burn care objectives cited earlier. Each objective may be met by providing the following care. With correct care, second-degree burns usually heal completely in two to three weeks.

## Care for Mild Second-degree Burn

1 Apply cold water.
2 Loosen or remove constricting clothing, shoes, or jewelry.
3 Call a physician or take the victim to an emergency room.

An external burn injures skin tissue. The depth of injury is classified as follows:

*First degree*: very superficial (similar to sunburn)

*Second degree*: moderately deep, with blistering. Usually heals without difficulty unless infected.

*Third degree*: deep, with total destruction of skin tissue. Often requires skin graft.

*Fourth degree*: deep, with destruction of skin, muscle, tendon, nerve, blood vessel, and bone. Requires surgery and skin graft.

After treatment in the Emergency Room, you SHOULD:

• Keep burn site elevated.

• Keep burn site clean and dry.

• Take all medication prescribed. FOLLOW LABEL INSTRUCTIONS.

• Be watchful for the following signs of infection:
  Localized redness at burn site
  Red streaks extending from wound
  Unpleasant odor from wound
  Pain, fever
  Abnormal drainage from wound
  IF ANY OF THESE SIGNS AND SYMPTOMS OCCUR, SEE YOUR PHYSICIAN OR RETURN TO THE EMERGENCY ROOM.

• See your private physician for follow-up care.

After treatment in the Emergency Room, you SHOULD NOT:

• Attempt to puncture blistered areas.

## GENERAL INSTRUCTIONS

☐ Change dressing in manner described by physician or nurse. Be as clean as possible.

☐ Do not change dressing.

  Do NOT drive or operate machinery while taking pain medications or muscle relaxants.

☐ You may return to work.

☐ You are advised not to work until released from your physician's care.

I have read and understand the above instructions.

_____

Patient or Guardian

_____

Date

**FIGURE 11.3**

Burn care instruction form

**Major burn injury** Second-degree burns of greater than 25% of body surface area (BSA) in adults (20% in children); third-degree burns of 10% of BSA or greater; all burns involving hands, face, eyes, ears, feet, or perineum; all inhalation injuries and electrical burns; burn injuries complicated by fractures or other major trauma; and all burns in poor-risk individuals (e.g., the elderly, those with chronic disease). These victims would normally enter the system at the site of the injury and be transported to a hospital with optimal facilities (burn unit or burn center) depending on distance and time, complications (respiratory shock), and bed availability. Direct communications and transfer agreements in this regard are extremely important. If seriousness of the injury dictates transportation to the closest effective emergency department of a special expertise hospital, transfer to a hospital with optimal facilities should be arranged after the cardiopulmonary system is stabilized and intravenous fluid therapy is started. Rehabilitation, including corrective surgery for cosmetic and functional deficiencies, completes the therapeutic circle.

**Moderate uncomplicated burn injury** Second-degree burns of 15% to 25% of BSA in adults (10% to 20% in children) with less than 10% third-degree burns and not involving eyes, ears, face, hands, feet, or perineum. Excluded are electrical injury, burn injuries complicated by fractures or other trauma, inhalation injury, and all injuries in poor-risk individuals.

**Minor burn injury** Second-degree burns of less than 15% of BSA in adults (10% in children) with less than 2% third-degree burns and not involving eyes, ears, face, hands, feet, or perineum. Excluded are electrical injury, complicated injuries, and all injuries in poor-risk individuals. Persons may be treated at the scene of the accident by emergency medical technicians and then transported to a hospital emergency department, where definitive care is initiated, including follow-up to complete recovery and discharge from the system. A similar course would be followed by any person self-admitted to the hospital emergency department for treatment. A primary care physician may function either in the emergency department role or as follow-up physician, or both.

**FIGURE 11.4**

American Burn Association guidelines: three categories of burn severity. (Adapted with permission of the American Burn Association, Phoenix.)

### Care for Extensive Second-degree Burn

1 Apply cold water.
2 Loosen or remove constricting clothing, shoes, or jewelry.
3 Give fluid as the victim requests (none to an unconscious person).
4 Cover the burned area with a sterile dressing.
5 Cover the victim with a clean sheet, when possible; keep the victim warm.
6 Take the victim to the hospital as quickly as possible.

## __Third-degree Burns

Third-degree burns involve deep damage to the skin and underlying tissues. The injury is characterized by great destruction of muscle, fat, and sometimes bone tissue. The surface may vary in appearance from white to charred or possibly dull gray. Areas radiating outward from the injury are red and usually the source of great pain (a main factor in the development of shock). The purplish appearance around the center of the burn indicates poor circulation, which often results in death of the tissue involved. Beyond this area is bright red, moist flesh that is sensitive to the prick of a pin.

Third-degree burns require surgical procedures, often involving skin grafting. Without skin grafting, nature will in all likelihood cause the skin to draw and limit the mobility of the involved areas. It is highly unlikely that third-degree burns will heal with only the body's natural healing ability.

The severity of third-degree burns and their depth readily exposes them to infection and contamination. Pain is almost always present, shock is quite likely, and loss of fluids is usually extensive. Special care must be given to the third-degree burn victim to relieve pain, reduce the severity of shock, and control the chances of infection or contamination. This is all the first-aider can do. The following first aid procedures should be carried out:

1 Treat for shock.
2 Remove obvious foreign matter when this can be done without increasing the victim's discomfort.
3 Cover the damaged area with a clean sterile dressing.
4 Give small sips of fluids to alert victims.
5 Keep the person warm and transport in a reclined position, the feet raised.
6 Take the person to the hospital or burn center as quickly as possible.

All persons with third-degree burns need medical treatment. Third-degree burns over 10% of the body or involving the hands, face, feet, or ears are considered major burn injuries (Figure 11.4).

## __Fourth-degree Burns

Fourth-degree burn is a classification most often used by burn specialists to indicate that the full thickness of each skin layer, deep muscles, tendons, nerves, blood vessels, and bone may be involved in the injury.

Fourth-degree burns are usually caused by exposure to intense heat. Fourth-degree burns are generally associated with blazing structures, spatterings or overflows from molten metal or plastics, nuclear explosions, use of flame throwers, and other activities involving extreme heat. Fourth-degree burns, like extensive third-degree burns, do not heal without surgery or skin grafting or both.

Injuries classified as fourth-degree burns cause shock in the victim. The principal aim of first aid care thus is to control shock. Fluids therefore are needed. The first-aider will have to seek help to determine the amount of fluid lost and the amount of fluid the victim needs to lessen the chance of dehydration. The most desirable fluid is blood plasma, but plasma and whole blood are not available to first-aiders. A combination of salt and water (a saline solution of one teaspoonful of salt per quart of water) or of sugar and water (one tablespoonful per glass of water) may be given by mouth. **Caution: The first-aider should not attempt to administer fluids to an unconscious person.**

If the burn is known to have been caused by an explosion or a sudden blast of extreme heat, care must be taken to ensure that the victim's airway is open. Oxygen may be administered if available. All fourth-degree burn victims should be rushed to a major hospital or burn center.

# ___TYPES OF BURNS BY SOURCE

## ___Chemical Burns

A chemical burn occurs when the skin comes into direct contact with a strong corrosive substance such as an acid or alkali. Chemical burns affecting large numbers of people commonly occur in industrial settings, while individual burns may happen at home, school, or industrial settings.

### First Aid Care

Chemical burns should be flushed with large amounts of water to dilute the chemical and avert the possibility of additional injury. Further damage to chemically burned areas is usually caused by attempts at neutralization rather than dilution. Harm may occur in one of three ways: (1) the counteracting agent may be too strong and may itself burn the tissue, (2) the reaction of the counteracting agent with the original chemical may create additional heat, thereby extending the amount of damage and possibly increasing the severity of the original burn, or (3) the reaction product of the combination of two chemical agents may be salt, which can damage tissue.

Any contaminated clothing should be removed. Medical help must be sought and the first-aider must also continue to flush the area until help becomes available. If the cause of the burn is a dry chemical, any powder on the skin should be brushed from the skin surface before the area is irrigated. Water added to dry chemicals may generate heat and result in severe burning.

### Chemical Burns of the Eyes: A Special Concern

All burns involving eyes are considered major burn injuries (Figure 11.4). Chemical burns of the eyes must be irrigated immediately to prevent serious damage. Extensive flushing of the eye with flowing water is essential (Figure 11.5). The head is positioned so that the water flows *away* from the nose. Also, care is taken not to wash the chemical into the other eye.

After the eye is flushed with clear tap water, a solution of one teaspoonful of salt added to a quart of water may be used to continue flushing. After flushing thoroughly,

**FIGURE 11.5**

Chemical burns of the eye must be irrigated immediately to prevent extensive damage. Care is taken not to wash the chemical into the other eye.

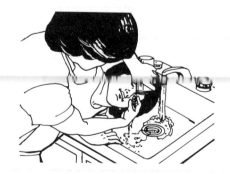

the first-aider closes the victim's eyelids, covers both eyes with a dry, sterile dressing, and obtains the services of an ophthalmologist. **Both eyes must be covered to prevent movement of the damaged eye** (refer to Chapter 9, Figure 9.10, p. 174).

## —Electrical Burns

Electrical burns are increasing in frequency. They now comprise over 3% of admissions to burn centers and hospitals. The increase in the number of persons being treated for electrical burns may be due to the greater use of high-voltage electrical equipment at home and at work sites. Electrical burns are also caused by lightning.

Electrical burns result from electricity being conducted through the body. The heat, which can be more than 20,000° C, devitalizes tissue along the pathway of the current. Electrical burns are far more serious than they appear initially. Their extent is directly related to the amount, duration, and frequency of the current and to the pathway involved. Electrical currents of very high frequency transfer to tissue as heat and cause extensive burns. Low-frequency current (AC) stimulates cardiac muscle, smooth muscle, skeletal tissue, and nerves. AC can create widespread destruction of these tissues.

Electrical burns are classified into three types.

1 *Type I* burns are characterized by tissue damage along the conduction route.
2 *Type II* burns result from arcing between a source of high current and the body. They are characterized by external skin damage with a small entrance wound and a large exit wound. There is charring, edema, and discoloration. Type II burns may cause deformity in limbs.
3 *Type III* burns have the characteristics of Type I and Type II burns plus the clothing and other flammable items worn by the victim ignite.

Because of the severity of electrical burns and the fact that the amount and type of damage they cause cannot be easily assessed, these burns pose a difficult problem for the first-aider. This does not mean that the first-aider cannot be of assistance. If the first-aider finds the victim still in contact with the source of electrical current, the following steps are recommended:

1 Disengage the victim from the source of electrical current. Use a long pole or other nonconductant tool (e.g., rubber gloves, dry wood) to remove the wire from the victim or the victim from the wire, or turn off the source of the current and then remove the source.
2 Once the victim is no longer in contact with the current, determine if the victim is breathing. When respiration and cardiac functions are not detectable, begin CPR (Chapter 6). Because of the possibility of extensive paralytic damage to the cardiovascular system, continue CPR until professional or medical assistance becomes available. External injuries of electrical burns may be treated as third-degree burns, and the victim should be closely observed until professional help arrives.

## __Sunburns

Sunburn is caused by long periods of direct exposure to the ultraviolet rays of the sun. A sunburn may be as severe as a second-degree burn or as minor as a first-degree burn. Research clearly indicates that exposure to ultraviolet rays for a long time (ten to twenty years) may cause skin cancer. This is especially so with individuals who have little pigmentation in the skin or a light complexion. In extreme cases of sunburn (second-degree burns), the damaged skin may become infected, the victim may become nauseous, and sun poisoning may occur.

First aid care for sunburn is consistent with first aid care for other first- or second-degree burns. For simple first-degree sunburn (red, painful epidermis), application of cold wet compresses or freshwater ice packs to the burned area has gained favor as the appropriate treatment. When used early enough, this treatment may prevent a first-degree burn from developing into a second-degree burn.

Should the sunburn progress to a second-degree burn, care may continue as for the first-degree burn with additional first aid steps such as:

1 Cleanse the skin of dirt or grease; pat gently to dry.
2 Cover the burned area, after it has cooled, with a bland lotion.
3 Continue use of cold, wet compresses.
4 Have the victim drink as much fluid as possible.
5 Have the victim take aspirin or similar pain killer as needed.
6 Seek medical help if needed.

Medical attention should be sought for cases of sun poisoning, nausea, or infection or when 10% of the body surface is involved.

## __Radiation Burns

Exposure to unsafe levels of radiation may cause burns. Accidents in nuclear energy plants and accidents involving trucks and trains transporting nuclear energy have given rise to increasing numbers of radiation burns in the United States and elsewhere. Individuals who work with or near radioactive materials usually wear badges designed to indicate dangerous levels of exposure. This precautionary measure aids in the protection of workers to a point, but the incidence of radiation exposure continues to increase.

The unit of measure for radiation is roentgens. The amount of radiation absorbed by the tissues determines the severity of the injury or damage. The radiation absorbed dose (RAD) is a measure of the amount of radiation energy absorbed by body tissues per minute. The higher the rad, the greater the amount of damage. Exposure to four rads per minute creates observable damage. An exposure of 2000 rad over a short period can cause death within a relatively short time. Exposure to low-level radiation from televisions, microwave ovens, and other household appliances does not normally create a threat of radiation burn. But even these appliances should be periodically checked for radiation leakage. Symptoms of radiation sickness after high levels of exposure include
  · Nausea and vomiting
  · Dehydration and diarrhea

- Loss of appetite
- High fever
- General discomfort
- Increase in heart rate

These symptoms are not restricted to persons exposed to overdoses of radiation, but if the first-aider has reason to suspect overexposure, he or she should look for such symptoms.

As with other burns, radiation burns are classified by degree. Burns caused by exposure to high doses of radiation or intense thermal flashes are treated in the same way as other burns of equal degree. The first-aider must take additional caution, however, to reduce the possibility of self-exposure to radiation. It must be acknowledged that the first-aider is limited in the care he or she can deliver to persons exposed to high doses of radiation, but the following procedures are helpful when adequate precautions are taken:

1 Do not enter the contaminated area. Should the exposed person leave the area, the first-aider should maintain a safe distance from the person until a protective zone can be established. This can be done by placing a radioactive sign outside the immediate area. Figure 11.6 illustrates a placard for showing the presence of radioactive materials.

2 If specially trained individuals are not available for care of the exposed person, call the nearest hospital or emergency care center. In addition, direct the victim to

a Flush the skin with copious amounts of water.

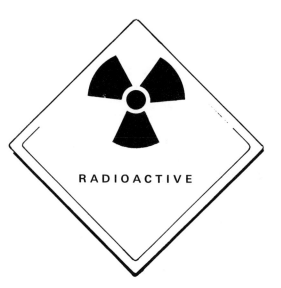

**FIGURE 11.6**

Placard to indicate the presence of radioactive materials

**b** Drink a solution consisting of one teaspoonful of table salt and one teaspoonful of baking soda in one quart of water. Drink as much of the solution as practical.

**c** Seek special medical assistance from a trained radiation specialist, usually at a hospital.

--------------------------- SUMMARY ---------------------------

The skin has several important functions that aid in the maintenance of homeostasis. It is the barrier between the external environment and inner tissues. When the skin comes into contact with excessive heat, a corrosive chemical, or radiation, it is burned. A burn that is restricted to the thin outer layer of skin (epidermis) is classified as a first-degree burn. First-degree burns cause reddening of the skin and tenderness. Second-degree burns result when the heat is great enough to destroy cells of the epidermis, creating blisters and pain. Third-degree burns result when the epidermis and the second layer of skin, the dermis, are charred. Muscle, fat, and bones may be involved. Fourth-degree burns involve all of the skin layers plus bones, muscles, and inner organs.

A victim with any of these burns may be attended to by a well-trained first-aider, if that person remembers the basic objectives of first aid: to prevent contamination, to prevent or treat for shock, and to relieve pain. Much of the pain and disfigurement resulting from burn injuries can be reduced with administration of appropriate first aid care.

--------------------- CHAPTER MASTERY: TEST ITEMS ---------------------

**True and False**                                                    Circle One

1. Burns to the epidermis that cause the skin to redden and become        T    F
   painful are classified as first-degree burns.
2. First-degree burns that do not receive first aid care may progress to  T    F
   second-degree burns.
3. A good index of the severity of a burn is the extent of pain.          T    F
4. Burns that involve deep dermal skin, making it appear dry and white or T    F
   sometimes a dull gray, are classified as fourth-degree burns.
5. First-degree burns should be treated with cold water or ice water.     T    F
6. Blisters caused by burns should be opened immediately.                 T    F
7. Third-degree burns that have entry and exit points are caused by       T    F
   extreme ultraviolet rays.
8. For estimating the percentage of the body surface involved in a burn   T    F
   accident, the rule of nines is useful.

9. Second-degree burns over more than 25% of the body surface of an adult should be considered a major burn injury and treated by a physician.  T  F

10. Fluids should be withheld from all burn victims until a physician's services can be obtained.  T  F

## Fill In the Missing Word(s)

1. First-degree burns involve only the _____ layer of skin, called the _____.
2. In addition to reddening of the skin, _____-degree burns are characterized by blisters and extreme tenderness.
3. Burns in which pain is often not perceived despite extensive skin, muscle, and bone damage are _____-degree burns.
4. Flushing with large quantities of water should be done for _____ burns.
5. Air should be kept from a burn to minimize _____.
6. When germ-laden articles touch a burn injury, _____ usually results.
7. The seriousness of a burn injury is determined by the _____ and depth of the burn.
8. A burn involving deep tissue destruction, which cannot heal by itself, is a _____ burn.
9. Electrical burns are caused by direct contact with electrical wires or _____.
10. Because of serious involvement of the circulatory and respiratory systems in _____ burns, CPR may be required for long periods.

## Multiple Choice (Circle the Best Answer)

1. Deep burns may not be painful because of
   a. shock caused by the injury.
   b. quick blood flow from the injury.
   c. nerve-ending destruction.
   d. the flight-or-fight syndrome.
   e. none of the above.
2. Chemical burns result when an individual
   a. comes in contact with strong acids.
   b. comes in contact with strong alkalies.
   c. attempts to neutralize corrosive substances with counteracting agents.
   d. adds water to powdered chemicals spilled on the skin.
   e. all of the above
3. Assessment of the severity of electrical burns is difficult due to
   a. the large size of the entry wound.
   b. limited burns beneath the epidermis.
   c. shock and incoherent behavior of the victim.
   d. the small size of the exit wound.
   e. damage to two areas, entrance and exit wounds.

4. The radiation absorbed dose (rad) is
   a. a measure of the amount of radiation energy absorbed by tissues.
   b. the unit of measure of radiation.
   c. the radiation detection material used in radiation badges.
   d. the lethal dose of radiation exposure.
   e. the radiation dose at which discomfort is experienced.

5. Long-term exposure to direct ultraviolet rays may
   a. cause first-degree burns.
   b. cause second-degree burns.
   c. cause cancer.
   d. lead to infection and nausea.
   e. all of the above

6. When a person gets a chemical(s) into one or both eyes, the first-aider should
   a. flush the eyes extensively.
   b. flush the eyes extensively, cover them, and transport the victim to an ophthalmologist.
   c. flush the eyes with a solution made of one teaspoonful of salt in a quart of warm water
   d. none of the above
   e. all of the above

7. All of the following are first aid procedures for first-degree burn **except**
   a. apply butter or oil immediately.
   b. apply cold water immediately.
   c. use a dry sterile dressing.
   d. apply antiseptic ointment to prevent drying of the skin.
   e. apply freshwater ice packs.

8. Appropriate and timely first aid for burn victims can
   a. reduce pain and suffering.
   b. reduce recuperation time.
   c. prevent further injury and/or complications.
   d. all of the above

9. All of the following are first aid procedures for third-degree burns **except**
   a. elevate the arms, feet, hands, and legs above the heart level.
   b. maintain the airway open.
   c. immerse the victim in cool water.
   d. use a mild ointment.
   e. cover the burned area with a dry sterile dressing.

10. In rendering first aid to a severely burned person, the step that would have the highest priority would be
    a. arrange for transportation to a burn facility.
    b. provide for psychologic reassurance for the victim.
    c. restore breathing if the victim's respiration has ceased.
    d. seek medical care immediately.
    e. cover the victim with a sterile clean dressing.

**Discussion Questions**

1. Working in a chemistry lab in school, a student has accidentally gotten an unknown chemical in her eye. She is in pain. What is the proper first aid response?

2. A young boy attempting to fill a lawn mower gas tank has been burned in a gasoline explosion. He has come running from the garage with his clothes on fire. What action should the first-aider take? What types of burns (by degree) are likely to be encountered? What first aid should be provided?

3. The first-aider has been asked to speak to a third-grade class regarding prevention of burn injuries. What should he or she tell these children?

————————————————— **BIBLIOGRAPHY** —————————————————

Annarino, A.A., and F. W. Kahma. *A Study Guide to First Aid, Safety and Family Health Emergencies.* Minneapolis: Burgess Publishing, 1979.

Barber, J. M., and S. A. Budassi. *Manual of Emergency Care.* St. Louis: C. V. Mosby, 1979.

Do Carmo, P. B., and A. T. Patterson. *First Aid Principles and Procedures.* Englewood Cliffs, N.J.: Prentice-Hall, 1976.

Judd, R. L., and D. D. Ponsell. *The First Responder—The Critical First Minutes.* St. Louis: C. V. Mosby, 1982.

Kirk R. H., and J. S. Ellison. *First Aid and Emergency Care.* Dubuque, Ia.: Kendall/Hunt Publishers, 1980.

Thygerson, A. L. *Accidents and Disasters.* Englewood Cliffs, N.J.: Prentice-Hall, 1977.

Wagner, M. M., *Care of the Burn Injured Patient.* Littleton, Mass.: PSG Publishers, 1981.

# 12

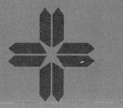

# Heat-related Disorders

GENE EZELL, ED.D.

After completing this chapter the student will be able to

- Describe the body's heat-regulating mechanism.
- Describe the causes of heat-related disorders.
- Portray the individual most at risk for heat problems.
- Differentiate between the signs and symptoms of heat cramps, heat exhaustion, and heatstroke.
- Demonstrate the proper first aid treatment for dehydration, heat cramps, head exhaustion, and heatstroke.
- Demonstrate the steps necessary to avoid heat-related problems.

## ____INTRODUCTION

Sustained exposure to heat and humidity can cause serious medical problems. In fact, each year thousands of people in the United States die from heat-related disorders. The human body is a phenomenal organism in which various systems interact efficiently to maintain a normal body temperature in most circumstances. However, sometimes the heat-regulating mechanisms can be overburdened. On these occasions the body's very sensitive heat-regulating mechanisms flash an "alert." The person who is aware of this signal can usually take preventive measures to avoid problems.

## ____THE ROLE OF BODY TEMPERATURE

The body is almost continually adapting to the ambient atmosphere in an attempt to keep the internal body temperature at 98.6° F or (37° C). The amount of heat produced by or reaching the body must equal the amount of heat it dissipates for normal temperature to be maintained. Heat is produced through oxidation of energy-producing sources, primarily food. Heat production occurs in the vital organs and muscles. The amount produced increases dramatically during vigorous activity. Heat reaches the body from the exterior through absorption from the surrounding air. The primary source of external heat is the sun's rays.

When the outside air temperature is lower than body temperature, the body loses heat through radiation from the skin. The blood brings the heat to the skin surface where it radiates to the air. When the outside air temperature is higher than body temperature,

**234**

the body loses heat through evaporation of perspiration. The greater the difference between outside air temperature and body temperature, the more fluid (perspiration) the body has to release to maintain homeostasis. The more vigorously muscles are used, the more fluid is lost. The body's ability to remove excess heat through sweating is limited. A normal person can sweat only up to about one quart an hour for one to two hours without problem. The relative humidity of the atmosphere has to be low for effective evaporation to occur. The higher the relative humidity, the slower the evaporation rate. The effective sweat evaporation rate (i.e., enough to cool the body) diminishes rapidly when the relative humidity rises higher than 60%; at about 75% sweat evaporation it stops (Bruch, Cade, and Tintinalli 1976).

A more detailed description of body temperature maintenance appears in Chapter 13.

# ____DISORDERS FROM EXCESS BODY HEAT

High body temperatures can result from heavy muscular work, prolonged sun exposure, fever, and anticholinergic drugs (Hafen and Karren 1980). The risk of high body temperature increases when heavy work or prolonged sun exposure, or both, is accompanied by the wearing of heavy dark clothing, low wind velocity, or high humidity. Excess body heat coupled with loss of body fluids through evaporation can result in dehydration, heat cramps, heat exhaustion, or heatstroke. Table 12.1 lists the causes, symptoms, and first aid care of the last three.

## ____Dehydration

When the rate of sweating increases to cool the body, dehydration can occur. Dehydration causes a decrease in total blood volume, which results in less blood to carry oxygen and heat. This syndrome overburdens the heart and lungs and results in difficult breathing, nausea, and an increase in body temperature.

Symptoms of dehydration can usually be abated through the intake of water. Some salt may be added to the water if the victim is not nauseated.

## ____Heat Cramps

Heat cramps are minor yet painful spasms or cramps in the muscles. They are caused by loss of excessive amounts of perspiration and salt, which results in an electrolyte imbalance in the body. Usually the large muscles in the arms, legs, and stomach are most affected. Heat cramps are fairly common in those who work or exercise for extended periods in hot, humid conditions and in overweight or out-of-shape persons who exercise vigorously. Cramps can also occur when water intake is high during exercise but salt is not replaced. Heat cramps are not considered an emergency; however, they are warning signals of potential danger.

**TABLE 12.1**

Comparison of heat-related conditions

| Condition | Causes | Signs and Symptoms | First Aid Care |
| --- | --- | --- | --- |
| Heat Cramps | Overexposure to heat; excessive perspiration and loss of salt | Muscle spasms; cool, clammy skin; normal body temperature; weakness; dizziness; possible nausea | Gently massage or apply ice to affected muscle; give sips of salted drinking water if victim not nauseated |
| Heat Exhaustion | Overexposure to heat; excessive perspiration and loss of salt; pooling of blood in blood vessels in skin | Possible muscle spasms; cool, clammy skin; normal or slightly elevated body temperature; weakness, dizziness; nausea; rapid, weak pulse; excessive sweating; fainting; shallow breathing; dilated pupils; blurred vision | Stop victim's activity; remove person to cool place; loosen or remove as much of victim's clothing as possible; give sips of salted drinking water if victim not nauseated; place person in lying position with legs elevated |
| Heatstroke | Cessation of sweating mechanism | Red, dry, hot skin; high body temperature; nausea; rapid, strong pulse; constricted pupils; convulsions; possible unconsciousness | Loosen or remove as much of victim's clothing as possible; lower the body temperature as rapidly as possible; obtain medical assistance. |

### Symptoms
Normally the only symptoms are the cramps themselves, but cramps are sometimes accompanied by a rapid and weak pulse, weakness, dizziness, nausea, and exhaustion.

### First Aid Care
First aid care for heat cramps includes the gentle massage or stretching of the affected muscle if this does not increase the pain. Ice may be applied directly to the muscle to relieve pain. The victim can be given sips of salted water (one teaspoonful of salt per quart) every fifteen minutes for a period of about one hour. Salt tablets should not be given, as they can cause severe abdominal cramping.

## __Heat Exhaustion

Another condition caused by overexertion in a hot, humid environment coupled with excessive perspiration and salt loss is heat exhaustion. Heat exhaustion can be considered an intermediate step in the progression from heat cramps to heatstroke. In other words, heat exhaustion is slightly more serious than cramps, but is not life threatening like heatstroke. People most at risk to heat exhaustion are those who engage in vigorous activities on hot, humid days or in a hot, industrial setting. The elderly are prone to heat exhaustion because of diminished thirst mechanisms that cause reduction in their intake of fluids even though dehydration may be occurring (Hafen 1981).

### Symptoms
Heat exhaustion (Figure 12.1) results from diminished blood flow to the heart, lungs, and brain. Specifically, the blood pools in the capillaries of the skin in an attempt to cool the body, resulting in less volume of blood to the vital organs. Heat exhaustion is character-

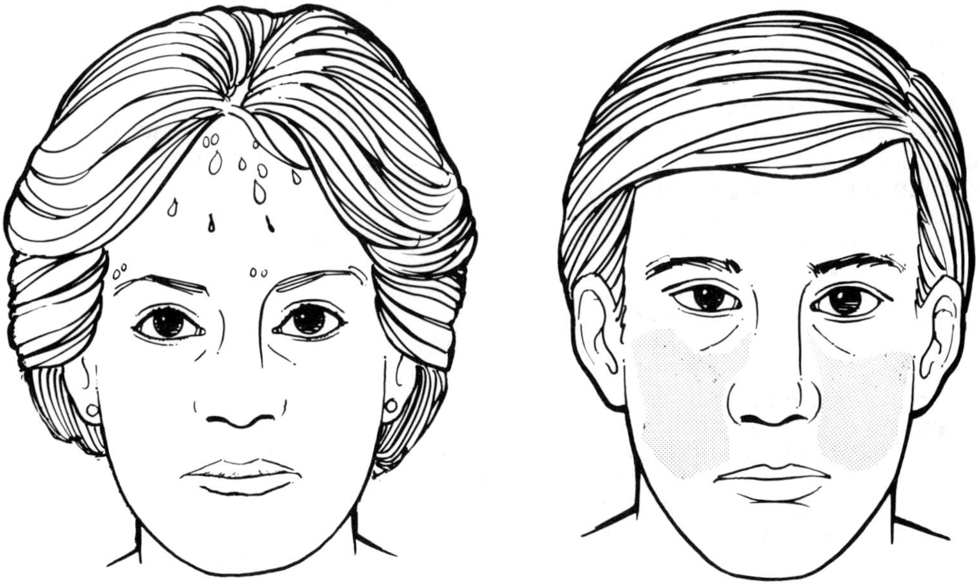

| Heat exhaustion | Heatstroke |
| --- | --- |
| Pale, cool clammy skin | Red, hot, dry skin |
| Excessive sweating | Cessation of sweating |
| Dilated pupils | Constricted pupils |
| Rapid, weak pulse | Rapid, strong pulse |
| Normal or slightly elevated temperature | High temperature (up to 110°F) |

**FIGURE 12.1**

Features that distinguish heat exhaustion and heat stroke

ized by pale, cool, clammy skin; normal or slightly elevated temperature; rapid and weak pulse; excessive sweating; generalized weakness; possible loss of consciousness; shallow breathing; headache; nausea; dilated pupils, muscle cramps; blurred vision; and extreme thirst. A victim of heat exhaustion may not exhibit all of these symptoms, but in most cases enough symptoms are present to enable the first aider to distinguish between this condition and simple fainting.

**First Aid Care**

A person with the described symptoms should stop all activity at once. He or she is removed to shade or a cool place. Clothing is loosened to aid in breathing and heat regulation; in fact, as much clothing as possible is removed. If the person is conscious and not nauseated, he or she is given sips of salted drinking water, as with muscle cramps. Heat can be dissipated somewhat by fanning and by placing cool, damp cloths on the victim. The victim is placed supine with the legs elevated to aid in blood circulation to the brain.

---

**☀ Protection Against Heat-related Disorders**

The best way to avoid heat-related disorders is to use proper preventive techniques:

• Minimize activity during the hottest part of the day, if possible. Try to do your work or exercise during early morning or late evening hours.

• Check the amount of sun, the atmospheric temperature, and the relative humidity when planning outdoor activities.

• Accustom yourself to the heat gradually by working or exercising only short periods during the first few days.

• Begin slowly when you work or exercise outdoors after you have been in a cool environment such as an air-conditioned house.

• Drink lots of fluids. Take sips of cool—not cold—liquids at regular intervals. Do not wait until you are thirsty to start taking in fluids.

• Wear light, loose clothing. Do not wear plastic or nylon sweat clothing, as these reduce evaporation of perspiration from the skin, thereby preventing appropriate heat loss. You may find a light hat helpful to reflect the sun's rays.

• Limit the amount of clothing you wear to expose as much skin as possible and thereby facilitate body temperature regulation.

• Rest periodically during work or recreation, preferably in a cool, shady area.

• Do not eat large quantities of food when anticipating work or exercise in the heat. Add salt to the foods that you eat unless you are on a low-salt or salt-free diet. If you are on such a diet, take special care during activity in the heat. Do not try to prevent heat-related disorders by taking salt pills, as they irritate the stomach and contribute to nausea and hypertension.

• Avoid consuming alcohol on hot days. Alcohol may cause the body to lose fluids, put a strain on the circulatory system, and interfere with the body's ability to regulate body temperature.

• Heed the early signals of heat-related problems described in this chapter. Stop all activity when these signals are noticed. If the symptoms persist, seek medical assistance. (Aaron et al. 1979; Hafen 1981).

---

Recovery from heat exhaustion can take several days to a week.

## ⎯Heatstroke

Heatstroke (Figure 12.1), sometimes called sunstroke, occurs when the body stops sweating and overheats. This condition does not happen as often as other heat-related disorders, but it is the most serious. Heatstroke can be life threatening or cause permanent damage; it should be considered a true emergency due to its detrimental effect on the brain and other vital organs. Heatstroke is seen most commonly in men, overweight individuals, infants, elderly persons, and alcoholics, but may occur in anyone of any age who is overexposed to heat.

### Symptoms
**Heatstroke is a serious, possibly life-threatening condition.** Symptoms are red, dry, hot skin; headache, rapid and strong pulse; dizziness; nausea; constricted pupils, possible cessation of perspiration; unconsciousness; and possible convulsions. Body temperature may reach alarmingly high levels—sometimes as high as 110° F.

**First Aid Care**

**The temperature of a person with heatstroke must be lowered as rapidly as possible to prevent heart and brain damage.** The victim should be moved to a cool, well-ventilated location and as much clothing removed as possible. After placing him or her on the back with shoulders and back elevated, one of the following procedures should be undertaken:

**1** Rub the victim with cloths soaked in alcohol or cold water.
**2** Cover the victim with sheets that have been soaked in cold water.
**3** Place the victim in a draft created by a fan or air conditioner.

If the victim does not have a preexisting condition that contraindicates the procedure, he or she can be placed in a cold shower or a tub of cold water. Ice should **not** be added to the water under any circumstances. Because this is a TRUE EMERGENCY, medical assistance should be obtained as soon as possible.

---

## SUMMARY

The body can easily regulate its internal temperature under most conditions; however, in some situations the body's heat-regulating mechanisms can be overburdened. Overexposure to the sun when temperature and humidity are high is a situation that can cause severe problems. Heat-related problems that can result from overexposure are dehydration, heat cramps, heat exhaustion, and heatstroke (heatstroke being the most severe). First aid care varies for each of these disorders, but its main objective is to restore normal body temperature through cooling and fluid intake (when advisable).

---

## CHAPTER MASTERY: TEST ITEMS

**True and False**                                                          **Circle One**

1. The body's ability to cool itself is unaffected by the relative humidity of   T     F
   the outside air.
2. Heat cramps are the result of an electrolyte imbalance in the body.          T     F
3. Overexposure to heat can be life threatening.                                T     F
4. Heat exhaustion is more serious than heatstroke.                             T     F
5. Elderly and overweight individuals are particularly at risk for heat         T     F
   problems.
6. Heat problems occur only when the atmospheric temperature is high.           T     F
7. The best preventive measure for avoiding heat problems is to take salt       T     F
   pills just before exercising.

8. Red, dry, and hot skin is a sign of heatstroke.         **T**     **F**
9. Periodic rests from activity can help prevent heat problems.    **T**     **F**
10. A heatstroke victim should be immersed in cold water.      **T**     **F**

### Fill In the Missing Word(s)

1. The symptoms of heat exhaustion are _____.
2. The best treatment for a victim of heat cramps is _____.
3. In heatstroke, the face is dry because _____.
4. For normal body temperature to be maintained, the heat lost from the body must equal _____.
5. High body temperatures can result from _____.
6. Dehydration occurs because _____.
7. The most serious heat-related disorder, heatstroke, occurs because _____.
8. Alcoholic beverages should not be given to a heatstroke victim because _____.
9. The best times of the day to exercise to avoid heat problems are _____ and _____.
10. The elderly are vulnerable to heat problems because _____.

### Multiple Choice (Circle the Best Answer)

1. The first thing to do for a heat reaction manifested by pale, cool skin; body temperature a little above normal; weak pulse; and shallow breathing is to
   a. place the conscious victim in a tub of very cold water.
   b. administer a stimulant.
   c. administer a salt solution.
   d. wrap the victim in wet, cold sheets.
2. The best first aid procedure for heat cramps is
   a. immersing the body in cold water.
   b. having the victim drink large amounts of cold water.
   c. administering a saltwater solution.
   d. gently massaging the affected muscle.
3. The best first aid procedure for heat exhaustion is
   a. elevating the upper part of the body.
   b. placing the victim in a cool place.
   c. letting the victim briefly rest before returning to normal activities.
   d. letting the victim drink as much water as desired.
4. Heatstroke is
   a. life threatening.
   b. serious, but easily treated.
   c. not as serious as heat exhaustion.
   d. brought on by working in the sun.

5. The purpose of all first aid measures for heat problems is to
   a. restore salt and water loss.
   b. relieve shock.
   c. prevent convulsions.
   d. lower the body temperature.

## Discussion Questions

1. While participating in a running road race, the first-aider notices that another participant has dropped out of the race. Her face is very red and her skin is dry. What should the first-aider do?
2. While watching a football practice during a hot afternoon at the local high school, a first-aider sees one of the players fall suddenly and hold his gastrocnemius (calf) muscle. On closer examination the muscle is observed to be taut, or "knotted up." What first aid procedures should be followed?
3. A friend's grandmother collapses while weeding the garden on a very hot day. Her skin is pale and moist. What are the proper first aid procedures?

—————————————— **BIBLIOGRAPHY** ——————————————

Aaron, J. E., A. F. Bridges, D. O. Ritzel, and L. B. Lindauer. *First Aid and Emergency Care.* 2d ed. New York: MacMillan, 1979.

Bruch, G. E., J. R. Cade, and J. Tintinalli. "Sorting Out the Heat Syndrome." *Patient Care* 10 (1 June 1976): 10.

Hafen, B. Q. *First Aid for Health Emergencies.* 2d ed. St. Paul: West Publishing, 1981.

Hafen, B. Q., and K. J. Karren. *First Aid and Emergency Care Workbook.* Englewood, Colo.: Morton Publishing, 1980.

# 13

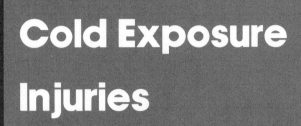

## Cold Exposure Injuries

DAVID M. WHITE, ED.D.

After completing this chapter the student will be able to
- Define frostbite.
- Define hypothermia.
- Explain the body's heat-regulating mechanism.
- Describe the signs and symptoms of frostbite.
- Explain and demonstrate appropriate first aid measures for frostbite (including frostnip).
- Describe the signs and symptoms of hypothermia.
- Explain and demonstrate appropriate first aid measures for hypothermia.
- Identify the prevention measures for cold exposure injuries.

# ___INTRODUCTION

During very cold weather, newspaper accounts of the tragic deaths of individuals stranded in stalled cars or of "street people" who faced the cold with little or no shelter are not uncommon. These people are victims of extreme weather conditions. However, cold exposure injury is not limited to extreme weather conditions or to an outside environment. Cold injury can even occur indoors (e.g., an elderly person living in a very poorly heated home). Although no formal studies show the incidence of cold exposure injuries, the cold winter weather that many face each year, along with the popularity of outdoor sports such as snow skiing, backpacking, and rafting, create a large group of people who run the risk of being injured by the cold.

Because of the potential seriousness of cold exposure injuries, it is very important for the first-aider to be able to recognize these problems and administer appropriate first aid care. The first-aider may have to deal with frostbite, a local injury, or with hypothermia, general overcooling of the body. Both hypothermia and frostbite can occur when the body's temperature-regulating mechanism is impaired by environmental or physiologic factors. To understand the care and prevention of problems created by the cold, it is important to understand the body's mechanism for temperature maintenance.

# ___BODY TEMPERATURE MAINTENANCE

The human body is very sensitive to temperature change because of the relatively narrow range of temperatures it requires for proper functioning. Body temperature is regulated through a system of heat production and heat loss.

## ___Heat Production

Body heat is the result of all of the body's metabolic processes. Energy is required for every metabolic process, and some of this energy is released in the form of heat. Changing food to energy produces heat. A working muscle produces heat. (This explains why humans tend to swing their arms or move about in very cold weather.) Shivering, another form of muscular activity, increases heat production. External sources, such as the sun, fire, and warm food and drink, give heat to the body passively.

## ___Heat Loss

Loss of body heat is affected not only by air temperature but also by direct contact of the body with something cooler (conduction), the speed of the air or water moving across the skin (convection), the wetness of the skin's surface from perspiration or rain (evaporation), respiration of cold air, and exposure of large surface-to-volume areas to surrounding cooler conditions (radiation).

### Conduction

Conduction is the transfer of heat from the body to a cooler object through direct contact. For example, touching a cold car door handle, immersing a bare foot into cold water, or sitting on the cold ground results in heat loss. Telephone lineworkers often relate instances of a near hypothermic condition after leaning against a cold telephone pole for only a short period. In this case the pole has absorbed a great deal of the worker's body heat.

### Convection

Convection is the transfer of heat to the cooler air or water moving across the body's surface. The more rapidly cold air moves past a warmer body, the greater the amount of heat lost. This mechanism of heat loss is often referred to as the windchill factor (Table 13.1). For example, a person exposed to 15° F in thirty-mile-per-hour wind would experience the same exposure as if the temperature were -26° F and there were no wind.

### Evaporation

Evaporation is the transformation of water or other fluid from a liquid to a vapor. Evaporation requires heat, and thus heat is lost during this process. Heat loss can be demonstrated by placing a volatile substance, such as rubbing alcohol, on the back of the hand. The hand will feel noticeably cooler as the alcohol evaporates. Evaporation of sweat from the body's surface is relatively slow compared with evaporation of other, more highly volatile liquids. This slow rate prevents rapid chilling. Also, the lower the humidity of the surrounding air, the more rapidly the water on the body's surface evaporates.

### Respiration

Respiration results in heat loss because the lungs transfer heat to the inspired air and the air is then exhaled.

**TABLE 13.1**

Wind Chill Factors

| Wind speed (mph) | Air temperature (°F) | | | | | | | | | | | | | | | | | | |
|---|---|---|---|---|---|---|---|---|---|---|---|---|---|---|---|---|---|---|---|
| | 45 | 40 | 35 | 30 | 25 | 20 | 15 | 10 | 5 | 0 | −5 | −10 | −15 | −20 | −25 | −30 | −35 | −40 |
| | Chill index* | | | | | | | | | | | | | | | | | | |
| 5 | 43 | 37 | 32 | 27 | 22 | 16 | 11 | 6 | 0 | −5 | −10 | −15 | −21 | −26 | −31 | −36 | −42 | −47 |
| 10 | 34 | 28 | 22 | 16 | 10 | 3 | −3 | −9 | −15 | −22 | −27 | −34 | −40 | −46 | −52 | −58 | −64 | −71 |
| 15 | 29 | 23 | 16 | 9 | 2 | −5 | −11 | −18 | −25 | −31 | −38 | −45 | −51 | −58 | −65 | −72 | −78 | −85 |
| 20 | 26 | 19 | 12 | 4 | −3 | −10 | −17 | −24 | −31 | −39 | −46 | −53 | −60 | −67 | −74 | −81 | −88 | −95 |
| | COLD | | VERY | | BITTER | | | | | | | EXTREME | | | | | | |
| 25 | 23 | 16 | 8 | 1 | −7 | −15 | −22 | −29 | −36 | −44 | −51 | −59 | −66 | −74 | −81 | −88 | −96 | |
| | | | COLD | | COLD | | | | | | | COLD | | | | | | |
| 30 | 21 | 13 | 6 | −2 | −10 | −18 | −25 | −33 | −41 | −49 | −56 | −64 | −71 | −79 | −86 | −93 | | |
| 35 | 20 | 12 | 4 | −4 | −12 | −20 | −27 | −35 | −43 | −52 | −58 | −67 | −74 | −82 | −89 | −97 | | |
| 40† | 19 | 11 | 3 | −5 | −13 | −21 | −29 | −37 | −45 | −53 | −60 | −69 | −76 | −84 | −92 | | | |

* Equivalent temperature in cooling effect on exposed flesh
† Wind speeds above 40 mph have little additional chilling effect.

*Source:* U.S. Department of Commerce, National Oceanic and Atmospheric Administration, National Weather Service.

### Radiation

Radiation is loss of heat through transfer to objects with which the body is not in direct contact. Body parts with large surface-to-volume ratios, especially the head, feet, and hands, are likely to lose a significant amount of heat through radiation.

## __Temperature Regulation

Temperature regulation is vital because the temperature of the human body must be maintained within a narrow range (77° to 113° F or 25° C to 45° C) for survival. In fact, for proper body functioning, the range is significantly narrower, within one or two degrees of 98.6° F or 37° C.

The foundation for the body's temperature-regulating mechanism is the division of the body into two distinct but connected parts, the core and the shell (Figure 13.1). The core contains the major body organs such as the brain, lungs, heart, liver, and kidneys. The core is a heat producer. The shell comprises the skin and its underlying layer of fat (subcutaneous fat), the skeletal muscles, and the peripheral nerves and blood vessels. The shell contributes to heat production, as through muscular activity, and also aids in temperature regulation by conserving or dissipating heat according to the body's needs. Because of the narrow temperature range in which proper functioning can take place, the body is constantly adapting to the internal and external environment to maintain a relatively constant temperature.

When the body needs to increase heat loss, the peripheral blood vessels dilate and allow more blood to circulate near the surface of the skin. This allows heat loss through both convection and radiation. This increase in blood flow created by enlargement of surface blood vessels is called *vasodilation*. The flushed face often seen after vigorous

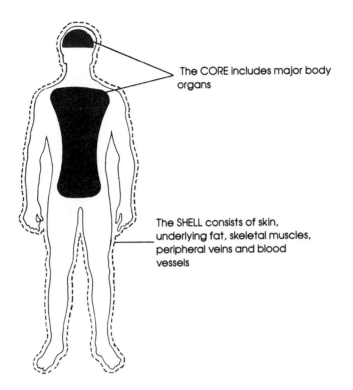

The CORE includes major body organs

The SHELL consists of skin, underlying fat, skeletal muscles, peripheral veins and blood vessels

**FIGURE 13.1**

The body's temperature-regulating mechanism comprises two distinct but connected parts, the core and the shell.

exercise is an example of heat regulation by vasodilation. Vasodilation is only one mechanism for heat loss. Evaporation of sweat is another important means of body heat dissipation.

In a cold environment, the body's need concerning temperature regulation is more likely to be for conservation rather than for dissipation. In this case the peripheral blood vessels of the shell constrict, thereby reducing blood flow near the skin's surface. This *vasoconstriction* allows less heat to be lost via convection and radiation and more heat to be conserved for maintenance of temperatures within the important organs constituting the core. Further, if the body is in direct contact with a cooler object, vasoconstriction reduces conductive heat loss. Two other methods of conserving heat for the core include involuntary muscular activity (shivering) and an increase in the basal metabolic rate, causing food and energy stores within the body to burn faster.

## ___INJURIES FROM COLD

When the temperature-regulating mechanisms fail, cold injury may occur. Such injury manifests itself primarily in two ways:

1 The core temperature is maintained at an adequate level but the shell temperature falls too low. The extent of injury can range from frostnip to deep frostbite.

2 Both core temperature and shell temperature drops and the body reacts to overcooling. This reaction is called hypothermia. Normal metabolic processes break down and death results if the condition is not reversed.

## __Frostbite

Frostbite is the condition of tissue being frozen. Fluids within the cells and the intercellular spaces crystallize, causing damage to blood vessels and often resulting in excessive blood clotting and a lack of oxygen to the affected area. The degree of frostbite can vary from very mild, such as the slight blanching of the cheeks of children walking to school on cold, windy days, to very severe, such as a frozen foot damaged to the extent that amputation is required. Medically, the degree of frostbite is evaluated after the frozen tissues are rewarmed. Estimating the extent of injury accurately is impossible when the area is still cold.

### Signs and Symptoms
The frostbitten tissue may be waxy looking and white, grayish yellow, or in severe cases, grayish blue in color. The affected area is numb. Blisters indicate greater severity and more problems in first aid care because of the increased risk of infection. The toes, fingers, nose, and ears are the body parts most commonly frostbitten. In fact, often the victim is unaware of a problem because of inability to see the frostbitten areas. Also, the site is numb and thus not painful, so the frostbite may easily go undetected while the victim remains in the cold. Once the area begins to thaw, however, the victim becomes painfully aware of frostbite.

The deeper frostbitten tissue is frozen, the more frozen it will feel when touched. Superficial *frostbite* (frostnip) feels hard on the surface but the underlying tissues feel soft. With deep frostbite both surface and underlying tissues are hard.

### First Aid Care
Light blanching, or frostnip, is not a serious injury. The tissue is white and feels soft to the touch. First aid care involves simply rewarming the tissue. Immersing the area in warm water until a flush returns is one appropriate measure. Lightly frostnipped fingertips may be rewarmed by placing them gently under the armpits or by blowing warm air on them. Numb feet may be warmed by placing them in the parka or on the abdomen of another person. Rewarming usually produces a tingling or burning sensation in the affected area. Immediate rewarming may avoid the development of a much more serious problem.

First aid care for frostbite that is more serious than simply frostnip depends on the severity of the injury, the areas affected, and the distance of the victim from warmth and shelter. Initially, the first-aider restricts all activity of the injured area. If the lower extremity is affected, the victim is transported by a stretcher or litter, if possible. The frostbitten area is freed from constrictive clothing and wrapped with loose, bulky dressings. Blisters must not be ruptured, and the area should not be rubbed or subjected to rough handling. Rubbing a frostbitten area with snow or massaging it may cause exten-

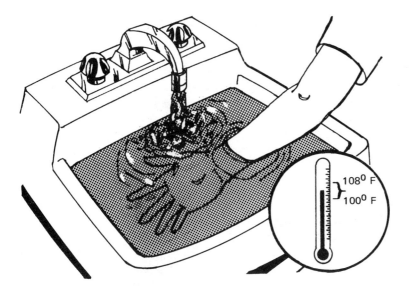

**FIGURE 13.2**

Frostbitten areas are rewarmed in water maintained at 100° to 108°F.

sive tissue damage. After the area has been immobilized and protected from further injury, the victim should move, or be moved, to a medical facility or shelter where rewarming can take place.

Rewarming is the only effective treatment for frostbite, and is best done at a medical facility. However, if transport is delayed, the frostbitten part should be promptly and thoroughly rewarmed. This is done in a waterbath with temperature carefully controlled at 100° to 108° F (38° to 42° C) (Figure 13.2).Water at this temperature feels warm but not hot to a warm hand (the hand must be warm). A good method for testing the water temperature if a thermometer is not available is to use a "warm" elbow (the elbow must be warm). Dry heat, such as a stove or portable kerosene heater, should be avoided as a source of heat for rewarming. The numb, frostbitten tissue can easily be burned by extremely hot water or hot temperature. The water container used for rewarming should be large enough so that the frozen part can be moved during rewarming without bumping into the sides. Warm water will have to be added periodically to keep the water temperature at the appropriate level.

Rewarming should continue until a flush has returned to the entire area. A flush may not appear, however, when the frostbite is so serious that permanent damage has resulted. This is not common. Rewarming usually takes about thirty minutes. The victim should be made aware that the process is very painful, especially the final ten minutes. **Caution: If the frozen area is subject to refreezing shortly after rewarming, it is best to delay rewarming until more permanent shelter can be reached.** For example, if a hiker notices frostbitten toes at camp but has to walk several miles to reach shelter, the frostbitten toes should not be rewarmed if the walk will be made soon. This is because tissue damage resulting from refreezing is significantly more severe than from initial freezing, and the pain involved with rewarming the toes at camp may make travel to shelter extremely difficult.

After rewarming, the thawed parts are very sensitive and prone to infection. Blisters should remain intact, and sterile gauze should be placed between the frostbitten fingers or toes. The victim should avoid exposure to cold or other activity that may cause injury. Even the slightest abrasion can result in a severe infection. Medical advice should be sought as soon as possible. One noteworthy result of rewarming a frostbitten area is its appearance. It is often mottled, swollen, and blistered and looks somewhat gruesome. The victim should be reassured and informed that the healing process will drastically improve the appearance of the area.

### Alcohol, Smoking, and Frostbite

Many people have images of huge St. Bernards carrying small kegs of brandy to victims stranded in the cold, but actually consumption of alcohol multiplies the problem of cold exposure. Heat loss increases because of the dilating effect alcohol has on surface blood vessels. More blood exposed to the surface of the skin means more heat is lost to the cold air. The victim also should not smoke. The nicotine in cigarette smoke causes surface blood vessels to constrict and may thus cause further lack of oxygen to the affected area. This in turn may increase the amount of tissue damage due to frostbite.

## ─Hypothermia

*Hypothermia* is defined as a core body temperature below 95° F (35° C). This condition is most commonly thought to result from sudden immersion in cold water or prolonged exposure to very cold temperatures. However, hypothermia can occur in susceptible individuals at temperatures well above freezing, even in the range of 45° to 50° F. Actually, air temperature is only one consideration, since wind velocity and moisture often play important roles in the development of hypothermia. Individual factors that contribute to its development include hunger (low blood glucose level and depleted energy stores), fatigue, and exertion. Alcoholics are often victims. As with other cold exposure problems, the elderly and the very young are most at risk because of problems with heat conservation: The elderly often have circulation problems and the young have a very high ratio of body surface to body core and thus much heat is lost via convection and radiation.

Hypothermia generally develops in stages, during which time the body goes through significant physiologic and metabolic changes. As core temperature drops, the shell reacts rapidly to conserve as much heat as possible. Peripheral blood vessels constrict, thus shunting warm blood toward the core. This causes a drop in the surface temperature of the skin. If existing conditions cause further heat loss, the body reacts by shivering. This attempt to generate heat is mild at first, but the shivering becomes intense as the core temperature drops below 95° F. Shivering alone is not effective in restoring core temperature to normal because the heat produced is not transmitted to the core. This is due to the curtailed transport of blood from the shell, where the shivering is producing heat, to the core, where the warmth is needed.

As the level of hypothermia increases (which it will unless something is done to reverse the heat loss process), shivering is replaced by muscular rigidity. However, shivering has been known to continue even as core temperature dropped to a level near 82° F. An unusual phenomenon, called "paradoxical undressing," occasionally occurs as the hypothermic state becomes more severe. The victim, obviously in a state of mental confusion, removes articles of clothing. This may cause those who discover the victim to assume mistakenly that an assault or rape has occurred. Researchers have hypothesized that, in the victim of severe hypothermia, control of peripheral blood vessel constriction has been lost, resulting in dilation of these vessels (Wedin, Vanggaard, and Hirvonen 1979). A rush of the warmer blood flows from the core to the surface, causing the victim to feel uncomfortably warm, and clothing is then shed.

As the core temperature drops to 86° F and below, the body's metabolic rate slows drastically. The need for oxygen decreases significantly, and breathing and heart rate slow. This slowed metabolic rate is important for decisions that must be made at the accident or emergency scene. The decision to begin CPR is an especially important one. When the heart rate and breathing rate are drastically decreased, the first-aider should allow a little extra time to determine whether the victim is breathing and has a pulse. **Also, in severe hypothermia the heart muscle is extremely irritable and arrhythmias may occur if the victim is roughly handled.**

The brain's oxygen requirement decreases in the hypothermic state. This, along with other slowing in metabolism, helps to explain cases in which a victim, deprived of oxygen for an extended period, has shown little to no apparent brain damage after resuscitation and rewarming. An experimental study on dogs showed that, for these animals, oxygen consumption is only 50% of normal when the core temperature is 84° F, and the safe period for total circulatory arrest at this temperature is eight to twelve minutes. When the dogs' temperatures were dropped to 61° F, oxygen consumption was only 12.5% of normal and the safe period for total circulatory arrest increased to thirty-two to forty-eight minutes (Gordon 1962). **Caution: In warm humans, the safe period for total circulatory arrest is is only four to six minutes.**

A case example of this slowed metabolic rate follows (Steinman 1983): In 1982, the Coast Guard rescued a 14-year-old boy from 37° F water. He was found floating face up under a pier. He had been missing overnight. He was unconscious, unresponsive, and had dilated, unreactive pupils (a sign of death). A physician on the pier examined him and, finding no pulse or respiration, was prepared to declare him dead. The Coast Guard rescuer swimmer was well versed in hypothermia. He felt the boy's carotid pulse for a full sixty seconds and found a heart rate of six beats per minute. The physician reexamined the boy and concurred. On arrival at the hospital, the boy had a core temperature of 62° F. Yet he survived. This example illustrates a very important point regarding hypothermia: **Victims who appear dead after exposure to cold should not be considered dead until their core temperature is near normal and they are still unresponsive to CPR.**

## Signs and Symptoms

The preceding section describing the body's reaction to overcooling (hypothermia) has indicated some important signs and symptoms of this heat-loss problem. These signs and symptoms generally appear as the hypothermia progresses through stages. The rate of progression depends on the conditions. For example, victims of cold water immersion may lose consciousness and drown after only twenty minutes of exposure (even excellent swimmers). On the other hand, hypothermia may progress slowly. It may take hours to develop in the hiker exposed to dampness, wind, and air temperatures in the 40° to 50° F range.

In the first stage of overcooling, the body attempts to generate heat by shivering. In the second stage, sluggish thinking and diminished coordination are evident. During this stage many individuals experience mood changes (notably, aggression). Apathy, sleepiness, and indifference may also be evident. The third stage is characterized by unconsciousness and a glassy stare. The pulse and respirations are very slow. If no measures are taken to reverse the overcooling process, the final stage, death, occurs.

Other signs and symptoms of hypothermia include a cold stomach, low blood pressure, a puffy face (waxy or oddly pink at times), and muscle tightening with difficulty in moving.

### First Aid Care

First aid care for hypothermia, whether the victim is wet or dry, on land or water, is essentially the same. Therefore, the following discussion of first aid procedures does not distinguish between chronic and acute or wet and dry hypothermia.

*In the victim of hypothermia, a rectal temperature is an important vital sign. Neither oral nor auxiliary (armpit) readings are valid indicators of core temperature.* The rectal temperature reading provides the closest approximation of the core temperature. Realistically, the average first-aider will seldom have access to a low-reading thermometer (regular thermometers do not record low temperatures and are probably dangerous in this emergency setting). Measurement of rectal temperature therefore probably has to be left to medical or paramedical personnel. The following first aid guidelines are not based on the victim's measured temperature.

At the very least, the first-aider must attempt to prevent further heat loss at the core. If the hypothermia is mild, passive rewarming may be sufficient. In a mild case the victim is fully conscious and alert, but cold and shivering. All victims of hypothermia should be treated very gently. Wet clothing is removed and replaced with dry clothing or dry coverings of some kind. The victim must be insulated from the cold. This may be accomplished by carefully wrapping the victim in a dry blanket or sleeping bag. Warm drinks (no alcohol) may be administered only if the victim is clearly conscious, able to swallow, not shivering, and showing some evidence of rewarming. Even in mild cases of hypothermia, medical advice should be sought.

If the hypothermic state is more serious, as when shivering has ceased and the victim is mentally confused or is semiconscious or unconscious, heat must be added. The term "added" is used rather than "rewarm" because often the victim is not actually made warmer with the addition of heat, but rather a further drop in core temperature is prevented or minimized. *Heat should be added gradually and gently.* Several means for adding heat may be available in the field. These include insulated hot water bottles, warm rocks wrapped in towels or clothing, and warm bodies. For example, several rocks may be placed near the fire until they are very warm, then wrapped in towels and placed

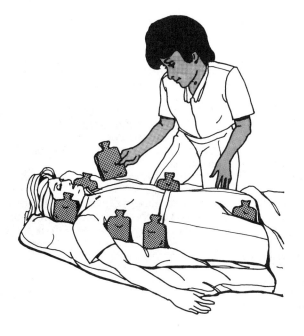

**FIGURE 13.3**
Warm objects are used to add heat to a person with hypothermia.

in the sleeping bag alongside the victim's head, neck, trunk, and groin (Figure 13.3). Or the first-aider's or another person's own body heat may be utilized by the person lying in the sleeping bag with the victim. Wet or bulky clothing is removed from both the victim and the person giving heat before they lie in the sleeping bag so that transfer of heat is efficient.

Several important "do-nots" apply to the first aid given for hypothermia:

1 *Do not rub or manipulate the extremities.* This will increase the likelihood of "afterdrop," which is a further drop in core temperature during or after rescue. It is caused by the return of cold blood from the peripheral circulation (especially from the arms and legs) to the core. Deep core afterdrop is probably the best explanation for postrescue collapse of a hypothermia victim.

2 Do not put the victim in a warm shower or bath. Although there is some controversy regarding the appropriateness of adding heat in this manner, most experts agree that warm water immersion promotes afterdrop. It should be noted that *first aid for hypothermia is distinctly different from that for frostbite with respect to warm-water immerson.* Uncontrolled warming techniques such as warm-water immersion can cause ventricular fibrillation, the typical cause of death from hypothermia, and metabolic imbalances that should be dealt with only in a hospital or clinical setting.

3 Do not allow the victim to drink alcohol or to smoke. These substances compromise blood flow throughout the body and thus should be avoided.

---

### ✳ Preventing Cold Exposure Injuries

Prevention of cold exposure injuries is based on the principles of heat loss and temperature regulation.

- Insulate the body with poor heat conductors, to prevent conduction and convection losses. Such materials include wool, Dacron, foam, and down.
- Wear several layers of clothing rather than a single thick layer. Air trapped between the layers is an excellent insulator, and layers may be removed or added as needed.
- Avoid wearing clothing that is wet from rain or perspiration.
- Always cover the head when exposed to the cold, as well as other areas of the body with large surface-to-volume ratios, such as the ears, hands, and feet.

- Use a protective, oil-based ointment on the nose, lips, and cheeks to reduce heat loss from these areas.
- Wear loose clothing. Tight clothing inhibits blood flow and increases the risk of frostbite. Gloves and boots in particular must fit loosely enough not to restrict blood flow.
- Warm numb hands and feet before extensive injury occurs.
- Avoid consuming alcohol and tobacco (smoked or chewed) in dangerously cold conditions. They interfere with circulation.
- Consume snacks and warm drinks. They enhance the body's ability to produce heat by providing energy.

---

The first-aider should always examine the hypothermia victim for other injuries such as fractures, soft-tissue injuries, and frostbite. These injuries may worsen the hypothermic state, while hypothermia may mask their usual signs and symptoms. The first-aider should examine the victim from head to toe and apply appropriate first aid for any associated injuries. *A medical emergency such as hypothermia may lead to accidental injury, just as an accidental injury may lead to a medical emergency like hypothermia.*

### CPR and Hypothermia

Although not mentioned in the preceding section, hypothermia protocol includes an initial examination for open airway, breathing, and heartbeat (the carotid or femoral artery is used for evaluation). This aspect is treated separately here because of the important considerations regarding CPR for the victim of severe hypothermia. As mentioned earlier, the cold heart beats slowly and is very irritable, and is thus highly vulnerable to arrhythmia if handled roughly. The breathing rate also may be very slow. This implies that more time can be devoted to assessment of breathing and heartbeat with the cold victim than can be with the warm victim. In fact, up to a full minute of assessment may be necessary. If both pulse and respiration are absent, CPR (Chapter 6) is begun. All victims of severe hypothermia should be transferred to a medical facility as soon as possible.

---
### SUMMARY
---

Cold exposure problems occur when the body's temperature is not adequately maintained. The body is constantly adapting to its internal and external environment by producing, conserving, and dissipating heat. Regulation of temperature is accomplished by dilation and constriction of surface blood vessels and by evaporation of sweat, shivering, and changing rates of metabolism. When the body is unable to conserve heat and its temperature drops, either of two types of injury may occur: frostbite (local injury) or hypothermia (systemic injury). Frostbite occurs when tissue is frozen, and hypothermia occurs when the core temperature drops to 95° F or below. Death occurs if the hypothermic condition is not reversed.

The degree of frostbite ranges from mild frostnip to severe frostbite. The color of the frostbitten area is white to yellowish gray and the area is waxy looking. The area is numb and may feel hard to the touch. The areas most commonly affected are the hands, feet, ears, and nose. First aid care for frostnip consists of rewarming, which may simply involve blowing warm air on the fingers. Deeper frostbite requires greater care. The activity of the victim is restricted and wet, constrictive clothing is removed. If transport to a medical facility must be delayed, the area is rewarmed in a warm-water bath. Rewarming usually takes about thirty minutes and the first-aider should warn the victim that it probably will be very painful.

Hypothermia generally progresses through several stages: shivering, mood changes, unconsciousness with a glassy stare, and, if no measures are taken to reverse the process, death. The first-aider should "think heat" with the hypothermic victim. Wet clothing should be replaced by dry coverings and the victim must be insulated from further heat loss. Hot water bottles, warm rocks, and "buddy warming" are recommended for adding heat to the victim. Warm water baths and massage of the extremities should be avoided because of the likelihood of afterdrop. The pulse and respiration rate of victims of severe hypothermia may be very slow. They should be assessed for up to a full minute, and then CPR administered if necessary. Rough handling can be very dangerous. A complete head-to-toe survey (see Chapter 2) is important for all cold exposure victims because associated injuries such as fractures and soft-tissue injuries may be masked by the cold. Alcohol and tobacco consumption compromises blood flow and should be avoided.

---

## CHAPTER MASTERY: TEST ITEMS

**True and False**

Circle One

1. Cold injuries can occur when the temperature is above freezing.    T    F
2. Shivering is a means of heat production.    T    F
3. Dilation of surface blood vessels is associated with an increase in body heat loss through both convection and radiation.    T    F
4. Hypothermia results when the body's "shell" temperature drops very low, but the "core" temperature remains at an adequate level.    T    F
5. Frostnip is usually characterized by whitish-colored skin, numbness, and tissue softness in the affected area.    T    F
6. Rewarming a frostbitten foot usually takes several hours.    T    F

7. The victim of cold exposure should consume a small amount of alcohol during rescue.  **T**  **F**

8. Rubbing a frostbitten area with snow may cause extensive tissue damage.  **T**  **F**

9. Shivering is generally effective in reversing the process of hypothermia.  **T**  **F**

10. A first-aider needs to assess the breathing and heartbeat of a person with severe hypothermia for more than twenty seconds.  **T**  **F**

## Multiple Choice (Circle the Best Answer)

1. A young boy begins shivering violently while outside. He has no hat and is sitting on the cold ground. The heat loss mechanisms causing his condition are
   a. conduction and convection.
   b. convection and radiation.
   c. evaporation and respiration.
   d. radiation and conduction.
   e. respiration and convection.

2. If a victim of hypothermia is placed in a tub of warm water,
   a. improvement is usually almost immediate.
   b. afterdrop may occur.
   c. the blood in the extremities will warm quickly and then flow to the body's core.
   d. improvement will be slow but sure.
   e. both a and c

3. A companion complains of a numb foot during a hike through snow. She removes her shoe and her toes are yellowish and waxy looking and the tissue feels hard on the surface. The first-aider should
   a. tell her to continue walking, exercise will help.
   b. have her place her foot inside the first-aider's parka.
   c. immediately clear an area, build a fire, heat some water, and rewarm the foot.
   d. return to shelter, helping her to not walk on the foot, if possible, and rewarm the foot when permanent shelter is reached.
   e. massage the foot until a flush appears, then return to shelter.

4. The sequence that best identifies the progression of the signs of hypothermia is
   a. shivering, sluggish thinking, unconsciousness, death.
   b. muscular rigidity, shivering, unconsciousness, death.
   c. sluggish thinking, unconsciousness, death.
   d. sleepiness, shivering, muscular rigidity, unconsciousness, death.
   e. sleepiness and apathy, muscular rigidity, shivering, unconsciousness, death.

5. Which of the following is a TRUE statement regarding appropriate first aid for hypothermia?
   a. The extremities should be massaged to encourage blood flow.
   b. Place the victim in a warm shower or bath as soon as possible.

c. Buddy-warming (lying in a sleeping bag with a hypothermia victim) is recommended.
d. A head-to-toe examination is usually not required.
e. The first-aider should add heat to several critical areas, namely, the feet, legs, and arms.

## Discussion Questions

1. Define hypothermia and describe the basic first aid procedures for the victim.
2. List and give an example of each of the body's five means of heat loss.
3. Identify the signs and symptoms of frostbite.
4. How should someone who will be working outdoors under extremely cold conditions dress to prevent frostbite or hypothermia?
5. Briefly explain why the condition of a victim of severe hypothermia may become worse if the victim is immersed in a warm bath.

## BIBLIOGRAPHY

Gordon, A. A. "Heat Exchangers as Hypothermia Inducers in Heart Surgery." *Annual Review of Medicine* 13 (1962): 75–86.

Steinman, A. M. "The Hypothermic Body: CPR Controversy Revisited." *Journal of Emergency Medical Services* 8 (1983): 32–35.

Wedin, B., L. Vanggaard, and J. Hirvonen, "Paradoxical Undressing in Fatal Hypothermia." *Journal of Forensic Science* 24 (1979): 543–553.

# 14

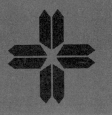

# Drowning and Other Water-related Accidents

GERALD C. HYNER, PH.D.

After completing this chapter the student will be able to
- Identify the major risks associated with water-related injuries.
- Differentiate saltwater from freshwater drowning in terms of pathophysiology.
- Cite the signs and symptoms of drowning.
- Describe specific rescue and resuscitation actions required for a water-related injury or drowning accident.

# ——INTRODUCTION

While the number of reported deaths due to drowning continues to decrease, the number of successful resuscitations and near-drownings is unknown. In spite of the encouraging decline in number of water-related deaths, drowning remains the third leading cause of accidental death for all ages after motor vehicle accidents and falls. It is the second leading cause of accidental death for victims between 5 and 44 years of age. Work and nonwork drownings, boating accidents, swimming mishaps, and falls into water claim nearly 6000 lives per year, most of the victims being between 15 and 24 years of age (National Safety Council 1985).

Nearly half of all adults in the United States are nonswimmers. Though swimming ability is certainly desirable, studies have shown that even skilled swimmers drown by miscalculating distances, hyperventilating before breath-hold diving, swimming while intoxicated, or attempting to test personal endurance.

Unattended children who fall into pools, streams, or canals account for a high proportion of accidental drownings each year. Most victims of boating accidents drown because of the lack of personal flotation devices, and alcohol-related boating accidents mirror the same unfortunate patterns seen on the nation's highways. With several hundred thousand scuba (self-contained underwater breathing apparatus) enthusiasts becoming certified divers each year, the potential for drownings and water pressure injuries has increased. Yet most of those injured or who die while scuba diving appear to have needlessly panicked or used poor judgment, reflecting lack of experience or disregard for safety procedures.

Clearly, the number of deaths and injuries due to water-related accidents could be significantly reduced. But as long as unsupervised children play near water and swimmers take unnecessary risks, training in water safety, rescue, and first aid for near drowning is necessary and justified. The first-aider can expect to encounter emergency situations that demand these skills.

# ___PATHOPHYSIOLOGY OF DROWNING

The biological consequences of drowning and near-drowning have been extensively investigated in animals. Understandably, human research is lacking, but survivors have provided anecdotal evidence and autopsies have offered pathologists a partial analysis. Several important findings are useful to the first-aider.

Regardless of the obvious signs and symptoms, no two drownings seem to be exactly alike. Much depends on the victim's general state of health and the circumstances surrounding the accident. The prognosis for recovery depends on at least three critical factors (Modell 1971, 1978):

- The length of time the victim has been underwater
- Whether the water is fresh or salt
- The amount of water the victim has taken into the lungs (aspirated)

Apparently only a small percentage of drowning victims die as a direct result of aspirated fluid. Many have a reflex spasm of the vocal cords and become unconscious due to lack of oxygen to the brain. Some drowning victims aspirate very little water into the lungs, while others take significant amounts into the stomach and lungs when the laryngospasm finally relaxes. Procedures aimed at evacuating fluid from the lungs are useless and unnecessary, even if the victim aspirated water.

The exact cause of death is usually considered asphyxia due to insufficient oxygen (hypoxia), which may be complicated by the aspiration of fluid into the lungs. If fresh (salt-free) water is aspirated, most of it is quickly absorbed into the circulation. Because blood is saltier than fresh water, many of the red blood corpuscles take in the water, expand, and rupture (hemolysis). Changes in blood chemistry and blood volume, the integrity of the corpuscles, and cardiovascular functioning depend on the quantity of aspirated fluid and the duration of the hypoxia. Interestingly, little fluid is found in the lungs of near-drowning victims in fresh water because the water is so quickly absorbed into the circulation. Frequently the alveoli of the lungs collapse; yet even this severe condition appears to be transient if the victim is resuscitated quickly.

Because salt water has the opposite effect of fresh water on the blood plasma, fluid is commonly found in the lungs of victims who have aspirated salt water. The alveoli are flooded and hypoxia is further aggravated. Both fresh- and saltwater drowning victims may expel frothy, blood-stained fluid. In saltwater drowning, more liquid accumulates in the airway than was aspirated. This secondary flooding of the lungs and subsequent risk of lung infection accounts for many of the deaths that follow apparently successful resuscitations. **All near-drowning victims must be taken to the hospital for observation, in spite of their relative well-being after rescue.** Respiratory distress (secondary drowning) can occur rapidly and requires immediate medical management.

A basic understanding of the pathophysiology of drowning and near-drowning in either fresh or salt water leaves the first-aider with four important concepts:

1 Attempting to remove water from the lungs is a waste of time, since reoxygenation is the first priority in all drownings.

2 All near-drowning victims need follow-up medical care, especially if water was aspirated.

3 The first-aider should inform medical practitioners as to the victim's vital signs at the time of rescue, the type of water, and the estimated duration of submersion.

4 The first-aider must realize that in spite of an apparently successful resuscitation, the victim may suffer severe, delayed effects that could not have been modified by the rescuer.

In spite of the serious pathological consequences of both freshwater and saltwater drowning, many of these changes are known to be transient and treatable if resuscitation is promptly and effectively initiated. Additionally, cases of successful resuscitation of young victims submerged for half an hour or more in cold fresh water have been reported. The potential for surviving total submersion in cold, fresh water (less than 70° F) for periods up to an hour has been attributed to the mammalian diving reflex (MDR). MDR is a typical response of mammals, especially dolphins and whales, to deep dives in cold water. During such dives the pulse rate drops and metabolism is greatly reduced. The function of MDR in humans may be overestimated; however, it appears to be important to survival during the first few minutes under water. Long-term survival, however, is probably a result of absorption of cold water into the circulation, with consequent rapid cooling of vital organs. Because of the potential for survival, the first-aider should aggressively pursue resuscitation, even when the victim has been under water for as long as sixty minutes. While the delayed effects of near-drowning are complicated and must be managed by a medical practitioner, the first-aider need only accomplish several important tasks to effect a rescue.

# ____FIRST AID CARE FOR DROWNING VICTIM

## ____Resuscitation

The drowning victim must be reoxygenated as quickly as possible. If the victim is not breathing, the first-aider should initiate mouth-to-mouth or mouth-to-nose resuscitation immediately, even if the victim has aspirated fluid and is still on the surface of the water. Forceful ventilation may be necessary, since aspiration of fluids can compromise resuscitative efforts. Maintenance of an open airway is difficult in the water; total airway obstruction will probably be due to failure to achieve an appropriate head tilt (hyperextension of the head; see Chapter 5), rather than to aspirated water.

For a victim without a pulse, CPR must await extrication of the person from the water to a hard, firm surface like the shore or a boat. A victim rescued from ocean surf should be positioned on shore with the top of the head nearest the sea. Because the shoreline usually slants downward toward the water, this position naturally lifts the legs and helps to hyperextend the head. Further, the hardest sand on the beach is usually near the water. The victim may have a substantial quantity of water in the stomach, and fluid commonly exits from the mouth as the first-aider attempts ventilation. Regurgitated debris should be quickly cleared to prevent aspiration and allow resumption of emergency ventilation. Mild pressure may be applied to the upper abdomen, and the

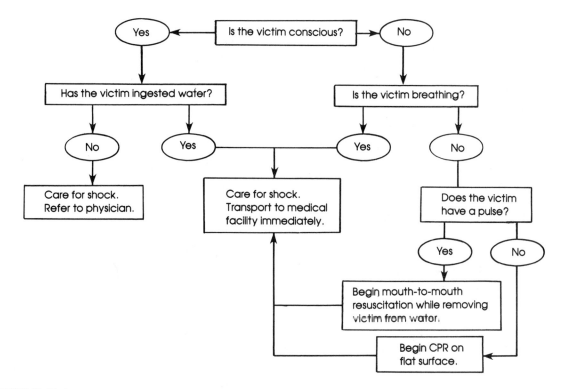

**FIGURE 14.1**

Steps in first aid care for drowning victims

entire body turned to the side for a few seconds to clear the airway. If spinal cord injury is suspected, **exceptional** care must be taken to roll the victim as a complete unit. **In no case should time be wasted trying to evacuate water from the stomach or lungs.** The first-aider must watch the rise and fall of the victim's chest for evidence of successful ventilation. The ventilatory rate is once every five seconds in the adult, more rapidly in children, and once every three seconds in the infant or young child (Chapter 5). Figure 14.1 is a flowchart of the first aid steps for drowning victims.

Techniques of aquatic rescue are complicated and require extensive training and practice; the interested reader is referred to the local Chapter of the American National Red Cross for courses in lifesaving and water safety. Unfortunately, each year well-intentioned first-aiders die attempting to rescue drowning victims. Whenever possible, the first-aider should try to assist a conscious victim by extending a pole or throwing a flotation device or rope before entering the water. A conscious, panicking victim may overcome the strongest first-aider if the person is untrained in the techniques of a swimming water rescue. While unconscious victims may not be struggling, the weight of the victim and the need for immediate reoxygenation make single-rescuer attempts difficult and dangerous. Only the first-aider can judge his or her ability to reach and rescue a victim who will likely drown without assistance.

## __Shock

All aquatic accident victims should be given care for shock (Chapter 4). Aspirated water may have adverse effects on blood volume, aggravating the shock that accompanies hypoxia. Cold water may quickly produce immersion hypothermia in the submerged individual, dissipating heat many times faster than air. The degree of shock can be affected by the victim's sensitivity to cold, the amount of body fat, the water temperature, and the duration of immersion.

In some people, sudden exposure to cold water produces symptoms similar to an allergic or hypersensitivity reaction. All drowning victims must be treated for hypothermia, a common complication and cause of shock in drowning victims. A detailed discussion of hypothermia and related first aid care is presented in Chapter 13. The usual procedures for the care of shock described in Chapter 4 should be maintained until the victim is given medical treatment.

# ____SPECIAL NOTE: HYPERVENTILATION

Special mention must be made of the extremely dangerous practice of purposeful hyperventilation before an underwater swim. By hyperventilating, the swimmer expels carbon dioxide from the lungs and thereby loses the normal stimulus for initiation of breathing. As oxygen becomes depleted, the swimmer may lose consciousness without warning. Such a condition is referred to as *shallow-water blackout.* The characteristic struggling behavior usually associated with drowning is absent. Rescued victims have reported a pleasant, carefree sensation before blackout. The victim may appear lethargic before losing consciousness, and water aspiration is common. Resuscitation of these victims is difficult because of rapid hypoxia and the aspiration of substantial quantities of water.

---

**Warning for All Swimmers**

To avoid shallow-water blackout, avoid hyperventilating, regardless of your aquatic skills. Public pools should post warnings about the dangers of hyperventilation, along with the traditional admonishments about running on wet decks and diving into shallow water.

---

# ____OTHER WATER-RELATED ACCIDENTS

## __Diving Board Accidents

The most serious injury associated with diving board accidents is one affecting the spinal cord. A victim who sustains a spinal cord injury and requires water rescue, resuscitation,

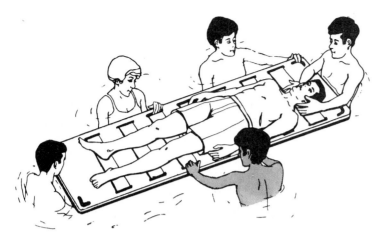

**FIGURE 14.2**
Positioning a backboard
under a person suspected
of spinal cord injury from
diving. One rescuer keeps
the victim's head and neck
aligned with the body.

and extrication from the water presents a most difficult problem. It is virtually impossible for one person to rescue such a victim efficiently. In a swimming pool, a backboard and cervical collar should be available and applied before the victim is lifted from the water (Figures 14.2 and 14.3).

To ventilate a victim with a suspected neck fracture, the mandible is displaced using the jaw thrust technique while the head is maintained in a neutral or fixed position (see Chapter 5). Clearly, in an unconscious, nonbreathing victim the first priority is reoxygenation in spite of possible spinal cord involvement. Nevertheless, if the first-aider

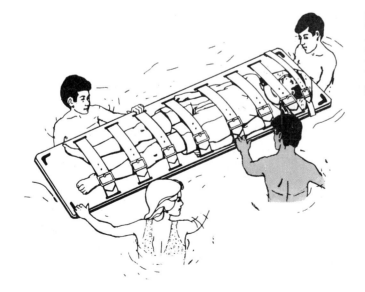

**FIGURE 14.3**
After the backboard and
cervical collar are applied,
the victim is secured to the
backboard, ready for lifting
from the pool.

witnessed the accident and noticed obvious trauma to the skull (or even suspects spinal cord trauma) rescue procedures should be quickly organized to deal with that possibility. The victim is handled without causing additional neck or back movement, the spine being kept in a straight line.

Similar injuries may also be incurred by surfboard riders who either are thrown from their board in shallow water or sustain injuries from the surfboard itself. Occasionally the rescuer may be able to use the surfboard like a backboard during extrication of the victim from the water.

## ▬Boating Accidents

Boating accidents present unique challenges to the first-aider. Trauma frequently accompanies drowning in boating accident victims. Hypothermia is common, since the victims may have unexpectedly been thrown into cold water. Unfortunately, most boaters fail to wear Coast Guard-approved flotation devices. Even experienced swimmers may be knocked unconscious in a boating accident, making the aquatic rescue more difficult. The circumstances that caused the accident may give clues to the types of injuries that can be expected. For example, boats traveling at high speed can sustain severe damage and quickly decelerate if they strike an underwater object like a sandbar or coralhead. Passengers then may be violently ejected from the boat or come into contact with propellers. Waterskiers are at particular risk of being struck by skis, other boats, or underwater objects. Individuals facing the stern (rear) of the boat watching the skier in tow may be launched overboard when the pilot quickly accelerates to lift the skier into the standing position. The possibility of propeller injury in this case naturally complicates the water rescue and the first aid care required. Aquatic rescue and resuscitation would be much simpler if sailors wore flotation devices that positioned them face up in the water; only a few of the commercially available life jackets do this. Consequently, for many boating accident victims the first-aider must be prepared to:

1 Begin ventilation procedures.
2 Control severe bleeding.
3 Care for spinal cord injuries.

## ▬Unexpected Falls

Rescue of drowning victims who have fallen into the water may be hampered by the victim's heavy clothing, trauma, or water currents. Fishermen wearing waders that accidentally flood can lose their footing and sink in deep water. Skaters and ice fishermen who fall through thin ice can seldom maintain consciousness for more than a few minutes after immersion in freezing water.

The swimming rescuer can avoid unnecessary hazards by taking a brief moment to assess the emergency situation before initiating the rescue. As in all drowning and water-related emergencies, multiple rescuers are preferred.

---

### ✤ Precaution for Ice Fishermen

• Always cut a triangular hole in the ice and slide the "cap" under the ice instead of attempting to lift it out. It is far easier to extricate yourself from a corner than from a rounded ice surface.

---

## — Snorkeling Accidents

Emergency procedures for snorkelers involve the same practices recommended for any drowning victim. Snorkelers may be in distress at a considerable distance from a potential first-aider. When their full attention is directed toward the view below them, they may lose a sense of their proximity to the diving boat or the shore. Snorkelers who dive beneath the surface while holding their breath may be at particular risk if they hyperventilate first on the surface. An unexpected wave that floods the snorkel can initiate panic. On the water surface, the first-aider can use the open end of the snorkel to inflate the victim's lungs as long as the head is hyperextended, the victim's lips are securely sealed around the mouthpiece, and the snorkel is free from water. Some snorkelers may be wearing a weight belt, which should be jettisoned; they may also be wearing an inflatable life jacket. If the snorkeler has such a jacket, it can be orally inflated by the first-aider, or, if available, a carbon dioxide cartridge can be activated which automatically fills the jacket.

## — Scuba Diving Accidents

The rescue and care of an injured scuba diver can be complicated, requiring specific training and recognition of unique water-pressure injuries (barotrauma). Scuba divers who drown are usually inexperienced or ignore the basic safety rules of the sport. Accidents are seldom associated with equipment failure or attack by underwater predators.

The first-aider who may be exposed by choice or by chance to scuba diving is referred to accepted training manuals (e.g., *The New Science of Skin and Scuba Diving* published by the Council for National Cooperation in Aquatics), which detail rescue procedures unique to this rapidly growing sport. Of particular concern is the scuba diver who suddenly surfaces from the depths suffering from a serious complication of diving that requires immediate first aid, "the bends." In a diver who has been breathing compressed air at depth and who rapidly ascends to the surface, bubbles may develop in the circulatory system, which act as clots interfering with blood flow to vital organs. Gas bubbles form when the water pressure is suddenly reduced by the scuba diver ascending more rapidly than one foot per second. Air in the lungs may quickly expand and rupture lung tissue. Smaller bubbles may accumulate in joints. The name "the bends" accurately describes the body positions assumed by many victims because of the pain. If some of the

**FIGURE 14.4**

The diving accident position for scuba divers with water pressure injuries. Oxygen is given, if available.

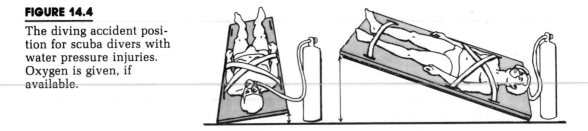

bubbles interfere with blood flow to the brain, permanent damage or death may result. Immediate first aid care is needed. If conscious, the victim may exhibit severe pain, numbness, difficulty in breathing, and decreasing consciousness. Victims should be put in the diving accident position (Figure 14.4) and given oxygen if available. They should NOT be allowed to sit up or stand. In a severe case, out-of-water recompression in a pressurized chamber is needed.

The Diving Accident Network (DAN) is a nonprofit group of physicians specially trained to advise a first-aider assisting a scuba diving victim. Its twenty-four-hour phone number (919-684-8111) can be called collect in emergencies. Since the symptoms associated with barotrauma may develop slowly, the alert first-aider should be ready to assist the victim should his or her condition suddenly deteriorate. Treatment for scuba diving-related injuries may require the skills of medical practitioners specially equipped to deal with underwater injuries.

---

## SUMMARY

Drowning is one of the leading causes of accidental death. The majority of cases are preventable. Near-drowning victims require prompt first aid care, since many require care for respiratory and circulatory arrest as well as shock. They should be referred to medical practitioners for care and observation. Drowning victims suffering from cold water exposure or trauma and persons with water-pressure injuries are at particular risk for severe complications.

Water is seldom found in the lungs of near-drowning victims, and even if fluid is in the respiratory tract, the highest priority must be given to airway maintenance and reoxygenation. Attempts to drain fluids are unnecessary and time consuming. Because of the unique physiologic effects that fresh water and salt water cause in drowning victims, the first-aider must be attentive to possible delayed effects, which can be life threatening.

—————————————— **CHAPTER MASTERY: TEST ITEMS** ——————————

**True and False**                                                       Circle One

1. Most drowning victims die as a result of fluid aspiration into the lungs.     T     F
2. First-aiders should attempt to evacuate water from the victim's lungs     T     F
   before beginning resuscitation.
3. Near-drowning victims should receive follow-up medical care, because     T     F
   complications are common.
4. Young children seldom survive prolonged submersion in cold, fresh     T     F
   water.
5. Mouth-to-mouth resuscitation should be attempted while the non-     T     F
   breathing victim is still in the water.

**Multiple Choice (Circle the Best Answer)**

1. All aquatic accident victims should be given
   a. CPR.
   b. care for shock.
   c. blankets to warm the extremities.
   d. warm drinks.
2. Hyperventilation syndrome or shallow-water blackout
   a. seldom affects experienced swimmers.
   b. occurs because the victim failed to take deep breaths before swimming
      underwater.
   c. can be recognized by the victim's struggling behavior in the water.
   d. results from the dangerous practice of hyperventilating before swimming
      underwater.
3. Victims with suspected cervical injuries
   a. should never be given mouth-to-mouth resuscitation while still in the water.
   b. require the same rescue procedures as any other drowning victim.
   c. can be ventilated by the jaw thrust method while the head is maintained in a
      fixed position.
   d. should be removed from the water before being placed on a backboard.
4. Treatment of victims who have been scuba diving
   a. may include transportation to a pressurized chamber.
   b. is seldom necessary as long as the victim is conscious.
   c. is not necessary unless the diver was in very deep water.
   d. will usually be for injuries caused by equipment failure or attack by marine
      life.

5. Near-drowning victims
   a. seldom have large quantities of water in their lungs.
   b. may require close medical observation after being successfully resuscitated.
   c. require immediate mouth-to-mouth respiration if they are not breathing.
   d. all of the above

### Discussion Questions

1. While walking along a crowded ocean beach, a first-aider notices a crowd at the water's edge. An adult is dragging a young, apparently unconscious adolescent from the surf. The first-aider is the only trained individual in the vicinity. Briefly describe the steps he or she should take to manage this emergency.

2. While relaxing at an unguarded hotel swimming pool, a first-aider overhears two youths discussing a challenge to swim the pool's length under water. Before they can be cautioned, they submerge and begin swimming. One youth surfaces, but the other is motionless under five feet of water. What may be wrong with the victim? How might this emergency have been avoided? Briefly describe how to manage this emergency.

—————————————————————— **BIBLIOGRAPHY** ——————————————————————

Council for National Cooperation in Aquatics. *The New Science of Skin and Scuba Diving.* Piscataway, N.J.: New Century Publishers, 1980.

Modell, J. H. *The Pathophysiology and Treatment of Drowning and Near-Drowning.* Springfield, Ill.: Charles C Thomas, 1971.

Modell, J. H. "Biology of Drowning." *Annual Review of Medicine.* 29:1-8, 1978.

National Safety Council. *Accident Facts: 1985.* Chicago: National Safety Council, 1985.

Pearn, J. H. "Secondary Drowning in Children." *British Medical Journal.* 281:1103-1105, 1980.

# 15

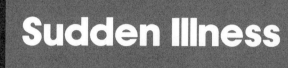

## Sudden Illness

FRANK E. SCHABEL, ED.D.

After completing this chapter the student will be able to

- Define sudden illness.
- Cite the signs, symptoms, and primary corrective factors associated with each type of sudden illness described in this chapter.
- Explain and demonstrate first aid procedures for immediate care of victims of sudden illness.
- Explain the limitations of the first-aider in rendering assistance to a person with sudden illness.

## ____INTRODUCTION

Since the beginning of this century, chronic diseases have replaced infectious disease as the number one health problem in the United States. Chronic diseases are the principal predecessors to potentially life-threatening sudden illnesses. Life-style plays a vital role in the development of many of these diseases and related sudden illness episodes. Life-style is estimated to be a 50% factor in heart disease and stroke, respectively the first and third ranking causes of mortality in the United States. If these two diseases and many others directly affected by personal life-style are to be brought under control, Americans are going to have to examine their health-related behaviors and modify them as necessary. Nonetheless, first-aiders must know how to both recognize the signs and symptoms of sudden illnesses resulting from a multiplicity of conditions and render appropriate assistance quickly and effectively.

The chapter describes signs, symptoms, and first aid procedures for a number of sudden illnesses.

### ⚕ Special Note

Additional sudden illnesses that the first-aider may encounter are discussed elsewhere in this text. Among them are heart attack in Chapter 6; internal hemorrhage in Chapter 7; concussion in Chapter 9; and alcohol and drug problems, anaphylactic shock, and food poisoning in Chapter 10. The first-aider should review the information presented on these conditions, including their first aid care.

# ___ANGINA PECTORIS

Angina pectoris literally means "pain of the chest." Victims often mistake this condition for indigestion. While angina is less severe than an acute heart attack, the first-aider must respond to the problem as he or she would to a major attack. Angina is typically chronic, and many persons with this condition carry prescribed medication for use as needed. If necessary, the first-aider may assist the victim with the administration of, for example, nitroglycerin tablets or the inhalant amyl nitrate. A person with a first attack of angina should see a physician as soon as possible. Delay will only postpone diagnosis of underlying coronary heart disease. First aid for victims of heart attack is discussed in Chapter 6.

# ___STROKE (APOPLEXY) OR CEREBROVASCULAR ACCIDENT (CVA)

A stroke, or apoplexy, is an interruption of the blood supply (and therefore oxygen) to a vital center in the brain. Stroke usually occurs in older people with high blood pressure and arteriosclerosis, although it may be caused by tumor or a cerebrovascular problem. Stroke is surpassed only by heart disease and cancer as the leading cause of death in the United States.

## ___Signs and Symptoms

A stroke victim may initially have dizziness, headache, and memory loss. Blackout sometimes occurs, followed by periods of imbalance and falling. A major stroke typically results in a combination of signs and symptoms including unconsciousness; defecation; urination; prominent neck veins; breathing difficulties; unequal pupil dilation; paralysis on one side or in parts of the body; and paralysis of one side of the face with frequently associated drooling, speech impairment, and loss of muscle tone (Figure 15.1). Many of these prove to be temporary. Lasting effects can include permanent brain dysfunction, paralysis, and speech impairment. A major stroke may even cause death.

## ___First Aid Care

A person who has had a stroke should be kept in a semireclining position. The first-aider cares for shock (Chapter 4) and loosens or removes any constrictive clothing around the person's neck. If breathing is difficult, the victim's head and chest are raised. No fluids are given. Reassurance is provided, and bystanders are kept away. The victim may appear unaware of surroundings and yet understand everything that is happening. Someone should be sent for emergency help right away. If it is needed, the first-aider gives artificial respiration (Chapter 5) or CPR (Chapter 6). *The most important first aid care is to maintain cardiopulmonary functioning and carefully watch the state of consciousness.*

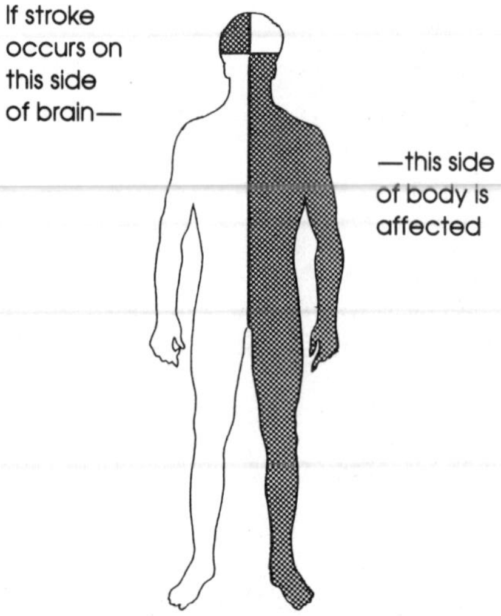

| | |
|---|---|
| If stroke occurs on this side of brain— | **Before stroke:** |
| | Bouts of dizziness, headache, memory loss |
| | Blackouts, periods of imbalance and falling |
| —this side of body is affected | **After stroke:** |
| | Unconsciousness |
| | Paralysis on one side of body |
| | Drooling, speech impairment |
| | Breathing difficulties |
| | Unequal pupils |
| | Diminished vision or loss of sight in one eye |
| | Loss of muscle tone |
| | Involuntary defecation and urination |
| | Prominent neck veins, often red face |

**FIGURE 15.1**

Signs and symptoms of stroke

## _____ METABOLIC EMERGENCIES

A metabolic emergency may result from radical or, sometimes, subtle metabolic changes in the body. Metabolic disturbances such as alterations in hormones, enzymes, acid-base balance, electrolytes, chemical substances, and especially glucose (sugar) level have a direct effect on the physiology of the human body.

A metabolic emergency can stem from drug overdose (especially from central nervous system depressants), from diseases that alter serum calcium level, and from distorted sodium levels. Usually the cause is diabetes, which alters blood sugar levels. Diabetes can lead to diabetic coma or hypoglycemia. The first-aider has to be able to recognize the signs and symptoms of an impending metabolic emergency so that he or she can give prompt and correct first aid care.

### Diabetic Coma

When the islets of Langerhans in the pancreas do not produce enough insulin for the body's needs, diabetes mellitus results. Insulin acts to allow transport of glucose from the bloodstream into cells, a process necessary for the maintenance of cell life.

With insufficient insulin, glucose is unable to pass from the bloodstream into cells, resulting in an increase in blood sugar levels (hyperglycemia). Hyperglycemia causes the kidneys to excrete large quantities of urine, which causes an enormous loss of body fluids. A resultant decrease of glucose within the cells develops further metabolic abnormalities, which cause an accumulation of a variety of acid end products in the body with a decrease of the pH of body fluids. The end result is a decrease in central nervous system functioning, which causes a decrease in consciousness and finally coma.

### Signs and Symptoms
The onset of diabetic coma may take several days. It may result from failure to administer needed insulin, administration of inadequate amounts of insulin, improper diet, or an infectious disease that alters the amount of insulin in the blood. Characteristic signs and symptoms are hunger, increased thirst and urination, labored breathing, a decrease in blood pressure, and an increase in heart rate resulting in a weak and rapid pulse. The breath may have a sweet, fruity odor (acetone). Other manifestations are a red, dry face; vomiting; abdominal pain; dimness of vision; headache; and restlessness that can merge into unconsciousness. Many of these signs and symptoms resemble those of alcohol intoxication; because of this, treatment is often delayed. Delay can yield irreversible and sometimes fatal results.

### First Aid Care
The first-aider checks the person with signs of diabetic coma for the presence of a Medic Alert bracelet or some other symbol of diabetic status. Such a symbol is helpful in determining what may be wrong.

The person going into or in a diabetic coma needs insulin. First-aiders are not trained in insulin administration; only skilled persons such as a nurse, a doctor, or a trained family member should administer it. The first-aider should quickly try to locate a family member who understands the problem and can give the needed insulin. If this is not possible, he or she arranges for transport or transports the victim to the nearest hospital or medical clinic. In the meantime, the first-aider attempts to maintain a proper airway, checks breathing and pulse status, and administers artificial respiration or CPR if necessary. If the victim is conscious, he or she may be offered oral glucose fluids such as orange juice. The addition of glucose will not cause the victim any additional harm and may benefit him or her greatly if the problem is indeed hypoglycemia (low blood sugar). **Caution: Fluids are given only when the victim is conscious.**

## —Hypoglycemia (Insulin or Diabetic Shock)

Hypoglycemia is caused by too much insulin in the blood. This can result from self-administration of an excessive amount of insulin or consumption of too little sugar to counteract the amount of insulin administered. The blood sugar level drops and insulin shock sets in. If hypoglycemia remains unresolved for some time, brain tissue begins to die. The person with diabetes can prevent insulin shock by controlling food intake (especially carbohydrates), avoiding excessive work, and controlling the amount of insulin administered to the body.

### Signs and Symptoms
The signs and symptoms of insulin shock include weakness; fatigue; a shaky, nauseous feeling; sweating; vomiting; paleness of skin; rapid heart rate; drooling; intense hunger; double vision (diplopia); and tremors. Many of these are caused by the body's attempt to raise the blood sugar level.

### First Aid Care

Because of the possibility of brain damage from insulin shock, the first-aider must be cognizant of its signs and symptoms and provide immediate first aid care. If the victim is conscious, the first-aider gives a sugar solution (e.g., orange juice or soft drink), candy, or sugar of any other kind. If the individual is unconscious, no liquids are given but sugar, a sugar cube, or another form of concentrated sugar is placed under the tongue for rapid absorption by the numerous capillaries located there. Artificial respiration is given if necessary, making sure that administered sugar substances do not block the airway.

## ___ CONVULSIONS

Convulsions are caused by unusual or abnormal stimulation of neurons in the brain. Convulsions are associated with a number of conditions, such as epilepsy, anxiety, low blood calcium level, lack of oxygen, fever, trauma, tumor, and various acute infectious diseases including measles and mumps. Convulsions may also be caused by drug usage, and sometimes by the development of toxemia in pregnancy (eclampsia).

Most commonly, convulsions are caused by epileptic seizures. Although many types of seizures exist, the first-aider should be particularly aware of the two principal forms, grand mal and petit mal.

*Grand mal seizures* are characterized by sudden loss of consciousness and (often) loss of bowel or bladder control or both, followed by gradual arousal. Convulsions associated with the seizure may affect part or all of the body and usually last only a few minutes. After the seizure the victim may show restlessness, incoherent speech, and mental confusion lasting up to a few days. The person often has forewarning (an aura) preceding a grand mal seizure.

*Petit mal seizures* last only a few seconds. The victim may stare into space, twitch the fingers, smack the lips, and speak incoherently. The victim returns to normal as soon as the seizure stops. Generally, petit mal seizures do not require emergency care. However, if the seizure is the first of its kind, it is strongly recommended that the person see a medical doctor.

## ___ Signs and Symptoms

Convulsions can last for a few minutes or even longer. Typically the muscles become rigid, and then jerky, spasmodic muscle contractions begin. The face may be bluish (cyanotic), especially around the lips, and loud hissing or deep utterances may be heard from the victim. Foaming and drooling from the mouth may occur and the victim may clamp the teeth shut, sometimes biting the tongue in the process. Loss of bladder or bowel control is possible. When the convulsions cease, the victim may be disoriented, tired, and irritable and may want to sleep.

Convulsions rarely cause death unless they occur repeatedly in close succession and the victim dies from exhaustion (major drug convulsions). The primary threat posed by convulsions is the circumstances in which they take place, for example, while the victim is driving a car or a boat or perhaps working with dangerous mechanical equipment. If death occurs, it probably stems from an injury incurred during the convulsion rather than from the convulsion itself.

## __First Aid Care

After recognizing a convulsion, the first-aider gently tries to lower the victim to the ground if he or she is standing or sitting. The person is not restrained, as this may result in torn muscles. Something soft is put under the person's head, and furniture is moved out of the way. The first-aider may gently attempt to cradle the person's head to protect it from injury. **Caution: Nothing is placed in the mouth.** Tight clothing around the neck is loosened or removed. Although rarely necessary, artificial respiration is given if breathing stops after the attack subsides.

Whether the convulsion is the first or one of a series of repeated attacks, medical attention is recommended.

# __ FAINTING (SYNCOPE)

Fainting is a mild, brief form of unconsciousness. It is usually self-correcting, because it causes the victim to fall, which in turn increases blood flow to the brain, arousing the person. Fainting may be caused by stress, nervousness, or possibly disease. Vasodilation (as in shock) of the venous circulatory system allows pooling of blood in the viscera, which causes a shunting of blood away from the brain. A lessened blood supply means a decrease in oxygen, and function. Fainting often happens to people standing at attention for prolonged periods. Nervous persons are also susceptible to fainting.

## __Signs and Symptoms

Fainting is sometimes preceded by nausea, ashen pallor, sweating, dilated pupils, and dizziness. Other typical signs include weak and rapid pulse, and irregular breathing.

## __First Aid Care

Because a decrease in blood volume to the brain causes fainting, circulation to the brain has to be increased. This usually quickly arouses the victim. If venous blood supply has pooled in the chest, abdomen, or lower extremities, treatment for shock, which includes lowering the body to a reclining position, is essential. If no head, neck, or back injuries are suspected, the legs are elevated to increase venous blood flow to the heart. An individual who feels faint is encouraged to either lie down or place the head between the knees while in a sitting position. Caution is needed in the latter case, because the person may still collapse and fall forward, possibly injuring the head or upper extremities.

**TABLE 15.1**

Organs located in the abdomen

| Solid | Hollow |
|---|---|
| Adrenal gland | Descending aorta and inferior vena cava |
| Kidneys | Esophagus |
| Liver | Large intestine |
| Pancreas | Small intestine |
| Spleen | Stomach |

# ____ACUTE ABDOMINAL EMERGENCIES

Acute abdominal emergencies include any acute intraabdominal disorder that is not associated with trauma. Types of acute pathological disorders that can occur in the abdomen are hemorrhage, inflammation, ischemia (inadequate blood supply), obstructions, and perforation. Many organs are located in the abdominal area (Table 15.1), and pain can occur in any of them. The particular location usually determines the type of problem. Pain in the lower abdominal area may be caused by infection; diarrhea often results. Upper abdominal pain may indicate indigestion or gastritis. **Caution: Only a physician should diagnose abdominal illness.**

## ___Signs and Symptoms

Table 15.2 lists general signs and symptoms of abdominal emergency and general first aid emergency procedures.

The first aider seeks answers to the following questions:

1 Is the pain worse when the abdominal area is touched?
2 Is there vomiting? (If so, part of it is saved for professional inspection.)
3 Is the stool, if present, bright red or dark?
4 Is there swelling in the abdominal area?

**TABLE 15.2**

General signs and symptoms of acute abdominal emergency and general first aid emergency procedures

| Signs and Symptoms | First Aid Care |
|---|---|
| Abdominal tenderness | Get medical attention immediately. |
| Vomiting of blood | Give psychological support. |
| Blood in stool | Keep victim comfortable, if possible. |
| Abdominal distention | Do not give medications, food, drink, |
| Abdominal rigidity | enema, or laxative. |

**5** Is the pain localized or spread throughout the abdominal area?
**6** Has the victim vomited blood?

This might be an appropriate time for the first-aider to review the subjective interview and objective examination of the secondary assessment, detailed in Chapter 2. The information acquired in the assessment is relayed to the medical personnel who subsequently take responsibility for the victim.

## —First Aid Care

The individual is not allowed to eat, drink, or take any medication. Bed rest often takes care of indigestion from overeating or from eating rich food. Persistent, severe abdominal pain is a medical emergency that cannot be remedied in the home. The first-aider should get the victim to professional medical help. If vomiting occurs, the first-aider ensures that the airway is open and, during transport, that the victim does not suffocate on stomach contents.

## ——SUDDEN PAIN

Pain, whether severe or slight, real or imagined, is always distressing. There are as many thresholds of pain as there are individuals. An illness in one victim may cause extreme pain, while the same illness in another may cause little or none. To the onlooker or first-aider, determining whether a person's problem is fear, panic, anxiety, external stress, or pain is quite difficult.

The first-aider attempts to make the victim relaxed, comfortable, and reassured. If injury is not apparent, he or she tries to determine, by questioning the victim, when the pain began, the exact location, and the type of pain (dull, burning, piercing, cramping). As much information as possible should be communicated to a medical professional, who then informs the first-aider whether the victim needs transport to a physician. Thus, the first-aider's major responsibility in a case of sudden pain is to seek and follow the advice of medical professionals.

## ——HEADACHE

Headache has many causes, including tension, injury, brain tumor, sinusitis, and hypertension. Other causes of head pain include eyestrain, premenstrual tension, and infection, such as the flu. Migraine headaches are common, but typically headache is caused by tension. Aspirin may alleviate headache pain, but if the pain persists over an extended period, a physician should be consulted for further diagnosis. Caution must be exercised in administering aspirin products to children and infants if viral infection is suspected. The wiser course is to use only nonaspirin products in children.

## \_\_\_\_EYE DISCOMFORT

Eye pain is often sharp and pulsating. If pain is accompanied by dimming and blurring of vision and halos are seen around lights, glaucoma may be developing. Glaucoma must be treated immediately, because this disease results in increased intraocular pressure, which may cause permanent blindness. Anyone over age 40 should have an annual eye examination. Eye specialists commonly check for glaucoma in every adult who has the eyes checked for visual acuity.

The first-aider should seek medical attention immediately for any person with sudden eye pain.

## \_\_\_\_EARACHE

Most earaches are very painful. Of major concern is middle ear infection leading to pressure on the eardrum. Pressure can cause rupture or perforation of the eardrum. Pressure can also result from high altitudes or scuba or skin diving.

If the eardrum has ruptured, the first-aider should not put any medication into the ear. If fluids of any type are draining from the ear, the first-aider should LIGHTLY place a sterile dressing over the affected ear, gently bandage it in place, and take the victim to a physician or medical facility immediately.

---

**Relief of Ear Pressure During Air Travel**

Pressure on the eustachian tube is increased during air travel, especially while the plane is descending. This pressure may be relieved by swallowing, chewing gum, or popping the ears. The last is done by taking a deep breath and holding it, pinching the nostrils, and attempting to blow through the pinched nose.

Some people have such intense ear pain that it radiates into the jaw, to the back of the neck, and even down the back. Persistence of pain for twenty-four hours or more calls for consultation with a physician.

---

## \_\_\_\_TOOTHACHE

Individuals with a sudden toothache should see a dentist as soon as possible. If care is delayed, perhaps due to distance, oil of cloves on a piece of cotton and placed on the tooth may relieve the pain. Aspirin or another pain reliever may help until a dentist can be seen. Again, caution is advised in the use of aspirin with children and infants. Little first aid can be offered the toothache victim except to clean the affected area, prevent air from contacting the tooth, and reassure the individual as much as possible.

## ___NECK PAIN

Most neck pain is caused by injury and overstretching of muscle fibers within the neck area. However, a number of infectious diseases that are prevalent in childhood, such as meningitis and poliomyelitis, cause neck pain. If neck pain is not relieved with the basic remedy of heat, the advice of a physician should be sought. Such advice is particularly important if the neck muscles become rigid and difficult to move (especially forward). This may result from serious infectious disease.

## ___BACK PAIN

Weak abdominal muscles are the single most common cause of back pain. Back pain causes short- or long-term disability in 60% of all men over age 40 in the United States, and is also very common in women. Back pain is often chronic. Sometimes it is caused by injury, especially from improper lifting of objects. Insufficient back support during sleep can cause early morning backache. Back pain could often be avoided if people diligently and correctly exercised their abdominal and back muscles.

Pain is most often experienced in the lower back or lumbar region of the musculoskeletal system. Muscle spasms may result from sudden twisting or lifting movements, and they may recur at the slightest provocation. With muscle strain injury, first aid initially consists of cold applications and later of heat in the form of warm baths and hot packs. Rest is also important for lower back pain. Emergency medical treatment is usually not needed for back injury unless it involves the spine itself. Injuries to the musculoskeletal system are discussed in Chapter 8, while those specifically related to the spinal column and spinal cord are presented in Chapter 9.

## ___RECTAL PAIN

Rectal pain is often caused by straining during bowel movements and constipation. Typical disorders are hemorrhoids, abscesses, and malignant or benign tumors. The pain is often intense because of severe muscle spasms in the rectum.

Hemorrhoids, like tumors, can be removed surgically if this is deemed necessary. First aid procedures for hemorrhoidal pain include baths and soothing ointments. Eating fresh fruits is often helpful, and the victim may use a mild laxative. The anal area must be kept clean. If intense pain or rectal bleeding persists, the person should consult a doctor. A person with hemorrhoids, abscesses, or benign tumors should consult a physician annually, especially if colitis (inflammation of the colon or large intestine) is a recurrent problem.

If a person is incapacitated from rectal pain, the first-aider should arrange for medical assistance.

## ___CHEST PAIN

Chest pain can result from numerous conditions including angina pectoris, pleurisy, pneumonia, bronchitis, infection, trauma, cancer, and psychosomatic problems. The pain may be located in the chest walls, ribs, heart, abdominal organs, or lungs, or a combination of these. Heart pain (heart attack) is discussed in Chapter 6.

### ___Signs and Symptoms

An individual with chest pain may describe the pain as dull, stabbing (sharp), or cutting. The pain may be exaggerated by lung expansion as a result of breathing or coughing. Sometimes the victim can lessen the pain by diminishing the expiration and by reducing the rate and depth of inspiration. Signs accompanying pain may include coughing, production of sputum, holding of the chest, fever, dyspnea (shortness of breath), increase in pulse rate, apprehension, and shock.

### ___First Aid Care

The first-aider should be cognizant of possible heart attack when aiding a person with chest pain. The first-aider puts the victim in a comfortable position, possibly a semireclining position, to allow easier breathing. If the first-aider can establish that the pain is not that of angina pectoris, fluids, and aspirin if there is fever, may be given. Adhesive strips (not directly on the skin) or an elastic strap can be placed around the rib cage to relieve the pain of breathing. If chest pain is still present in 24 hours, the victim should consult a medical professional.

## ___HERNIA

Hernia occurs when a weak area of the abdominal wall allows a loop of intestine to protrude through or against the wall. This may happen to anyone but is more common in obese persons. Healthy people can cause hernia by lifting a heavy object or by sudden exertion. Hernia is potentially dangerous, especially if the intestine becomes constricted and blood flow is cut off to that portion of the bowel.

Hernia should receive medical attention quickly. A protrusion in the abdomen should not be pressed or forced inward. The victim should avoid vigorous activity and not do any lifting. The victim may be comfortable on the back with pillows under the knees. If this position is painful, the victim is put in the knee-chest position (Figure 16.15c). No food, water, heat, or cold should be given.

## ___LEG PAIN

At times sudden pain occurs in the legs due to muscle cramping or trauma. First aid procedures include heat, gentle massage, and stretching of muscles. Muscle cramps are related to heat problems and possible lactic acid buildup.

Circulatory complications may cause leg pain, and in this case a doctor should be consulted.

## ____SHORTNESS OF BREATH (DYSPNEA)

Decreased respiratory function, cardiac and circulatory problems, emotional problems, and injury all can contribute to lack of oxygen, which in turn causes shortness of breath. Other causes of dyspnea include high altitude, exercise, and a variety of diseases leading to a reduced oxygen supply. Emergency resuscitation procedures should be followed (Chapter 5) if breathing stops or cyanosis (blue color) is observed in the victim. A semireclining position is best for shortness of breath because it allows easier lung expansion. The victim should seek medical care if the condition persists.

## ____ASTHMA ATTACK

An asthma attack is an allergic reaction that causes a panting, wheezing, high-pitched sound when the individual breathes. Typically the victim has had previous attacks and possesses medicine to alleviate the condition. Other signs and symptoms of asthma include coughing and spitting up of mucus. If an attack is severe, the victim may have cyanosis around the lips and under the fingernails. The first-aider can administer the needed medicine (usually antihistamine), keep the person in a sitting position, reassure the person, give warm liquids to drink, and, if possible, provide warm, moist air to breathe. The source of the allergic response should be removed (or the victim moved to an allergy-free environment). Medical attention should be sought when the attack is severe, especially in young children. Hospitalization may be required.

## ____EMPHYSEMA

Emphysema is a disease strongly associated with smoking cigarettes for many years. Alveolar tissues are ruptured and destroyed in this debilitating disease. The damage done to the lungs can never be repaired; however, the disease can be arrested by eliminating the cause of the disease. The individual with emphysema has trouble performing any physical activity and often needs to have supplemental oxygen to survive. He or she finds exhaling extremely difficult. An upright position is needed; even during sleep the person must not lie flat. If breathing should stop, resuscitation efforts should begin immediately.

## ____PALPITATIONS OF THE HEART

Extreme fluttering or throbbing of the heart may be quite severe; medical attention is required. Tachycardia, or rapid heartbeat, is recognized by an extreme increase in the number of heartbeats (200 beats per minute or more) without apparent reason. Typically the rapid heartbeat returns to normal in a short time. The tachycardia victim may experience nervousness, which causes weakness, breathlessness, and possibly fainting. No first aid, except reassurance, is required unless fainting occurs.

---

## SUMMARY

Whereas infectious diseases were once the leading causes of mortality in the United States, they have been surpassed by diseases that manifest themselves through sudden illness. Heart attack and stroke (sudden illnesses caused by cardiovascular disease) are respectively the number one and number three killers in the United States. Many other sudden illnesses are life threatening but usually do not require the basic life support that is indicated for these two conditions.

Diseases such as diabetes and epilepsy can cause emergencies that might result in death without proper first aid care. Many others require only a modest amount of care from the first-aider and do not pose a serious threat to the victim. No matter what the sudden illness is, the first-aider needs to be able to recognize the signs and symptoms and then quickly provide whatever first aid care is indicated.

---

## CHAPTER MASTERY: TEST ITEMS

### True and False

| | | Circle One |
|---|---|---|
| 1. Most sudden illnesses are caused by infectious disease. | T | F |
| 2. Amyl nitrate and nitroglycerin are drugs used by epileptic victims. | T | F |
| 3. Paralysis of one side of the face and unequal pupil dilation may be signs of apoplexy (stroke). | T | F |
| 4. Diabetics need a special diet to help control the disease. | T | F |
| 5. Loud hissing sounds, cyanosis around the lips, and drooling are signs of a petit mal seizure. | T | F |
| 6. A person with symptoms of acute abdominal pain may have appendicitis. | T | F |
| 7. Victims of sudden illness should immediately be placed in a supine position for examination. | T | F |
| 8. A first-aider should hold the tongue of a victim experiencing a grand mal seizure. | T | F |

### Fill In the Missing Word(s)

1. A person with frequent bouts of dizziness, headache, and memory loss is probably experiencing _____.

2. When physiologic processes are disrupted, metabolic balance is lacking, causing frequent urination, fatigue, excessive thirst, and possibly unconsciousnes. This manifestation can be called _____.
3. Unusual, abnormal stimulation of neurons within the brain, which may result from injury, infection, fever, or oxygen reduction, leads to _____.
4. Grand mal seizures in many victims may be preceded by an unusual _____.
5. Another term for shortness of breath is _____.
6. A disease characterized by difficulty in breathing and associated with long-term use of cigarettes is _____.
7. A heart rate above 200 beats per minute may be caused by _____.

**Multiple Choice (Circle the Best Answer)**

1. The *leading* cause of death in the United States today is
   a. cancer.
   b. heart attack.
   c. stroke.
   d. epilepsy.
2. First aid for epilepsy includes
   a. restraining the victim to prevent convulsion.
   b. placing a blunt object in the mouth to prevent tongue swallowing.
   c. removing furniture from the victim's surroundings.
   d. placing the victim in a warm tub of water.
3. When too much insulin is available in the blood for the body's supply of blood sugar, the condition is termed
   a. insulin shock.
   b. diabetic coma.
   c. hypoglycemia.
   d. a and b
   e. a and c
4. First aid care for insulin shock might include the administration of
   a. an emetic.
   b. insulin.
   c. orange juice.
   d. water.
5. When confronted with a person suspected of having a diabetic problem, the two critical questions to ask are
   a. Does your stomach ache? Do you have diarrhea?
   b. Have you eaten today? Have you taken insulin today?
   c. Have you had any alcohol? Have you taken any diet pills?
   d. Have you taken any water? Have you had a bowel movement?

6. One sign of a major stroke is
   a. dilated pupils.      c. unequal dilation of the pupils.
   b. bloodshot eyes.      d. constricted pupils.

7. A victim experiencing insulin shock appears
   a. cyanotic.      c. pale.
   b. flushed.      d. alert.

8. A person with signs or symptoms of diabetic coma is apt to
   a. mimic the actions of a drunk.      c. collapse suddenly.
   b. have a pale skin.      d. have increased blood pressure.

9. A person who has had a stroke should be placed in a
   a. sitting position.      d. semireclining position.
   b. standing position.      e. prone position.
   c. supine position.

**Discussion Questions**

1. While camping in the mountains, a first-aider and a friend find a semiconscious individual alone in an isolated camping area. The victim has a red, dry face and a sweet, fruity breath odor. What might the problem be? What can and should the first-aider do for this person?

2. Carol's new roommate informs her that she is taking medication for epilepsy and that she hasn't had a grand mal seizure in six months. What first aid care should Carol be prepared to provide?

3. An elderly man suddenly complains of shortness of breath. He falls to the floor, unconscious. After examining him, the first-aider finds that he has unequal dilation of the pupils, irregular breathing, and has also lost bowel control. Describe the first aid care that should be administered.

———————————— **BIBLIOGRAPHY** ————————————

American National Red Cross. *Advanced First Aid and Emergency Care.* Garden City, N.Y.: Doubleday, 1979.

Hafen, B.Q., and B. Peterson. *First Aid for Health Emergencies.* St. Paul: West Publishing, 1977.

Henderson, I. *Emergency Medical Guide.* New York: McGraw-Hill, 1978.

Parcel, G.S. *Basic Emergency Care.* St. Louis: C.V. Mosby, 1982.

Thygerson, A.L. *The First Aid Book.* Englewood Cliffs, N.J.: Prentice-Hall, 1982.

# 16

# Emergency Childbirth

CHRISTOPHER L. MELBY, D.H.SC., M.P.H.

After completing this chapter the student will be able to
- Explain the process of fertilization and fetal development.
- Describe the role of specific maternal organs and tissues which accommodate normal fetal growth and development.
- Describe the characteristics of the first, second, and third stages of normal labor and delivery.
- Describe the physical and emotional changes characteristic of each of the three phases of first-stage labor.
- Demonstrate an understanding of the major responsibilities of the first-aider toward the expectant mother in first-stage labor.
- Identify the criteria used to decide whether to transport the expectant mother to a medical facility or prepare for the birth at her present location.
- Explain the birth attendant's responsibilities in second-stage labor.
- List the important steps in the proper care of the infant immediately after birth.
- List the steps in assisting the mother during and after the birth of the placenta.
- Describe the major delivery complications and the appropriate care for these emergencies.

# ____INTRODUCTION

Childbirth has a certain mystique and excitement. For the first-aider, assisting at an emergency birth is far less common than providing immediate care for a broken bone or laceration. Splinting a fracture or dressing a wound is fairly routine in comparison with involvement in bringing a seven-pound, fragile-appearing, slippery new human being into what seems to be a foreboding environment. In today's society, it is uncommon for childbirth to take place outside an established medical institution, complete with sophisticated equipment and highly trained staff. Thus, the delivery of a baby in an environment such as the backseat of a car or a bedroom at home, far removed from fetal monitors, intravenous lines, sterile gowns and gloves, and a sure-handed obstetrician or midwife, is often fraught with anxiety and insecurity for both mother-to-be and the attending first-aider. However, the vast majority of births throughout history have occurred outside the medical care setting, and maternal labor and delivery are entirely normal functions, *usually* proceeding routinely and without complications.

The first-aider involved in providing emergency care for an expectant mother should take comfort in the knowledge that most births are not dire emergencies requiring the latest in medical equipment and training. Women with a high-risk pregnancy or prolonged or obstructed labor usually get to the hospital in time. It is women with short, uncomplicated labor who are more likely to deliver unexpectedly at home or in their own car, a taxicab, an ambulance, or a police car. The attendant at an emergency birth, if acquainted with a basic body of knowledge and some practical skills, can be invaluable in aiding and supporting the expectant mother to carry out her normal role in giving birth to her child. The purpose of this chapter, then, is to provide the first-aider with a basic understanding of the labor and delivery process in childbirth, and to provide opportunity to develop the insights and skills needed to aid in an emergency birth necessarily outside of a medical setting.

## ——NORMAL PREGNANCY AND CHILDBRITH

Pregnancy begins when a *spermatozoon*, or sperm cell, from a male unites with the *ovum*, or egg cell, of the female. This union is called *fertilization* and usually occurs in the *oviduct*, or fallopian tube, of the female. Figure 16.1 illustrates the reproductive organs of the nonpregnant female. The fertilized ovum undergoes cell division as it migrates toward the *uterus*, or womb, and implants in the uterine lining approximately

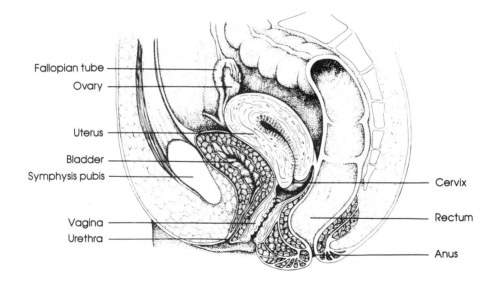

**FIGURE 16.1**

Anatomy of female reproductive system

**FIGURE 16.2**

Anatomy of pregnant woman at full term. Note attachment of umbilical cord to placenta.

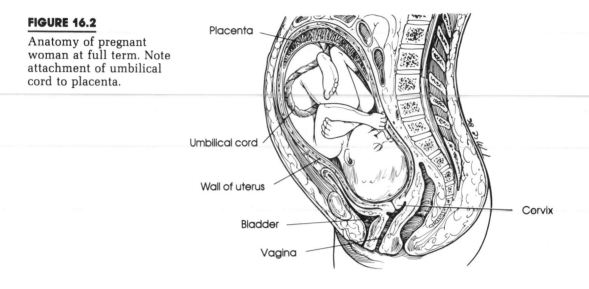

Placenta

Umbilical cord

Wall of uterus

Bladder

Vagina

Corvix

seven to ten days after fertilization. The mass of cells, now called an *embryo*, that eventually becomes the fetus is soon enveloped within the fluid-filled space, the *amniotic cavity*, lined with a smooth membrane, the *amnion*. The *amniotic sac*, also called the bag of waters, has a number of important functions: it provides a medium in which the fetus can move and develop, it affords a protective cushion against injury, and it provides a constant internal temperature for the fetus.

The entire growth and development of the fetus occurs in the uterus, which progressively enlarges to accommodate the increasing size of the fetus (Figure 16.2). The mouth of the uterus, called the *cervix*, opens into the vagina. The cervix is closed during pregnancy with a thick mucous plug. By the third month an organ unique to pregnancy, called the *placenta*, has developed and is firmly attached to the uterine wall. The placenta serves as an exchange station between mother and fetus. Oxygen and nutrients diffuse into the placenta from the maternal circulation and are transported to the fetus via the umbilical cord. The pathway is reversed for carbon dioxide and other fetal waste products; they diffuse into the placenta from the umbilical cord and enter the mother's system from which they are eliminated. At full term (completion of approximately forty weeks of pregnancy) the placenta weighs between one and two pounds. It, along with the umbilical cord, is completely expelled after the birth of the baby.

Striking changes occur as the embryo develops. Starting from a one-celled zygote after fertilization, it usually grows into a highly differentiated six- to nine-pound baby approximately twenty inches long at birth. The duration of pregnancy is approximately 265 days, although the range is 240 to 280 days. Some fetuses apparently need a shorter time, others a longer time for full in-utero development. Babies born before the thirty-seventh week of pregnancy are considered preterm (premature), usually weigh less than a full-term infant, and are at higher risk for development of health problems after birth.

**FIGURE 16.3**

Three stages of labor

| First stage: cervical dilation | |
| --- | --- |
| Early phase* | Cervix dilates 1 to 4 cm.<br>Uterine contractions last 30 to 45 sec.<br>Contractions are 5 to 15 min. apart. |
| Active phase | Cervix dilates 4 to 8 cm.<br>Contractions last 45 to 60 sec.<br>Contractions are 3 to 5 min. apart. |
| Transitional phase | Cervix dilates 8 to 10 cm.<br>Intense contractions last up to 2 min.<br>Contractions are 2 to 3 minutes<br> apart. |

| Second stage: birth of baby |
| --- |

| Third stage: expulsion of placenta |
| --- |

* All measurements for phases of the first stage of labor are
approximate and vary from person to person.

Full-term infants who weigh less than 5½ pounds are considered low-birth-weight babies and are also at higher than average risk for postpartum complications. Adequate weight gain and good nutrition during pregnancy are important factors in the delivery of a healthy, normal-weight infant.

At the end of approximately nine months of pregnancy, maternal changes prepare the fetus for expulsion from the uterus, in a series of events termed *labor*. The amount of time spent in labor varies from woman to woman, ranging from just a few hours to more than twenty-four. Usually labor during the first pregnancy is longer than that of subsequent pregnancies. The labor period can be conveniently examined in three stages (Figure 16.3).

## ___First Stage of Labor

The exact mechanisms that initiate the process of labor are not entirely understood, but probably hormonal changes and the physical pressure of the fetus on the walls of the uterus are involved. The first stage of labor allows the baby to move into the vagina as the cervix dilates, or opens. The cervix must dilate to approximately ten centimeters (four inches) to accommodate the passage of the baby. The three muscle layers of the uterus contract, pushing the fetus toward the cervix, and they also pull the sides of the uterus up, resulting in the "extrusion" of the baby. When the muscles relax they do not release to their original length, thereby drawing the cervix open and creating progressively more mechanical pressure on the fetus to descend.

**FIGURE 16.4**

Early labor. The cervix
begins to dilate but the
amniotic sac is still intact.

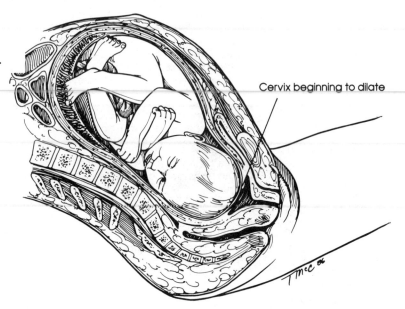

Cervix beginning to dilate

The first stage of labor is subdivided into three periods: the early phase, the active phase, and the transitional phase. The early phase is characterized by dilation of the cervix (Figure 16.4) from one to four centimeters and uterine contractions lasting approximately thirty to forty-five seconds spaced approximately five to fifteen minutes apart. During this early phase, uterine contractions do not usually cause great discomfort, but the mother-to-be recognizes that labor has begun and usually initiates a call to her physician or midwife to communicate her present labor status.

The active phase of labor is characterized by further dilation of the cervix from four to eight centimeters, and contractions of forty-five to sixty seconds in length spaced approximately three to five minutes apart. The uterine contractions during this phase are more intense and may produce a great deal of discomfort. Usually, midway through the active phase of first-stage labor the expectant mother is in the labor room of the hospital or birth center.

The final phase of the initial stage of labor is almost always the most difficult for the mother. Contractions are very intense, lasting up to two minutes and occurring in rapid succession so that there is little time to rest between them (sometimes less than one minute). The cervix becomes completely dilated (to approximately ten centimeters) to accommodate the baby's head, which usually enters the vagina first (Figure 16.5). This phase is characterized by severe discomfort and sometimes extreme mood changes including anger, panic, fear, or apathy. A small amount of bleeding often occurs as the cervix become fully dilated. The amniotic sac may rupture before the initiation of labor or anytime during the first stage. Rarely does the sac remain intact until delivery.

In summary, the first stage of labor is called the dilation stage and begins with the first symptoms of true labor and ends with the complete opening of the cervix. The time

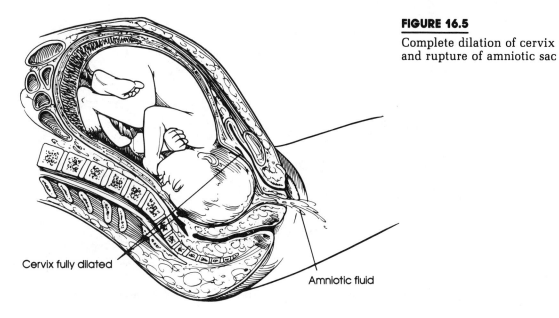

**FIGURE 16.5**
Complete dilation of cervix
and rupture of amniotic sac

Cervix fully dilated

Amniotic fluid

of progression from the early phase to the end of the transitional phase varies from person to person and pregnancy to pregnancy. During the early phase, contractions are sometimes sporadic but usually settle into a consistent pattern by the middle of the active phase. The uterine contractions that accomplish cervical dilation are often feared by the expectant mother. Such fear may actually prolong labor and intensify the discomfort experienced. Methods of helping the mother cope with the fears and discomforts will be discussed later in the chapter when the responsibilities of the attendant first-aider are described. However, if the mother is still in the early phase of the first stage of labor, there is usually ample time to transport her to a medical facility.

## Second Stage of Labor

Second-stage labor begins when the cervix is fully dilated and ends when the baby is born. It normally lasts thirty minutes to one hour, but may last as long as two hours. Certain signs and symptoms mark the beginning of this stage, and these must be watched for by the first-aider. Typically the woman in this stage of labor will have a strong urge to push the baby out, which she may mistake for the need to have a bowel movement. This urge results from the baby's head pressing down on the floor of the maternal perineum, the area between the vagina and the anal opening. The baby continues down the vagina or birth canal with each contraction, often aided by the pushing or bearing down of the mother. During this stage the mother is usually in a reclining position with her torso elevated above her pelvis, her legs apart and knees drawn up toward her chest, as shown in Figure 16.6. As the first part of the baby, usually the head, reaches the end of the birth canal, the perineum begins to stretch and the baby's head becomes visible (Figure 16.7).

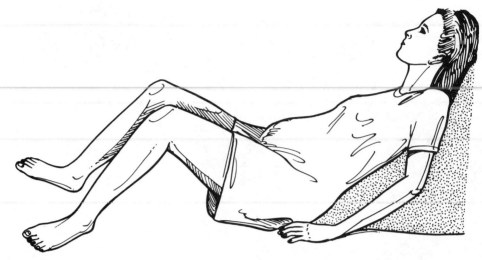

**FIGURE 16.6**

Bearing down is easier for the mother if her torso is elevated above her pelvis and her knees are drawn up.

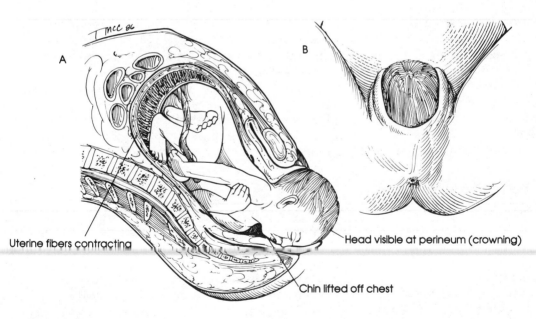

Uterine fibers contracting

Head visible at perineum (crowning)

Chin lifted off chest

**FIGURE 16.7**

The baby's head crowns (appears at the vulva); labor is nearly over. (*A*) Cross section. (*B*) External view.

This is called *crowning* and signals that birth is imminent. As the infant's head stretches the vaginal opening, pushing may be less intensive, to prevent tearing the perineal tissue.

The baby is usually born in the anterior position, or face down. Once the head is outside the birth canal, the infant rotates laterally to allow the upper shoulder to descend through the widest portion of the pelvis, follwed by the bottom shoulder. The torso and legs then descend quite quickly and the baby enters the world, still attached by the umbilical cord to the placenta, which remains in the uterus until the third stage of labor. In a hospital birth, the umbilical cord is tied off and cut, usually within a few minutes of birth, before the third stage of labor begins.

## — Third Stage of Labor

The third stage of labor is initiated by the return of uterine contractions following the birth of the baby. The purpose of these contractions is to expel the placenta, which usually occurs within thirty minutes of the baby's birth. This stage is characteristically signaled by a small gush of blood from the vagina, resulting from separation of the placenta from the uterine wall. After the placenta is delivered, the uterus begins slowly to return to normal size.

From this overview of the birth process, the first-aider should have a firm understanding of the sequence of events that normally occur in labor and delivery. A detailed procedural guide follows to enable the first-aider to assist properly in childbirth. Ideally the birth would be attended by a physician or midwife and would occur in a facility capable of handling any complication that might arise. However, this may be impossible, and the first-aider may be forced to serve as the primary birth attendant. The important responsibilities of a first-aider from early labor until the mother and newborn child are stable or in the hands of trained medical personnel are described in the following sections. The first-aider should recognize that contact with the mother may begin or end at any time during the course of delivery, depending on the situation.

## —— NONEMERGENCY AID (FIRST STAGE OF LABOR)

When confronted with a woman in labor, an untrained person (often the husband) is prone to panic and hurry her off to the hospital. While such action may be warranted, an initial evaluation of the situation is a prudent measure to ensure that the best possible decisions are made.

If the woman is in first-stage labor, there is usually time to transport her to the chosen medical facility. Often labor appears to have started, only to stop a short time later. This may be *false labor* and is difficult to distinguish from the real thing. True labor is characterized by steady continuous contractions that increase in intensity despite any change of position by the woman. If the woman has contractions while in an upright position, she should be encouraged to lie on her side for a time to see if the contractions continue. Similarly, if she is lying down when contractions begin, she should stand and walk around. If the contractions stop due to a change of position, this may indicate false labor. Loss of the mucous plug, evidenced by a slight blood-tinged mucous discharge from the vagina, normally accompanies or slightly precedes onset of labor. Sometimes the amniotic sac ruptures, causing a rush of fluid from the vagina. Rupture may occur before the onset of labor or as late as stage two. The attendant should time the length of and the interval between contractions to determine the woman's progress in first-stage labor. The first-aider can detect each contraction by placing a hand on the woman's abdomen and feeling the increasing firmness as the uterus contracts and the softening as the uterus relaxes. *Generally, when contractions are steady and spaced approximately five minutes apart, the physician or midwife should be notified and the woman transported to the place where she has planned to give birth.*

During the early portion of first-stage labor, the woman should be encouraged to carry on any normal activities in which she was engaged when contractions first started. Some women make the mistake of lying down immediately when labor begins. Unless the woman is checking for false labor by changing positions, lying down is probably unnecessary. Relaxing in a chair with a good book, or doing some light work or other nonvigorous activity, can help the expectant mother take her mind off the discomfort she may be feeling.

As labor progresses and the contractions become longer and more intense, the woman should be encouraged to find a position that affords her the most comfort and enhances her ability to relax during and between contractions. During contractions, she should try to relax her whole body so that muscles in her arms, legs, back, neck, face, and other regions are not tense. The first-aider can enhance the mother's relaxation by being calm and praising her for the progress she is making and by controlling her environment as much as possible by dimming the lights, adjusting the room temperature for comfort, and minimizing distracting noise. The first-aider can also help the mother by identifying points of muscular tension such as a furrowed brow, clenched fist or jaw, or tightened neck muscles. This tension during labor is frequently unnoticed by the woman, but contributes to discomfort, pain, and fatigue. Between active contractions she should rest, but not sleep. The rationale offered for the latter is that being awakened by a uterine contraction may result in panic and fear, leading to a subjective intensification of pain. While resting, the woman may find back rubs, leg massages, or sponge baths helpful. She should be encouraged to urinate frequently, since a full bladder can impede labor.

Usually most women are in a medical care setting by the time the transitional phase of labor begins. However, if this is not the case, the first-aider should be able to recognize from signs and symptoms that the woman's cervix is almost completely dilated. During the transitional phase, the woman may panic, become extremely fearful, and entertain negative, foreboding thoughts as to her ability to cope with labor and actually deliver her baby. This type of reaction, while not uncommon, must be controlled as much as possible. The attendant first-aider remains calm, appears confident, and helps the woman regain control. This is best accomplished by grasping her wrists with both hands, looking her directly in the eyes, and empathetically and firmly communicating words of praise and support. *The woman must be encouraged to take one contraction at a time.* Helping her focus on the immediate task of relaxing through the present contraction is essential. The first-aider should refrain from making any negative comments. Fortunately, by the time contractions are of sufficient intensity to cause panic, the first stage of pregnancy is usually almost over.

Other signs and symptoms indicative of the transitional phase include extreme mood swings, anger, frustration, nausea, vomiting, belching, hot flashes, and lack of desire to communicate. This is a difficult time for the woman, and she must be empathetically supported. By recognizing the hallmarks of the transitional period, the attendant can inform her that labor is almost finished, thus rekindling her hope and optimism.

Development of the urge to push or have a bowel movement often signals the end of first-stage labor and the start of the second stage, in which the baby moves through the cervical opening into the birth canal. Ideally, a woman at this stage would find herself in a cozy environment attended by highly trained and experienced obstetric personnel. However, if for any reason this is not the case, the first-aider must quickly make some important decisions. Transportation to a nearby hospital may be feasible, either by private car or by ambulance depending on the stage of delivery of the mother. If an ambulance staffed by paramedics can arrive quickly, this alternative is better than the first aider trying to transport the woman to the hospital in a private automobile.

If an ambulance is unavailable, the first-aider must elicit information that will aid in the decision either to transport the expectant mother or to provide assistance at her present location. The attending first-aider should

1 Ask the woman if this is her first baby. Usually second-stage labor is longer for first births than for subsequent ones.
2 Ask the woman if she feels an urge to push or to have a bowel movement.
3 Determine if the baby is crowning. This may be difficult and embarrassing for both the first-aider and the woman but is necessary to determine how far labor has progressed. The first-aider requests permission to check the woman's progress, and then carefully removes or shifts her clothing to visualize the perineum. If the vagina is bulging or the top portion of the infant's head is visible, then indeed the baby is crowning and birth may be just minutes away. When examining the woman for crowning, the first-aider should communicate the purpose of this to the woman and protect her privacy to the extent possible (particularly when bystanders are at the delivery scene).

If this is the expectant mother's first childbirth experience, if she has no urge to push or to have a bowel movement, and if the baby is not crowning, most likely she should be transported to a nearby medical facility, if possible, by private auto if an ambulance is not immediately available. Even if this is not the first childbirth for the woman, if there is no urge to push or any sign of crowning there still may be time for transport. The mother should be transported in a reclining position or one that she finds particularly comforta-

**TABLE 16.1**

Useful Supplies for Emergency Childbirth

- Plastic bags or sheeting to protect bedding or car upholstery
- Newspapers for padding and protection of bedding
- Clean towels
- Clean sheets for privacy of mother
- Blankets for mother and baby
- Pillows
- Sterile ties for umbilical cord
- Sterile razor blade for cutting cord
- Rubbing alcohol (70% isopropyl alcohol) for sterilization of supplies if boiling water is unavailable
- Sanitary napkins for mother
- Diapers (disposable or cloth)
- Safety pins
- Scissors
- Large container for placenta
- Disposable underpads
- Bulb syringe for suctioning infant's nose and mouth
- Washcloths
- Soap and water

ble, with a clean sheet or blanket under her buttocks. Preferably the father, a friend, or another first-aider should sit with her to provide comfort and encouragement on the way to the hospital. At this stage the woman should not be allowed to go to the bathroom for a bowel movement, and she should not attempt to delay the delivery in any way. **She should not cross her legs or hold her knees together, because this is extremely dangerous for the baby!**

If either the baby's head is visible or the woman is intent on pushing, it is too late for transport. Hurrying off to a hospital at this point will only ensure that the woman delivers in the confined quarters of an automobile rather than indoors in a setting more conducive to comfort and relaxation.

When special circumstances dictate that a birth must occur outside of a hospital or birth center, preparations must be made for the mother to deliver wherever she is. The supplies listed in Table 16.1 should be available if at all possible for the emergency childbirth. If at home, the supplies that require sterilization should be put in boiling water for at least ten minutes or completely soaked in isopropyl alcohol for a minimum of twenty to thirty minutes. These include the scissors; the single-edged razor blade; and the rope, shoelaces, or sterile gauze to be used for tying and cutting the cord. If the materials cannot be sterilized, they should be made as clean as possible. The first-aider also thoroughly cleans his or her hands and arms with soap and hot water, if possible.

# ___PREPARING THE WOMAN FOR BIRTH (SECOND STAGE OF LABOR)

The woman should remove all underclothing that could interfere with delivery. She should lie in a semireclining position on a sturdy, flat surface such as a table or bed, preferably the latter if she is at home. If a table is used, it should be padded with blankets to provide the most comfort possible. A clean sheet should be placed under the woman's buttocks. A plastic bag or waterproof pad can be used under the sheet to protect the mattress or blankets from being soaked with the fluids that accompany delivery. To enlist the aid of gravity in the birth process, pillows and supports are used to elevate the woman's torso above her pelvis. If in a car, the woman can slump down sitting in the back seat and deliver the baby over the edge of the seat into the hands of the first-aider. If on a country road in warm weather, the delivery could occur outside the car on newspapers or blankets spread on the ground. Clean newspaper or clothing can take the place of a clean sheet under the buttocks.

It two attendants are available, one should be stationed at the expectant mother's head to provide encouragement and physical support and to assist in gently turning the woman's head if she begins to vomit. The other should be in a position to support and guide the baby from the birth canal.

A large pan should be positioned near the place of delivery to receive the placenta during the third stage of labor. A dishpan or large pot serves the purpose well. Clean sheets or other materials should be used to drape the expectant mother without obstructing the perineal area.

As the time of birth approaches, the woman is kept as calm as possible and is given affirming feedback. The first-aider can enhance the birth process by developing a strong rapport with her and communicating in a positive manner what is happening and the joy they will soon experience. As the contractions intensify and the urge to push is felt, the woman should be in position to give birth, usually in a semireclining position with the legs apart and knees drawn upward. If the woman has a strong urge to bear down she may do so, but should not unduly strain herself. The uterus will continue to contract and push the baby down through the birth canal. The vagina will stretch to accommodate the baby, but some tearing of the perineum near the vaginal opening may occur as the head is pushed out. This should not be of immediate concern to the first-aider. Any tearing can be medically treated later.

As the baby's head appears, the first-aider places one hand immediately under the vaginal opening and with a clean cloth or sheet protects the baby's head from coming in contact with the mother's anal area. The other hand is placed on the infant's head to prevent its "explosive" delivery (Figure 16.8). When the head emerges from the vagina it should turn naturally to one side or the other. **Caution: the baby's head should never be forced or pulled.**

Usually after the head is delivered the mother can be encouraged to relax for a minute or two. During this time the first-aider checks to make sure the umbilical cord is

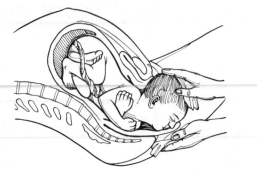

**◀FIGURE 16.8**

As the baby's head appears, the first-aider protects the face with a clean cloth and positions his or her hands to prevent rapid expulsion.

**FIGURE 16.9▶**

If the umbilical cord is wrapped around the infant's neck, the first-aider uses the index finger gently to remove it.

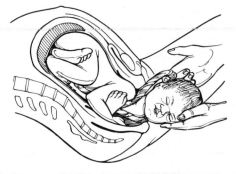

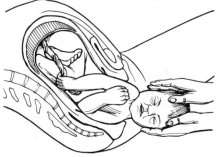

**◀FIGURE 16.10**

The first-aider supports the baby's head as the upper shoulder is delivered.

**FIGURE 16.11▶**

The baby's head is guided upward to help delivery of the lower shoulder.

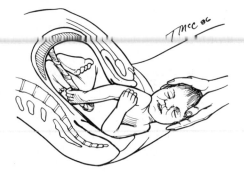

not wrapped around the infant's neck. If it is, it is removed by inserting an index finger between the baby's neck and the cord and *gently* slipping the cord over the infant's head (Figure 16.9).

After the emergence and rotation of the baby's head to one side, the shoulders are naturally positioned to pass through the maternal pelvic opening. Since the shoulders are too wide to pass through together, the upper shoulder is usually delivered first. The first-aider continues to support the head, and on delivery of the initial shoulder (Figure 16.10), guides the baby's head upward to assist delivery of the second shoulder (Figure 16.11). The mother delivers the baby—the first-aider simply assists the mother by guiding the baby out. **The baby should never be pulled!**

With the head and shoulders delivered, the rest of the infant's body usually follows quickly. Great care is needed in handling the infant, as a newborn is very slippery and difficult to hold. After delivery, the baby should be held with the head slightly lower than the body and the face turned sideward to permit drainage of any mucus that may be in the nose or throat. A sterile gauze or cloth may be used to wipe blood and mucus away from the baby's mouth and nose. If a clean rubber suction bulb is available, the first-aider uses it to remove excess oral and nasal mucus by compressing the bulb, inserting the tip into the infant's mouth and nose, and releasing the bulb to draw mucus into the syringe (Figure 16.12).

Normally the baby begins to breath a few seconds after delivery. The baby may be somewhat ashen or white at birth but usually turns pink within minutes after commencement of breathing. The baby is placed on a clean sheet and kept warm or is given directly to the mother, covered, and cuddled on her abdomen or breast.

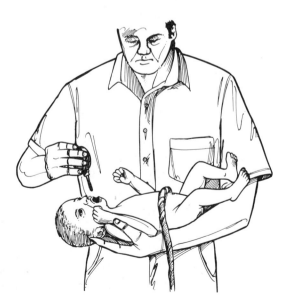

**FIGURE 16.12**

After delivery, the infant's head is held lower than its body to allow drainage of mucus. A suction bulb can be used to remove excess.

**FIGURE 16.13**

Sterile laces are tied on the umbilical cord after pulsation ceases to stop the flow of blood. The cord is cut with a sterile scissors or razor blade.

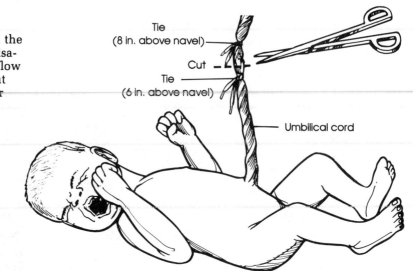

In handling the newborn, the first-aider should ensure that the umbilical cord is not pulled or stretched, since the baby is still attached by way of it to the placenta, which remains in the mother's uterus. The umbilical cord usually appears as a fat, pale-blue cord; it continues to pulsate for a few minutes after delivery and then stops, becoming thinner and more pale. The cord need not be cut immediately after birth or even at all by the first-aider if the mother is to be transported to the hospital. The procedure can be performed at the hospital with the proper sterilized supplies by trained medical staff. **If, however, transport is out of the question, the first-aider should cut the umbilical cord only after it stops pulsating.** The cord should be cut in the following manner: Two sterile ropes or laces are tied in two places on the cord, two inches apart and the first one approximately six to eight inches from the infant's navel, as shown in Figure 16.13. The ties should be tight enough to stop the flow of blood through the cord, but not so tight that the lace actually cuts the cord. Using a sterile razor blade or scissors, the first-aider cuts the cord between the two ties. The cut ends are then examined to make sure they are not bleeding. **If the cord is not tied off completely the baby could bleed to death.** If the cord is found to be leaking blood from the tied end, another sterile tie is placed just below the first (closer to the baby). **No attempt should be made to loosen and retie the initial ligation.**

After the cord has been appropriately tied and severed, the infant is wrapped in warm blankets, approximately as many layers as required by the adults present, and placed on the mother's breast or abdomen. If possible the first-aider records the time of delivery.

## THE AFTERBIRTH (THIRD STAGE OF LABOR)

Shortly after delivery, uterine contractions resume with the purpose of expelling the placenta. Typically the placenta is delivered within thirty minutes of the birth of the baby. The placenta detaches from the uterine wall and is delivered through the vagina with considerably less work than that required for delivery of the infant. The mother may assist with its delivery by gently bearing down after it detaches. **Caution: The umbilical cord should NEVER be pulled in an effort to speed things along.** Pulling may tear the cord or damage the uterus, thus provoking hemorrhage and fatal blood loss by the mother. The delivered placenta is placed in a large pan previously positioned for this purpose.

Once the placenta has been delivered, the first-aider gently massages the mother's abdomen, which will stimulate the uterus to contract and stop the bleeding. The mother should encourage the infant to suckle her breast at this time, because breast feeding causes the release of a hormone that also stimulates the uterus to begin contracting to its normal size, thus aiding in the control of bleeding. As noted, the placenta is normally delivered intact and should be placed in the designated container and kept for inspection by a physician or midwife.

After expulsion of the placenta, a moderate amount of bleeding is to be expected, possibly as much as two cupfuls. The first-aider can minimize the amount of blood loss and lessen the possibility of shock by firmly massaging the mother's lower abdomen every five minutes or so. When bleeding has slowed, the perineum can be gently washed with clean soapy water and a sanitary napkin or pad placed over the vaginal opening. The mother should be kept warm and comfortable. She is encouraged to drink liquids such as orange or apple juice to replace fluids lost in bleeding and to replenish her energy supply. The attending first-aider might also help the mother wash her hands and face and comb her hair, to be refreshed after completion of an exhausting task. She should be given an opportunity to sleep if she desires, confident that her baby will be well cared for by the husband, relative, friend, or first-aider.

Figure 16.14 shows the steps for assisting at an uncomplicated delivery.

# ___DELIVERY COMPLICATIONS

While the birth of most babies is routine and relatively straightforward, some situations seriously complicate the birth process. The first-aider should have enough knowledge to recognize a true emergency childbirth, so that appropriate steps can be taken to transport the mother to a hospital.

## ___Breech Presentation

Occasionally the infant's buttocks or feet, rather than the head, emerge from the birth canal first (Figure 16.15, inset). This is called a *breech presentation* and is one of the most common complications of delivery. A breech presentation should, if at all possible, be handled by trained medical personnel. However, if the woman is away from the hospital, the birth is imminent, and it is not possible to secure skilled medical personnel, the attending first-aider must provide assistance.

The infant's buttocks, legs, and torso are usually spontaneously delivered. The attending first-aider places one hand between the baby's legs and extends the hand forward to support it. While support for the infant is firm, the legs are allowed to dangle,

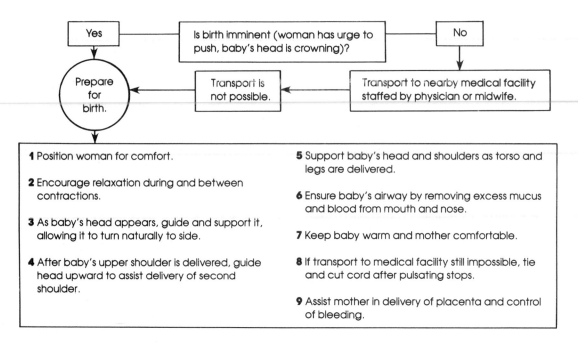

**FIGURE 16.14**

Steps in assisting at an uncomplicated delivery

so that gravity can aid delivery of the head. The infant's legs and torso are kept warm before delivery of the head to minimize the stimulation to breathing caused by cold air. The baby may be facing up or down in a breech presentation. Regardless of position, the infant's torso must be supported to allow safe and rapid delivery of the head.

The baby's head usually delivers on its own within a few minutes of the buttocks and torso. The mother is encouraged to bear down with contractions to expedite the process. **If the head takes longer than three minutes to emerge from the birth canal, a dangerous condition may develop.** The circulation in the umbilical cord may be impeded as it is squeezed between the birth canal and the baby's head. This can result in the baby receiving inadequate oxygen. Another possible consequence is that the infant will begin spontaneous breathing before its head clears the birth canal. The pressure of the vaginal wall on its nose and mouth may render breathing impossible. Thus, quick action is needed if the infant's head is not delivered within three to four minutes of the buttocks.

Whether the infant presents face up or face down, the first-aider must ensure that the infant has an airway. He or she thus inserts one hand into the mother's vagina (with the palm toward the infant's face), placing the index finger on one side of the nose and the middle finger on the other side (Figure 16.15). Pressure is then exerted by the back of the fingers on the vagina, to lift it away from the baby's face. **The baby should not be**

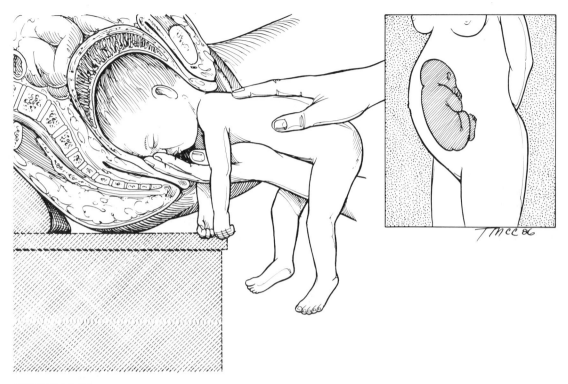

**FIGURE 16.15**

Management of breech presentation. If the baby's head does not deliver within three minutes, the first-aider makes an airway with the index and middle fingers.

**pulled from the vagina by the legs or torso**. Delivery of the head should occur spontaneously as a result of uterine contractions and strong pushing by the mother.

If the head does not deliver within three minutes of establishing an airway, the mother should be quickly transported to a hospital, the first-aider maintaining the baby's airway until the head is delivered or until the medical staff at the hospital takes charge of the birth.

## ▬ Multiple Births

The birth of twins is usually no surprise to a woman who has been receiving good prenatal care, although occasionally the presence of twins within the uterus is unknown even to the expectant mother's physician or midwife. Twins are delivered in the same manner as a single baby, one right after the other. After the first baby arrives, uterine contractions continue, and the second baby is usually born within minutes.

If the first-aider is aware that a second child is to be born, the umbilical cord of the first infant is tied to prevent hemorrhage of blood from one infant to the other. The same procedures for tying and cutting the cord can be followed for both babies. Since twins are often smaller than a single baby, special care must be taken to keep them warm and protected.

## ___Baby Not Breathing

If the baby does not initiate breathing on its own within thirty seconds after delivery, quick action must be taken. The first-aider makes sure that all excess mucus has been removed from the mouth and nose. The baby is stimulated by slapping the soles of the feet and rubbing the back (or both) while its head is kept lower than its trunk. If stimulation does not initiate breathing, mouth-to-mouth-and-nose resuscitation should be started, as described in Chapter 5. If resuscitation is unsuccessful after two minutes and no pulse is detectable, CPR must be started immediately (Chapter 6). The infant and mother should be transported to the hospital quickly, with the first-aider continuing CPR efforts.

Some babies are born dead and resuscitation is not indicated. Usually the first-aider can determine such an occurrence by the disagreeable smell and the appearance of large blisters on the skin of the infant. This is an especially difficult situation, and the first-aider must provide as much emotional support as possible to the grieved mother or both parents.

## ___Prolapsed Umbilical Cord

Occasionally the umbilical cord emerges from the birth canal before the baby (Figure 16.16). The danger of this complication is similar to that in the breech birth, where

**FIGURE 16.16**

Prolapsed umbilical cord. (*A*) The baby's head squeezes the cord and impairs circulation. (*B*) Pressure is relieved by gently pushing the infant's head up two or three inches. (*C*) The mother is transported to the hospital in the knee-chest position to keep the baby's weight from bearing down on the cord.

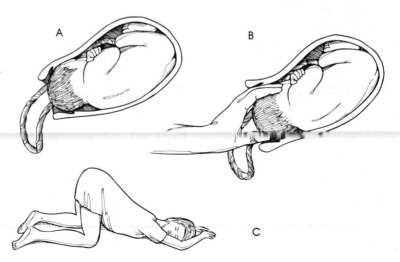

circulation in the cord is impaired as a result of its being squeezed between the vagina and the infant's head during crowning.

In this situation the first-aider must get the expectant mother to a hospital. In the meantime, she must be positioned so as to elevate the vaginal opening above the uterus, to prevent the weight of the baby from pushing down on the vagina and the protruding umbilical cord. Placing the mother in the knee-chest position (Figure 16.16C) is probably the best procedure, although an exaggerated shock position (the legs and pelvis elevated above the head) may also be used.

If the first-aider has access to a sterile glove, he or she should insert a hand into the vagina and gently push the baby's head up two or three inches to relieve pressure on the cord (Figure 16.16B), and should maintain this position until hospital personnel assume command. The first-aider should not attempt to return the cord to the vagina, but should loosely wrap it with a sterile towel and if possible keep it moist with sterile saline solution on the way to the hospital.

## Limb Presentation

Infrequently an infant shifts position during birth so that an arm, a leg, or a shoulder, or a combination, is the first part of the baby to present in the vaginal opening. In this situation the only first aid action to be taken is to **transport the expectant mother to a medical facility immediately!**

## Premature Birth

A baby who is born before the seventh month of pregnancy or weighs less than 2500 grams (5½ pounds) is considered premature. The mother usually knows the expected due date so that the degree of prematurity can be computed. A premature baby, identified by the mother's information or the small size of the infant or both, must receive special care. The infant is especially susceptible to infection and must be protected accordingly. Enroute to the hospital it should be kept warm, wrapped snuggly in a blanket, positioned in an area free of drafts, and kept from contact with all but the mother and the first-aider who has assisted in delivery.

## Spontaneous Abortion (Miscarriage)

A spontaneous abortion (miscarriage) is defined as delivery of the fetus and placenta before the twenty-eighth week of pregnancy, before the fetus can normally be expected to survive outside the womb on its own. Any bleeding from the vagina during pregnancy may indicate a possible spontaneous abortion, and the woman should immediately be evaluated by her physician. In a spontaneous abortion, the woman is in danger of excessive blood loss and must be cared for as though in shock. Sterile napkins or cloths should be placed over the vaginal opening in an effort to control bleeding. Nothing should be inserted into the uterus, and the cord or fetus must not be pulled. The woman should be quickly transported to a medical facility. *Any tissue delivered from the vagina should be saved and given to the physician for examination.*

_____ **SUMMARY** _____

Labor and delivery usually proceed in a routine manner without complications. The mother delivers her baby and the first-aider provides assistance. The person attending an emergency birth must be able to evaluate the situation quickly to determine if transport to a medical facility is possible. If birth is imminent, preparations for childbirth must be made regardless of the setting. The first-aider provides confident support and encouragement for the woman, attends to her needs, and enables her to cope effectively with the discomfort of uterine contractions. During birth, the first-aider guides the delivery of the infant but does not force or pull the baby in any way. He or she provides immediate care for the newborn and enlists the help of friends or family of the mother, if available. The first-aider needs also to know what to do for unusual deliveries or complications, so that the mother and child receive the best possible care.

_____ **CHAPTER MASTERY: TEST ITEMS** _____

**True and False**                                                                          **Circle One**

1. Labor and delivery in most pregnancies are accompanied by complications.                      T          F

2. In the first stage of labor, the cervix dilates to approximately ten centimeters to accommodate passage of the baby into the birth canal.    T          F

3. During the early phase of first-stage labor, uterine contractions are usually very intense and prolonged.    T          F

4. In active labor, fear of expected pain associated with childbirth may prolong labor and intensify the discomfort experienced by the pregnant woman.    T          F

5. Second-stage labor ends with the birth of the baby.                                         T          F

6. Real labor is easy to distinguish from false labor.                                         T          F

7. When labor first begins, the expectant mother must cease other activities and lie down.    T          F

8. The transitional phase of first-stage labor is often characterized by the mother-to-be experiencing anger and extreme moodiness.    T          F

9. The best way of coping with the discomfort of labor is for the woman to grit her teeth and tightly grip the first-aider's hand.    T          F

10. Proper care of the umbilical cord by the birth attendant is important for the well-being of both mother and infant.    T          F

## Fill In the Missing Word(s)

1. The function of the placenta during pregnancy is _____.
2. Babies born before the thirty-seventh week of pregnancy are considered _____, while full-term infants who weigh less than 5½ pounds are called _____.
3. True labor is characterized by steady contractions that remain _____ despite changes of _____ by the mother.
4. The first stage of labor ends when the cervix has completely _____.
5. The bulging of the maternal perineum due to the downward pressure of the infant's head (visible in the vaginal opening) is called _____.
6. In deciding whether to transport the expectant mother in labor or to provide assistance at her present location, the first-aider should elicit the following information: _____, _____, and _____.
7. The infant's buttocks emerging from the birth canal first is called a _____ presentation.
8. If the newborn does not initiate breathing on its own within thirty seconds of delivery, the first-aider should _____.
9. In handling the newborn, the first-aider should ensure that the _____ is not pulled or stretched, since the baby is still attached by way of it to the placenta.
10. In an effort to prevent undue distress, the first-aider should encourage the mother-to-be to handle one _____ at a time and focus only on the immediate task at hand.

## Multiple Choice (Circle the Best Answer)

1. During the transitional phase of first-stage labor, the first-aider should
   a. leave the woman alone.
   b. encourage the woman to breast feed the infant when it arrives.
   c. provide strong emotional support and encourage the woman to relax.
   d. encourage the woman to slow down labor by holding her legs together.
   e. encourage the woman to stand and walk during the uterine contractions.
2. Breast feeding of the infant after delivery of the placenta
   a. increases maternal blood loss.
   b. is impossible for most mothers.
   c. makes the baby cold.
   d. helps contract the uterus and control bleeding.
   e. prolongs third-stage labor.
3. When the umbilical cord emerges from the birth canal prior to the baby,
   a. the situation is called a breech birth.
   b. the mother should be positioned so as to elevate the vaginal opening above the uterus.
   c. the first-aider should not be concerned, since this is a common occurrence.
   d. the first-aider should pull on the cord.
   e. the mother should be encouraged to push.

4. All of the following indicate that real labor has begun EXCEPT
   a. loss of the mucus that plugs the cervical opening.
   b. consistent uterine contractions despite changes in physical position by the expectant mother.
   c. rupture of the amniotic sac.
   d. contractions increasing in intensity.
   e. active fetal movement within the uterus.

5. In preparing the mother for second-stage labor, the first-aider does all of the following EXCEPT
   a. allow her to go to the bathroom for a bowel movement when she feels the urge to do so.
   b. examine her for evidence of crowning.
   c. help her remove all clothing that could interfere with the birth.
   d. provide calm, affirming encouragement and support.
   e. position her so that she is comfortable, preferably with the torso slightly higher than the pelvis.

## Discussion Questions

1. A first-aider receives a telephone call from a next-door neighbor who is pregnant for the first time and thinks she may be in labor. She doesn't want to go to the hospital if it is false labor, but wants to make sure she gets there in time if her labor is real. How might the first-aider help her determine if and when she should go to the hospital?

2. While driving along a street in a residential area, a woman sees a man run out of his house. He frantically waves at her. She stops her car and is informed that the man's wife is in labor and that his car won't start. The first-aider accompanies the man into the house to assist him in getting his wife and her belongings into her car for the trip to the hospital. She discovers that the woman is on her way to the bathroom with an uncontrollable urge to have a bowel movement. What should the first-aider do?

3. A first-aider is providing care at an emergency childbirth. The expectant mother in active labor panics and begins screaming hysterically. What should the first-aider do to help her regain her composure?

4. During an emergency childbirth, a first-aider notices that the baby's buttocks are crowning, rather than the head. What procedures should be followed in assisting with the birth of this baby?

5. A first-aider is assisting at an emergency childbirth. The umbilical cord emerges from the birth canal before the baby does. What should be done?

## BIBLIOGRAPHY

Bradley, R. A. *Husband-Coached Childbirth*. New York: Harper and Row Publishers, 1974.

Brewer, G. S., and J. P. Greene. *Right from the Start*. Emmaus, Pa.: Rodale Press, 1981.

Grant, H. D., R. H. Murray, and J. D. Bergeron. *Emergency Care*. 3d ed. Bowie, Md.: Robert J. Brady, 1978.

Hafen, B. Q. *First Aid for Health Emergencies*. 2d ed. St. Paul: West Publishing, 1981.

Reeder, S. J., L. Mastroianni, and L. L. Martin. *Maternity Nursing*. 14th ed. Philadelphia: J. B. Lippincott, 1980.

White, G. J. *Emergency Childbirth: A Manual*. Franklin Park, Ill.: Gordon R. Carson Police Training Foundation, 1978.

# 17

# Bandaging

STEPHEN H. STEWART, DR.P.H.

After completing this chapter the student will be able to
* Differentiate between a bandage and a dressing.
* Identify appropriate materials for use as bandages and dressings.
* Demonstrate the ability to apply a dressing properly in a first aid situation.
* Demonstrate the ability to apply the appropriate bandage properly in a first aid situation.

## ___INTRODUCTION

Application of bandages is one of the primary skills of first aid. It is also the most frequently used skill. The skill has two distinct aspects: application of a *dressing* (alternately called a *compress*), and application of a *bandage*. Techniques for the application of both are based on the type of injury encountered, the supplies available, and the skill of the first-aider.

The dressing is the covering placed directly on the wound. The dressing should, if at all possible, be sterile at the time of application and should provide an effective cover for the wound, to prevent contamination. It also assists in controlling hemorrhage and absorbing blood and other secretions. Dressings can be made of any absorbent lint-free material. Those most commonly used are sterile, prepackaged, multilayer gauze units. These are readily available in various sizes, most commonly two-by-two inches, three-by-three inches, and four-by-four inches. Alternatively, sterile dressings can be prepared by wrapping the dressing material in foil and heating it to 350° F for three hours.

A bandage is any material used to hold a dressing in place. Its purposes are to provide pressure, which controls bleeding and reduces swelling, and to immobilize and support the injury. Since the bandage does not directly contact the wound, sterile material is not required; however, the material should be clean. Bandages can be classified as *roller*, *triangular*, or *adhesive*.

In addition to the kinds of bandages and dressings just described, prepackaged sterile dressing–bandage combinations are available commercially (Figure 17.1). The most common of these is the *adhesive compress* (Band-Aid) commonly used for small wounds. More commonly used in emergency situations is the *bandage compress*. This includes a gauze dressing centrally attached to a long tail of gauze or muslin. It is available in various standard sizes. The *general purpose dressing* is a large, very thick sterile dressing that may or may not have tails or be waterproof. It is a multipurpose unit commercially available in several sizes, and is of value in covering both large wounds and burns.

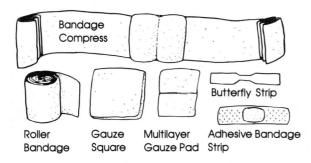

**FIGURE 17.1**
Common commercial bandages and dressings

# ___GENERAL GUIDELINES FOR APPLICATION OF DRESSINGS AND BANDAGES

## ___Dressings

In selecting and placing a dressing, the first-aider should follow certain rules:

1 Select a dressing that will extend an inch beyond the wound in all directions.
2 Avoid contaminating the dressing either by touching that portion of it that will be placed on the wound or by coughing or breathing on it.
3 Lower the dressing directly onto the wound rather than sliding it on.
4 If the first dressing becomes saturated with blood, add another dressing on top without disturbing the original.

**Once placed, a dressing should not be disturbed.**

## ___Bandages

In selecting and placing a bandage, the first-aider should follow certain rules:

1 The bandage need not be sterile but should be clean.
2 Place the bandage so that it covers the entire dressing.
3 Place the bandage snugly enough so that, once in place, it will not slip, but not so snugly that it interferes with circulation.
4 Leave extremities exposed, if possible, so that signs of decreased circulation such as swelling, discoloration, and coldness can be observed. If this occurs, loosen the bandage and reapply it without disturbing the dressing.
5 Take particular care if a gauze bandage has become wet. A wet gauze bandage will shrink as it dries, causing interference with circulation. If a gauze bandage must be applied while wet, allow sufficient room for shrinkage.
6 Do not place bandages of materials that do not stretch, such as tape, completely around an injured part, as any swelling will then cause the bandage to decrease circulation. Never place a circular bandage around the neck.

**Andrew Carnegie Library
Livingstone College
701 W. Monroe St.
Salisbury, N.C. 28144**

## ____ TYPES OF BANDAGES

### ___ Roller

As the name implies, roller bandages are strips of material commonly distributed in roll form. The two types most readily available are *gauze* bandages and *elastic* bandages. These come prepackaged in various widths, most commonly one, two, three, and four inches. Gauze bandages are ten yards long, while elastic bandages come in various lengths. The first-aider needs to choose the width appropriate for the application. For example, the first-aider would not want to use four-inch-wide gauze to bandage an injured finger or one-inch-wide gauze to bandage the adult arm.

Gauze bandages have a tendency to slip when applied; to avoid this, the bandage must be properly anchored (Figure 17.2):

1 Start the bandage with the end positioned on the bias.
2 Encircle the injured part, allowing the biased end of the bandage to protrude.
3 Fold down the protruding end.
4 Circle the part again.
5 Bandage as required.

When bandaging is completed, the first-aider needs to secure the gauze. If neither a pin nor tape is available, the gauze must be tied off. One of two methods may be selected.
Split-tail method (Figure 17.3):

1 Cut the gauze off far enough beyond the last turn to assure adequate material for tying (normally, one half the circumference of the body part plus six inches).
2 Split the end lengthwise back to the last turn.
3 Pass one split-tail clockwise around the body part and one split-tail counterclockwise.
4 Tie off the tails, preferably with a square knot.

Loop method (Figure 17.4):

1 Take the gauze beyond the injured body part approximately one half its diameter.
2 Pass the gauze around the figure in such a way as to form a loop.
3 While holding the loop, pass the gauze back around the member in the reverse direction.
4 Tie the loop and the end together.

When using elastic bandages, the first-aider should be wary of overstretching the bandage. This common error can cause interference with circulation. Given this simple caution, the elastic bandage may be the easiest of all bandages to apply, since its elasticity allows it to conform to the injured part. To apply the elastic bandage, the first-aider should

Andrew Carnegie Library
Livingstone College
701 W. Monroe St.
Salisbury, N.C. 28144

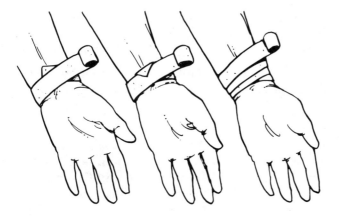

**FIGURE 17.2**
Anchoring a roller bandage

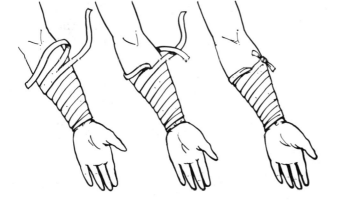

**FIGURE 17.3**
Split-tail method of securing a gauze bandage

**FIGURE 17.4**
Loop method of securing a gauze bandage

1 Begin at the lower end of the area to be covered.
2 Take two circular turns around the injured part.
3 Bandage as required.

When the bandaging is completed, the elastic bandage can be clipped (clips are usually provided with each bandage), pinned, or taped.

## __ Triangular

The triangular bandage (Figure 17.5) is one of the most versatile tools available to the first-aider. It is a large piece of material, normally muslin, cut in an isosceles triangle approximately forty inches on a side, with the hypotenuse being fifty-five inches. In its full unfolded condition, the triangular bandage can be used as a sling or as a covering for extensive wounds to the trunk, scalp, or other large area.

## __ Adhesive

The adhesive bandage is one of the most easily used of all bandages. When applied properly it should not interfere with circulation. Special adhesive strips called *butterfly* bandages (see Figure 17.1) are especially valuable in closing small lacerations. In applying an adhesive bandage, the first-aider should hold the wound shut and slightly overlapped, so that on relaxation after the bandage is applied it will return to correct alignment. Excessive pain is an indication of improper application. If pain persists the bandage should be reapplied.

# __ APPLICATION OF BANDAGES

The following deals with the application of bandages to various parts of the body. Use of the triangular bandage and the cravat is illustrated; other appropriate bandages are listed. When the cravat or triangular bandage is not the most appropriate, the preferred alternative bandage is illustrated. The type of bandage selected depends on the site and the extent of the injury involved. In all cases, a dressing must be in place before the bandage is applied.

## __ Bandages of the Head and Scalp

### Scalp Wounds

A triangular bandage is used to bandage scalp wounds. It is applied as follows (Figure 17.6):

1 Fold a two-inch hem lengthwise along the bias of the bandage.
2 Place the bandage over the head with the base, hem side out, across the forehead just above the eyes and the tail extending across the scalp and down the neck.

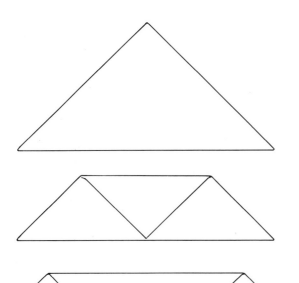

**FIGURE 17.5**
The triangular bandage, shown open and folded as a cravat, is the first-aider's most versatile tool. It can be used as a sling or to cover extensive wounds.

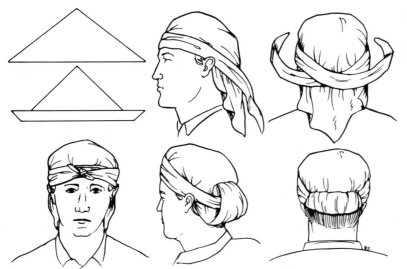

**FIGURE 17.6**
Application of the triangular bandage for a scalp wound

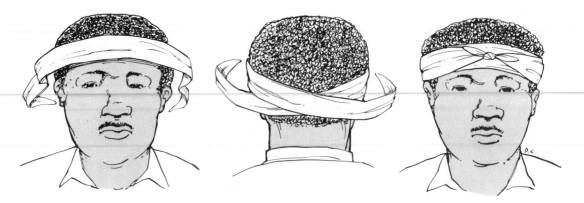

**FIGURE 17.7**

Application of the cravat for a forehead wound

3 Cross the two ends of the base over the tail and below the protrusion of the skull at the back of the head.
4 Tie the two base ends together in the middle of the forehead.
5 While gently holding the scalp area of the bandage, pull the tail of the bandage until it is snug over the entire scalp area.
6 Tuck the tail into the base at the rear of the skull.

### Forehead Wounds

To bandage forehead wounds, the first-aider may use either the cravat or any roller bandage. This bandage may also be used for eye or ear wounds. It is applied as follows (Figure 17.7):

1 Center the cravat over the wound.
2 Pass the tails around the skull and bring them back over the wound.
3 Tie directly over the wound (except in the case of eye injuries, when the tie will be above the bridge of the nose).

### Cheek Wounds

To bandage cheek wounds the first-aider may use the cravat or any roller bandage. This bandage may also be effective for wounds to the ear, the side of the forehead, or the chin. This bandage, in effect, **holds the mouth shut.** The first-aider should be wary of applying this bandage if the victim is in danger of vomiting, and it should never be applied if the person is unconscious. The cheek-wound bandage is applied as follows (Figure 17.8):

1 Center the cravat vertically over the injury (except in the case of a chin injury).
2 Pass the tails over the scalp and under the chin.
3 Meet the tails on the side of the skull away from the wound and above the level of the eyes.
4 Cross the bandage and bring the tails around the forehead and the back of the skull.

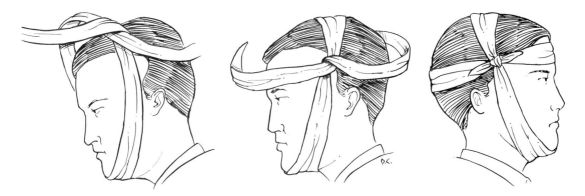

**FIGURE 17.8**

Application of a bandage for a wound to the cheek, ear, side of forehead, or chin

**5** Tie directly over the vertical strip of the bandage on the injured side. Tie with a bow to allow easy release should the victim begin to vomit.

### Chin Wounds

To bandage chin wounds, the first-aider uses a gauze bandage or another material. The chin-wound bandaging technique also works for wounds to the nose. The bandage is applied as follows (Figure 17.9):

**1** Cut off about three feet of four-inch gauze.
**2** Split both ends, leaving intact a center area large enough to cover the wound adequately.

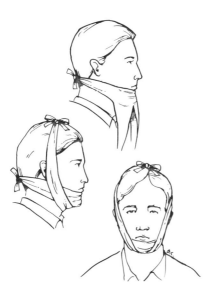

**FIGURE 17.9**

Application of bandage for a chin wound

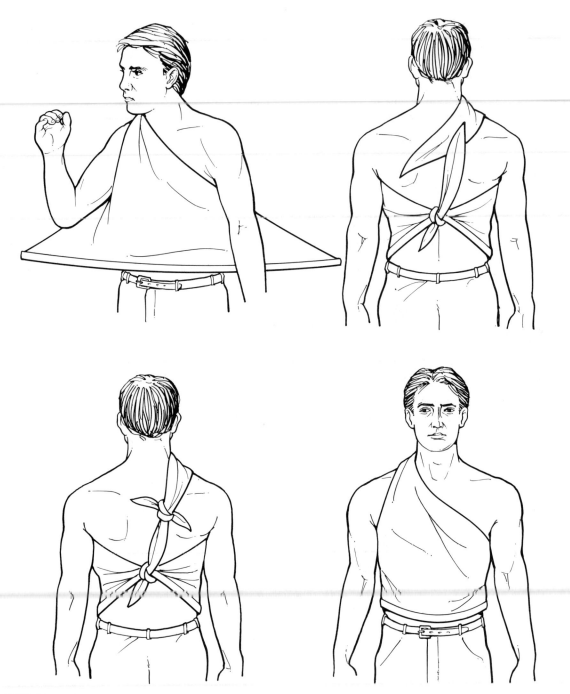

**FIGURE 17.10**

Application of a triangular bandage for burns or a large wound

**3** Center the bandage over the wound.

**4** Pass the two upper tails around the skull and tie in back below the level of the ears.

**5** Pass the two lower tails upward and tie at the top of the skull. Tie with a bow to allow for easy release should the victim vomit.

## ⎯ Bandages of the Trunk

Bandages of the trunk should be applied so that they do not interfere with respiration. Adhesive bandages applied to the dressing are, in most cases, adequate. However, in the case of burns or large wounds, a triangular bandage may be used to secure the dressing (Figure 17.10). The bandage is applied as follows (Figure 17.10):

**1** Place the point of the bandage over the shoulder on the injured side.

**2** Place a one-inch hem in the base and pass around the body.

**3** Tie off the two ends of the base on the opposite side of the body, leaving one end longer than the other.

**4** Tie the point to the longer tail of the base. If the point and base cannot be tied, tie a second cravat between the point and base to bridge the space. Secure the bandage.

## ⎯ Bandages of the Arms and Legs

### Shoulder/Hip Wounds

To bandage the shoulder (or the hip), both a triangular bandage and cravat or roller bandage are used. These bandages are applied as follows (Figure 17.11):

**1** Roll the point of the triangular bandage around the cravat several times to secure.

**2** Place the cravat over the neck on the injured side and under the armpit on the uninjured side. The triangular bandage should be centered over the injured shoulder. (For the hip, the cravat is placed around the waist).

**3** Tie the cravat just in front of the armpit.

**4** Fold the base of the triangular bandage to the desired length.

**5** Pass the ends around the arm (or leg) and tie.

### The Sling

The sling is not a bandage per se but is used as a support for an injury to the shoulder or arm. The triangular bandage is used as follows (Figure 17.12):

**1** Place the base of the triangular bandage vertically down the front of the chest with one end over the shoulder of the uninjured side.

**2** Bend the arm and place the point of the bandage behind the elbow on the injured side.

**3** Pick up the other end of the bandage and bring it upward over the neck on the injured side, picking up the lower arm in the process.

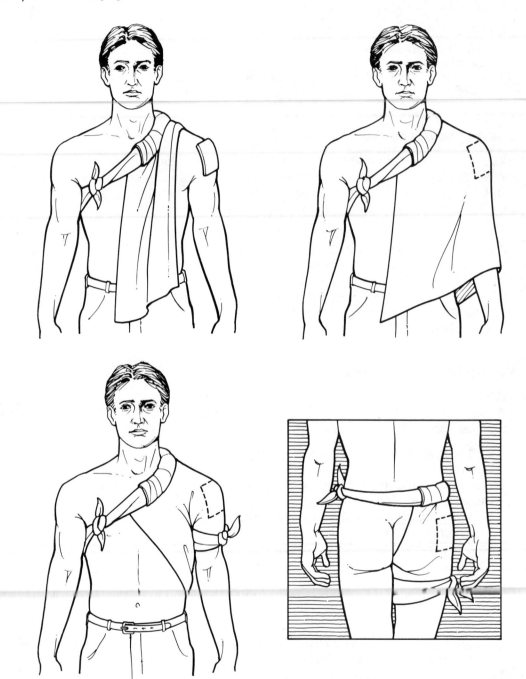

**FIGURE 17.11**

Application of both triangular and cravat bandages for a shoulder or hip wound

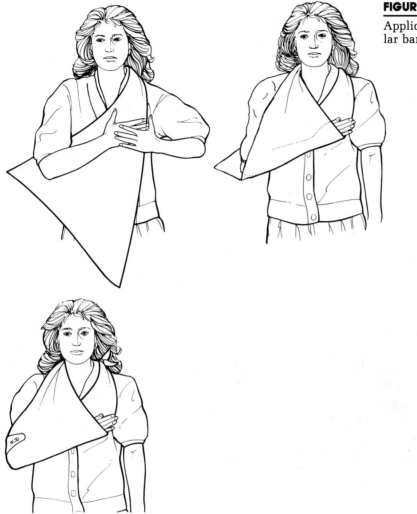

**FIGURE 17.12**
Application of the triangular bandage as a sling

4 Tie the base ends together so that the knot is not resting directly on the spinal column in the back.
5 Make sure that the hand within the sling is elevated approximately four inches, above the level of the elbow. If not, readjust the knot.
6 Make sure the fingertips are exposed and that the hand is in a thumbs-up position within the sling.
7 Twist the point of the bandage and tuck it in at the elbow, or pin the point to the body of the sling.

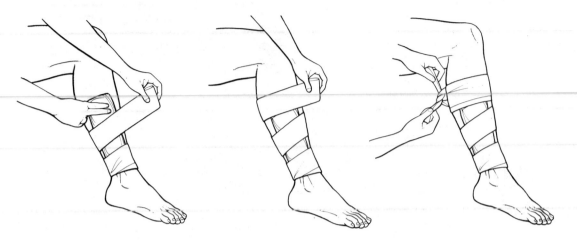

**FIGURE 17.13**

Application of the open spiral wrap

**Spiral Wraps of the Limb**

Spiral wraps are used on the long bones of the arm or leg. Either the cravat or a roller bandage works adequately. However, a roller bandage, especially elastic, is preferred. The bandage is applied as follows (Figure 17.13):

1 Anchor the bandage.
2 Spiral the bandage upward to cover the wound. The spiral is said to be *open* when the turns do not overlap (this is valuable in anchoring large dressings or splints), or the turns may overlap approximately three fourths of an inch, in which case the wrap is said to be *closed*.
3 Tie off the bandage as previously described.

## ___Bandages of the Knee or Elbow

Bandages for the knee and the elbow are developed to allow some motion in the joint. Either the cravat or roller bandage may be used. The bandage is applied as follows: (Figure 17.14):

1 Bend the elbow or knee slightly.
2 Center the cravat over the injury and carry the ends around the limb.
3 Pass the ends around to the site of the injury, with one end overlapping the upper margin of the bandage and one end overlapping the lower margin.
4 Continue around the limb, and tie off at the outside of the limb.

A

B

C

D

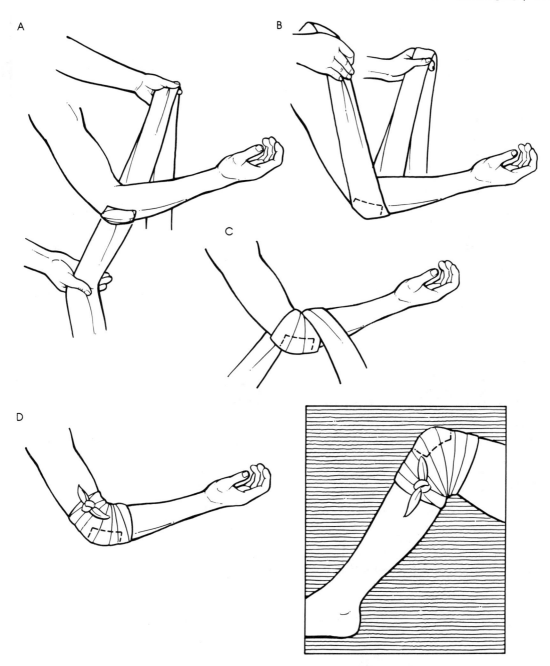

**FIGURE 17.14**

Application of a bandage (either cravat or roller) for an elbow or a knee wound. Some motion of the joint is needed.

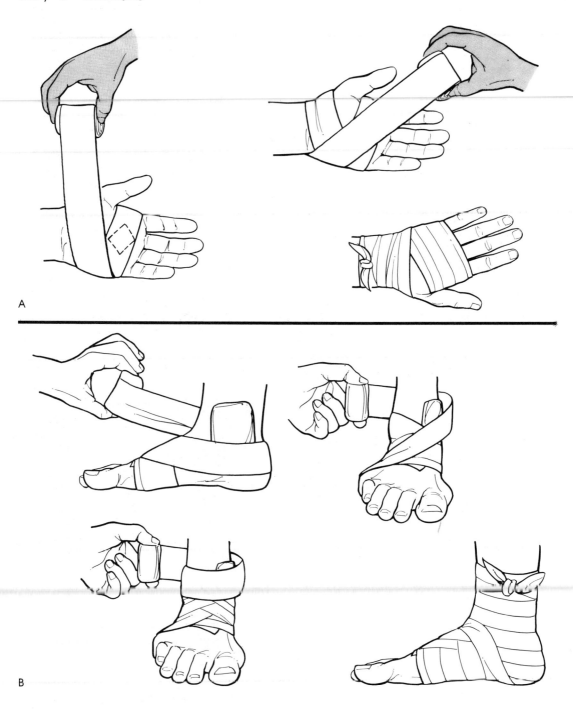

**FIGURE 17.15**

Application of a figure-eight bandage to the hand (*A*) and ankle (*B*)

# —Bandages of the Hands and Feet

### Figure-Eight Bandage for the Hand or Foot
The figure-eight bandage is used to secure a dressing to the foot or hand, and also to support the ankle and wrist. The roller bandage is preferred for this wrap.

**For the hand,** the figure-eight bandage is applied as follows (Figure 17.15*A*):

1 Anchor the bandage near the fingers and take two additional turns around the palm.
2 Carry the bandage across the back of the hand, around the wrist, and back across the palm.
3 Complete several turns, overlapping each by about two thirds of the bandage width.
4 Make two additional turns around the wrist, and tie.

**For the foot,** the figure-eight bandage is applied as follows (Figure 17.15*B*):

1 Anchor the bandage at the instep and make two or three turns around the instep and heel.
2 Make several figure-eight turns by taking the bandage diagonally across the front of the foot, around the ankle, and again diagonally across the foot and under the arch.
3 Make additional turns around the ankle, and tie.

### Pressure Bandage for the Hand
This bandage is used only in cases of severe bleeding and only for short periods. The cravat is the bandage of choice, but a roller bandage will suffice. The bandage is applied as follows (Figure 17.16):

1 Have the victim squeeze a dressing tightly in the fist.
2 Center the cravat over the palm side of the wrist.
3 Pass one end behind the wrist and up over the clenched fist at the little-finger side.
4 Pass the other end behind the wrist and up over the fist at the thumb side.
5 Pull down firmly.
6 Cross the ends in opposite directions around the wrist and tie at the side.

### Fingertip Bandage
This bandage is of value for wounds to the fingers or toes; it is difficult to apply, however. One-inch roller gauze is the material of choice. The bandage is applied as follows (Figure 17.17):

1 Make several folds of gauze approximately twice the length of the injured part.
2 Center the folds over the part.

**FIGURE 17.16**

Application of a pressure
bandage to the hand

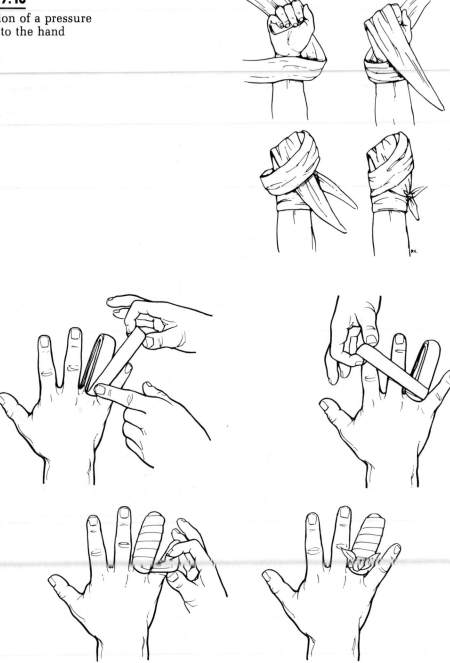

**FIGURE 17.17**

Application of a fingertip bandage with finger tie-off

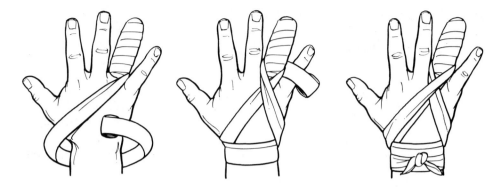

**FIGURE 17.18**
Alternate tie-off at the wrist for the fingertip bandage shown in Figure 17.17

**3** Spiral the gauze over the folds to the end of the injured part and then spiral back to the base.
**4** Pass the bandage around the part and make a split-tail tie-off at its base.

An alternate method of holding the fingertip bandage in place on a finger is to use a figure-eight turn as follows (Figure 17.18):

**1** After spiraling the gauze over the folds to the base of the injured finger, pass the bandage across the back of the hand, around the wrist twice, and back across the back of the hand to the finger, forming a figure eight.
**2** Pass the bandage around the finger and repeat the sequence as necessary.
**3** Make a split-tail tie-off at the wrist.

## SUMMARY

Bandaging is one of the crucial skills developed by the first-aider. Bandaging includes application of both dressings and bandages. The dressing, which should be sterile if possible, is applied directly to the wound, and the bandage covers it completely. The first-aider must select the proper bandage, on the basis of knowledge of the site and type of injury and of the materials available for bandaging. The proper techniques bandage application can be learned only through repeated practice.

## CHAPTER MASTERY: TEST ITEMS

**True and False**                                                                                     **Circle One**

1. The dressing is used to hold the bandage in place.                    T    F
2. To secure a dressing to the arm, wrap tape completely around the limb.    T    F

3. Use of the elastic bandage presents no hazard.          **T**     **F**
4. In most situations, dressings need to be clean but not sterile.     **T**     **F**
5. Only a physician should loosen a bandage.          **T**     **F**

**Discussion Questions**

1. In each of the following situations, how should the first-aider bandage the injury? (Be specific as to dressing selection and technique of bandaging.)
    a. A woman falls on a bottle and incurs a severe lesion of the palm.
    b. A young girl falls off her bike and has a four-inch laceration of her right forearm.
    c. A man falls while motorcycling and severely lacerates his chin.
    d. A young woman falls while skiing and severely lacerates her thigh.
    e. A man cuts his right index finger severely while fixing dinner.
2. Define each of the following:
    a. Bandage
    b. Dressing
    c. Gauze bandage
    d. Combination bandage
    e. Triangular bandage

―――――――――――――――― **BIBLIOGRAPHY** ――――――――――――――――

American Academy of Orthopedic Surgeons. *Emergency Care and Transportation of the Sick and Injured*. Menasha, Wis.: George Banta Co., 1977.

American National Red Cross. *Advanced First Aid and Emergency Care*. Garden City, N.Y.: Doubleday, 1979.

Breyfogle, N.D. *The Common Sense Medical Guide and Outdoor Reference*. New York: McGraw-Hill, 1981.

Hafen, B.Q., and K. J. Karren. *First Aid and Emergency Care Skills Manual*. Englewood, Colo.: Morton Publishing, 1982.

Henderson, J. *Emergency Medical Guide*. New York: McGraw-Hill, 1978.

# 18

# Transportation, Emergency Rescue, and Extrication

NEAL R. BOYD, JR., ED.D.

After completing this chapter the student will be able to

- Explain the rationale for moving a victim from an accident scene.
- Demonstrate techniques for transporting persons with mild injuries.
- Explain and demonstrate the following transportation techniques: one-person carry, chair carry, fore-and-aft carry, fireman's drag, two-hand or four-hand seat, direct ground lift, and three-person hammock carry.
- Explain and demonstrate the use of a blanket for transporation.
- Demonstrate three ways to improvise a stretcher.
- Demonstrate the technique for moving victims by stretcher.
- List the tools needed by a first-aider to gain access to a trapped victim.
- Explain the procedure for gaining access to victims of motor vehicle accidents.
- Explain when to use the cervical collar.
- Demonstrate the procedure for use of the backboard (short and long) to remove a victim from a wrecked motor vehicle.
- Explain the procedure for removing a victim from a vehicle on its side, an upside-down vehicle, the seat of a vehicle (front and back), the floor of a vehicle (front and back), an elevation or excavation, a cave-in, a machine accident, a structural collapse, and a toxic or oxygen-deficient atmosphere.

## INTRODUCTION

Accidents do not always take place in locales that are easily accessible to proper and immediate care. Therefore, first aid skills, in addition to those for psychological and physiological care, must include techniques for transporting the injured, gaining access to those difficult to reach, and removing the injured when necessary.

In most accident situations, trained emergency personnel are quickly dispatched to the scene. These rescuers are prepared to handle transportation and extrication of the injured. In these situations the first-aider should not attempt to move the accident victim unless a life-threatening circumstance exists at the emergency scene. Movement of the victim by an untrained person can cause further injury. The first-aider should give attention to first aid care where the injured person lies.

## ___TRANSPORTATION

As discussed in Chapter 2, the initial challenge encountered by the first-aider is whether the injured or ill individual should be moved. **A basic principle of first aid practice is to not move the victim from the emergency scene unless such movement is required to protect the safety of the victim or that of the first-aider.** The determination of safety is first made as a part of the initial emergency scene assessment. The decision is reviewed again as a part of the secondary emergency scene assessment. The first-aider then continuously monitors the emergency scene until relieved of responsibility for the victim by more sophisticated medical personnel. It would be wise for the reader to review again the initial and secondary assessment procedures detailed in Chapter 2. If the dynamics of the emergency setting require moving the victim (or if moving is required to get the person to medical care), the move should be carefully planned and executed with minimal disturbance to the victim.

## ___TRANSPORTING THE AMBULATORY VICTIM

If a person is not seriously injured, he or she often can walk to safety with some assistance (Figure 18.1). The following method is used in giving this assistance:

1 Help the victim to his or her feet.
2 Place one arm around the victim's waist.
3 Place the victim's arm over your shoulder and secure it firmly with your free hand in the chest or shoulder area.

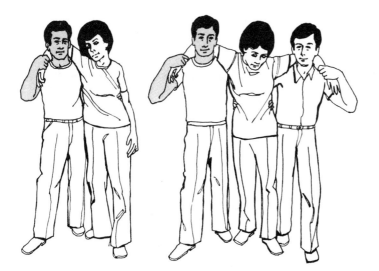

**FIGURE 18.1**
A person with minor injuries can be helped to safety by one or two first-aiders.

A second first-aider, if available, can assist in like manner from the opposite side. **Caution: A person with a suspected heart attack should not be allowed to walk.**

# TRANSPORTING THE NONAMBULATORY VICTIM

In a motor vehicle accident in which the victim is still inside the vehicle and the vehicle is on fire, the obvious action is to pull the injured person from the vehicle and move him or her to a safe area. This action would have to be undertaken quickly and at some risk of spinal cord injury to the victim. First aid for any life-threatening condition present would have to be delayed until after rescue. In the event that a rescue effort of this type must be attempted, the first-aider should remember that **any movement of the victim should be in the direction of the long axis of the victim's body.** The victim also should be moved in the supine (lying on the back) position, if possible, to protect the spine. (It may not be possible, however, to protect the victim's spine.) If the person is already in the supine position, the risk is somewhat reduced. The person can be dragged to safety by tugging on the clothing or using a blanket. If the person is unconscious, the arms (hands) should be secured (if possible) across the front of the body. No accident victim should be lifted or moved until he or she has been assessed for neck and spinal cord injuries, unless absolutely necessary.

After moving the victim to a safe place, the first-aider gives care immediately. If the person needs medical attention, the first-aider continues any needed life support until a proper transportation unit arrives on the scene.

## Techniques of Transportation

First-aiders should be experienced in transportation techniques even if the experience is in the nature of simple practice. A stretcher is of course preferable. However, a stretcher is not always available, and a manual carry may be the only resort.

### One-Person Carry
A person without serious injuries or wounds who is lightweight can be carried to safety by one first-aider. He or she supports the victim with one arm under the knees and the other arm under the upper back and armpit.

### Chair Carry
If two persons are available and the accident victim has sustained no spinal cord, neck, or leg injuries, a chair carry can be used. The victim is seated in a chair, which should be strong enough to support him or her. One first-aider grasps the chairback supports, while the second grasps the front legs of the chair from a squatting position. They lift the chair simultaneously and carry it with the victim by marching to the designated destination (Figure 18.2). To assure coordination of effort and thereby minimize the possibility of further injury to the victim, the forwardmost first-aider issues a series of signals or commands for each movement (e.g., "Ready?" "Prepare to lift." "Lift." "Forward." "Halt." and "Lower.").

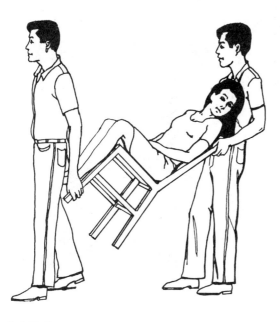

**FIGURE 18.2**
Chair carry

### Fore-and-Aft Carry

If the injured person has sustained no fractures or all fractures have been splinted, two first-aiders can employ the fore-and-aft carry (Figure 18.3). Both first-aiders kneel, with first-aider A at the victim's head and first-aider B beside the victim's knee. A places the hands under the victim's shoulders while B holds the victim's wrists. B then pulls the victim to a seated position with the help of A, who pushes the victim's shoulders and supports the victim's back and head against his or her own body. A then places the arms under the arms of the victim and grips the victim's wrists. Facing forward, B reaches down and positions the hands under the victim's knees. Both first-aiders rise from their squatting position on signal from A ("Ready?" "Prepare to lift." "Lift."). The victim is now ready to be moved, and A continues to be responsible for the signals ("Forward." "Halt." "Lower.").

### Fireman's Drag

In many accident situations, an unconscious victim must be moved from a limited space, such as a tunnel, or from an area where staying low is crucial to obtaining sufficient oxygen. One means of movement under these conditions is the fireman's drag (Figure 18.4). The accident victim is placed on his or her back and a cravat or some other improvised material, such as a belt, is looped over the victim's head and down underneath the armpits. The first-aider then kneels astride the victim and loops the cravat around his or her own neck. By lifting with the upper body, the first-aider can crawl and at the same time drag the victim. The victim's hands may be tied with another cravat and placed over the first-aider's head and neck. This allows the first-aider to move the victim more conveniently and securely. **Caution: The fireman's drag should not be used with a victim with spinal cord injury.**

**FIGURE 18.3**

Fore-and-aft carry

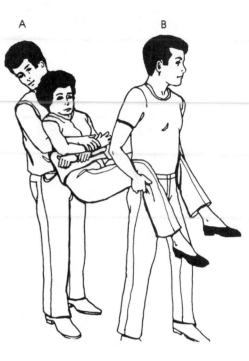

## Two-Hand or Four-Hand Seat Carry

In many accident situations, injuries are slight and the victim is conscious. If the victim is able to cooperate, two first-aiders may use either a two-hand or a four-hand seat for transportation. To form a two-hand seat, one first-aider places the right hand on the second's left shoulder, and the second places the left hand on the first's right shoulder. (Figure 18.5). This provides support to the victim's upper body. Next, the victim's arms are placed across the first-aiders' shoulders, and the two first-aiders grasp each other's wrists to form a seat under the back of the victim's thighs. The victim is then lifted and

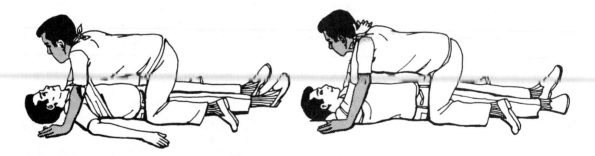

**FIGURE 18.4**

Fireman's drag. (*Left*) A cravat is placed under the victim's armpits and around the rescuer's neck. (*Right*) Victim's wrists are tied together to form a loop of the arms.

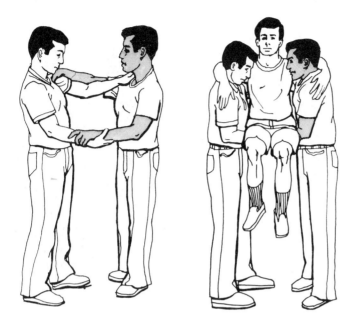

**FIGURE 18.5**

Two-hand seat carry

carried to safety. Again, a series of action-coordinating signals is given by one of the first-aiders.

With the four-hand seat carry, two first-aiders place their hands together to form a seat (Figure 18.6). The victim is then lifted and carried on this seat. The victim places his or her arms around the necks of the two first-aiders, to support the upper body.

**Direct Ground Lift Carry**

When the spine has not been injured, a direct ground lift is possible (Figure 18.7). At least two first-aiders, and preferably more, are needed to execute this lift. All first aiders align themselves on the uninjured side of the victim, who is placed on the back. Then each drops to the knee (the same knee for all) that is nearer the feet of the victim. First-aider A, located at the victim's head, becomes the lead rescuer and gives the signals to initiate lifts and moves. First-aider A places one arm under the victim's neck and shoulders and cradles the head. The other arm is placed under the victim's upper back. First-aider B places one arm under the victim's lower back and the other arm under the thigh area. First-aider C places one arm under the victim's knees and the other arm under the victim's ankles.

When all first-aiders feel they have a firm grasp of the victim, first-aider A signals by saying, "Ready? Prepare to lift." This signal is followed by the command, "Lift." At this command all lift the victim to their knees, and then roll him or her to their chest. Now a signal to stand is given, and all stand. The victim is now moved to safety, again with coordinating commands to walk and halt being given by first-aider A. When the injured person is to be placed on a stretcher, the procedure is reversed. Usually if a fourth first-aider is available, he or she places the stretcher or cot for the victim.

**FIGURE 18.6**

Four-hand seat carry. This carry provides a better seat than the two-hand carry, but the victim must support his or her own back.

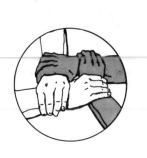

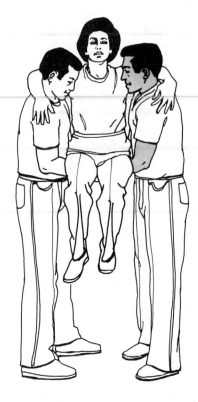

If six first-aiders are available, the direct ground lift carry can be executed with three first-aiders on each side. All drop to the knee nearer the feet of the victim and gently place their palms under the person. The hands of all should rest at the midline of the victim's body (Figure 18.8). The lead first-aider then signals to prepare to lift. At the command, "Lift," all first-aiders rise to their knees while lifting the victim, and then they stand at the signal to stand. Again, if the victim is to be carried any distance, coordinating commands to walk and halt are given by the lead first-aider. To lower the victim to a stretcher, or the ground, the procedure is reversed.

**Three-Person Hammock Carry**

When an accident victim is found in the supine (lying on the back) or prone (lying on the face) position and spinal cord injury is not suspected, first-aiders may use a technique called the three-person hammock carry (Figure 18.9). First-aiders A and C are on one side of the victim and B is on the other. To execute this carry, all drop to the knee closer to the victim's feet. First-aider A places the arm closer to the victim's head under the head and shoulders of the victim to form a cradle. The other arm is then placed under the victim's lower back. First-aider B places the arm closer to the victim's head above first-aider A's lower arm. He or she then places the other arm below the victim's buttocks. First-aider C places the arm nearer the victim's head under the person's thighs (above

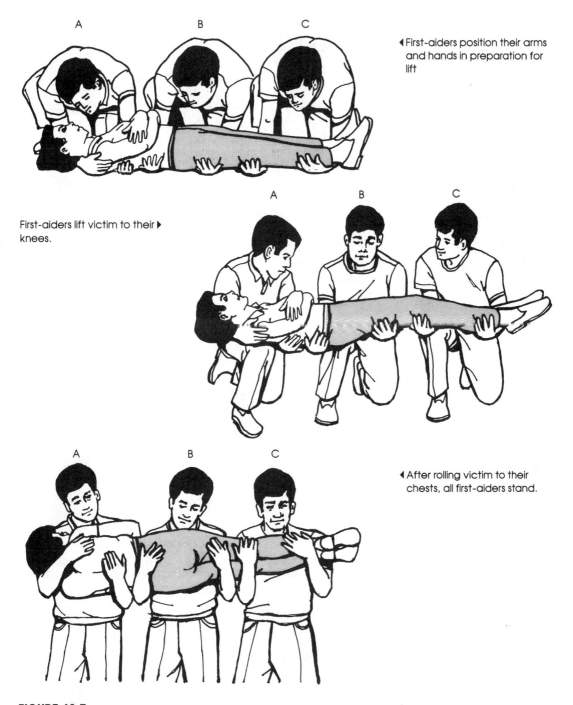

◄ First-aiders position their arms and hands in preparation for lift

First-aiders lift victim to their ▶ knees.

◄ After rolling victim to their chests, all first-aiders stand.

**FIGURE 18.7**

Direct ground lift carry with three rescuers

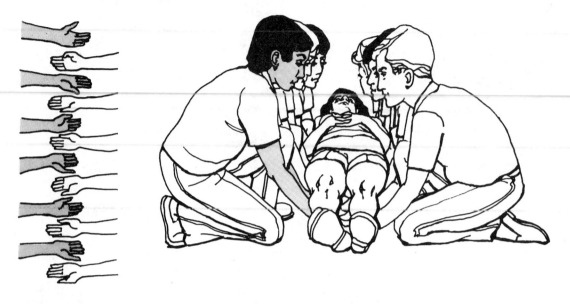

**FIGURE 18.8**

Direct ground lift carry with six rescuers

the lower arm of first-aider B) and the other arm under the victim's knees. First-aider A then gives the signal to prepare to lift, followed by the command to lift. The victim is lifted to the first-aider's knees and is rested there. The hands are moved under the victim to the point where they can be rotated to form two interlocking grips, as shown in Figure 18.9 (inset). When these grips are secure, first-aider A signals to prepare to stand and then to stand, at which time all first-aiders stand (Figure 18.9). Commands to walk and halt follow. The procedure is reversed to lower the victim.

## The Blanket as a Transportation Tool

Many accident situations call for a victim to be moved by a carrying device known as a litter. However, dangerous circumstances may dictate that the person be moved before a litter is available. In such cases a blanket can be used (Figure 18.10). Certain precautions are associated with the use of a blanket for this purpose. If a blanket is the only alternative for moving a person suspected of having neck or back fracture, the person's head must be held steady and in a manner that provides traction in a straight line away from the injured trunk. Should the victim's body need turning, it should be turned as a unit, avoid twisting the neck and back.

The blanket is pleated and placed alongside the supine victim. The first-aider leans over the victim and places one hand and arm over the far shoulder and the other over the hip and gently rolls the victim onto the side nearer the first-aider. The leading edge of the blanket is then wedged tightly against the victim's body. The first-aider then gently

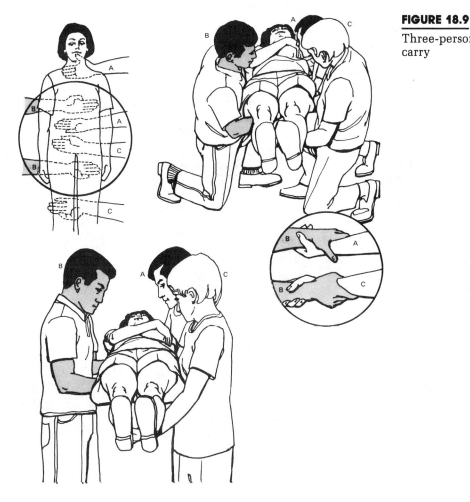

**FIGURE 18.9**
Three-person hammock
carry

returns the victim to the supine position. Placing one hand and arm over the near shoulder and the other over the hip, the first-aider rolls the victim to his or her other side. The leading edge and several pleated portions of the blanket are now visible and readily reached. Continuing to support the victim with one hand at the shoulder, the first-aider pulls the blanket through and extends the pleats. Again supporting the shoulder and lower back, the first-aider returns the victim to the supine position. This should place the person in the middle of the blanket. The blanket can be rolled from the sides and used to lift the victim. Everyone available should assist.

Often only one first-aider is at an accident scene. If this person cannot lift and carry the victim alone, he or she can use a *blanket (mattress) drag* as transport to safety. In this drag, the first-aider places the victim on a blanket in the supine position and then drags the blanket from the head end (Figure 18.11). To ensure that the victim's head is not

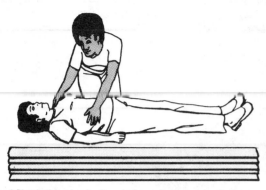

**1** Blanket is pleated and placed alongside victim.

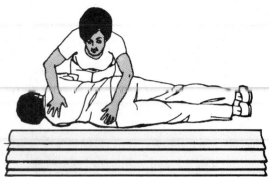

**2** Victim is rolled on side toward first-aider. Leading edge of blanket is secured against victim.

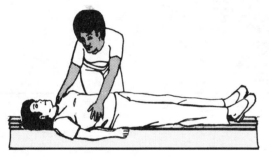

**3** Victim is returned to supine position.

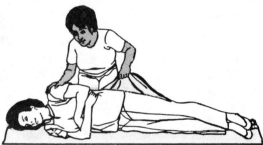

**4** Victim is rolled on side away from first-aider. Edge of blanket is pulled through.

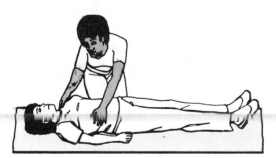

**5** Victim is returned to supine position. Blanket is fully extended on either side.

**FIGURE 18.10**

Steps in placing a blanket under an injured person. A second person must stabilize the head if fracture of the neck or back is suspected.

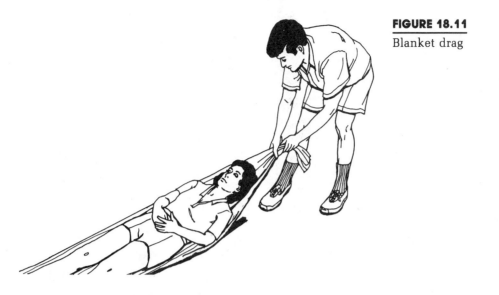

**FIGURE 18.11**
Blanket drag

bumped during this move, the head and shoulders are raised **slightly** (the minimum amount needed to initiate the drag). A mattress is an alternative to the blanket. However, to lift and drag a victim onto a mattress usually requires at least two first-aiders. The blanket/mattress drag should not be used with a victim of spinal cord injury unless life-threatening circumstances at the emergency scene necessitate immediate movement and no more suitable transportation alternative exists.

## ___Stretchers

First-aiders must often improvise stretchers for moving accident victims. A house door removed from its hinges is suitable. A stretcher can also be constructed from two poles and a strong piece of material such as a blanket, robe, rug, sheet, or tarpaulin. The pole is placed lengthwise on the material about a foot from the center, and the short side of the material is folded over it. Then the second pole is placed parallel to and about two feet from the first pole (on a double thickness of the material) (Figure 18.12). The remaining material is placed over the second pole. The victim's weight secures the folds. Another stretcher can be improvised from two poles and two jackets. A person wearing a jacket grasps two poles and leans forward. A second person removes the jacket from the first by pulling the jacket from the lower back area over the person's head and onto the poles (Figure 18.13). The first person then does the same to the second and the "jacket stretcher" is ready.

If strong material is available but nothing that can be utilized for poles, the material can be used alone for the stretcher if several people are available. The victim is placed in the supine position lengthwise in the center of the material and the long ends are then rolled inward toward the victim and grasped for carrying (Figure 18.14). Four or more

**FIGURE 18.12**

Improvising a stretcher
with two poles and a
blanket

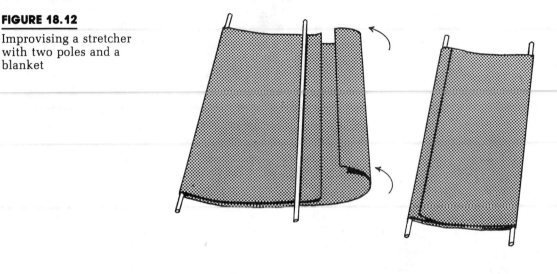

first-aiders are preferable. As a precaution, the improvised stretcher should be tested
before being used: A first-aider about the same size as the victim should lie on the
stretcher and allow the other first-aiders to lift him or her.

Sometimes first-aiders rush into a building or cave, improvise a stretcher to remove
the injured victim, and then find that the stretcher is too large to carry out of the small
space. Therefore, any stretcher, whether improvised or manufactured, should be carried
to the victim along the same path by which it will be removed.

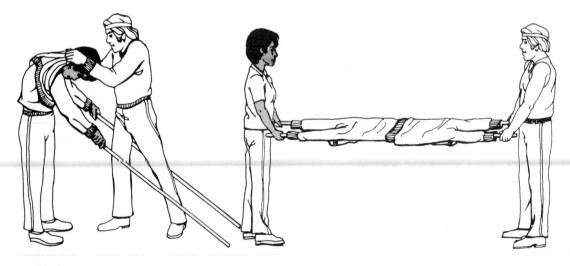

**FIGURE 18.13**

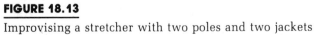

Improvising a stretcher with two poles and two jackets

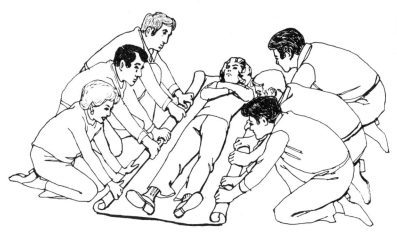

**FIGURE 18.14**

Using a blanket as an improvised stretcher when poles are not available

First-aiders must take care in placing a victim on a stretcher. All involved work together and lift and move at the signal of the leader to ensure that the victim does not suffer unnecessary pain.

The three-person direct ground lift carry (p. 339 and Figure 18.7) is utilized, with a fourth first-aider assisting in both lifting the victim and placing the stretcher (Figure 18.15). Three first-aiders align themselves on the same side of the victim, one (A) at the shoulder, one (B) at the hip, and one (C) at the knee. The fourth first-aider (D) takes a position opposite and facing B at the hips. All drop to the knee closer to the victim's feet.

A places the hands under the victim's neck and shoulders, B and D alternate their hands under the pelvis from the upper leg to the small of the back, and C places the hands under the knees and ankles. A gives the signal to prepare to lift, followed by the command to lift. When this command is given, all four first-aiders slowly lift the victim to rest on the aligned knees of A, B, and C. D places the stretcher under the victim and then resumes the role of a lifter, returning to his or her place opposite first-aider B. **If a spinal cord injury is suspected, the victim is lifted only as high as necessary to quickly place the stretcher in position.** At a signal from A, all four first-aiders lower the stretcher (Figure 18.16).

Once the victim is secured, the first-aiders assume positions as follows: A at the head, B and D on each side of the stretcher, and C at the foot. A signals all to squat and grasp the stretcher. Once the carriers have a firm grip, A signals for the lift to a standing position. One last signal is for a shift to stabilize the stretcher for transport. In this shift the two carriers along the sides of the stretcher each slide one hand toward the front to support the stretcher as the first-aider at the foot turns to face the direction in which the stretcher will be carried. The victim is carried feet first, unless bleeding is severe, in which case he or she is carried head first on the chance that tranportation up an incline or steps is necessary. A gives a marching command so the carriers march in unison. To this end, C at the foot of the victim and B and D at the sides step out on the left foot, while A at the head steps out on the right foot. This type of marching prevents the stretcher from swaying.

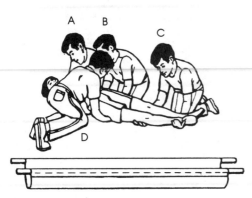

**1** First-aiders align themselves and prepare to lift.

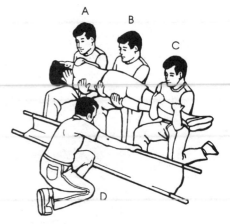

**2** Victim rests on knees of A, B, and C while D places stretcher.

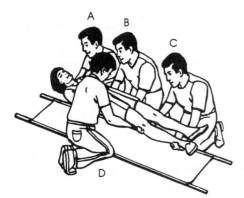

**3** D assists in lowering victim to stretcher.

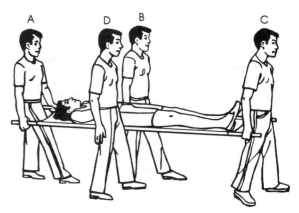

**4** Victim is carried feet first. A starts on right foot, B, C, and D on left.

**FIGURE 18.15**

Procedure for placing an injured person on a stretcher and the method of march

## _____ GAINING ACCESS TO THE VICTIM: GENERAL PRINCIPLES

Sometimes a victim of injury or illness is trapped or found in a relatively inaccessible location. To give care, or to move the person from a dangerous situation and then give care, the first-aider must gain access to the person as quickly as possible. He or she must thus have some knowledge about methods of quick access and the skills to accomplish it.

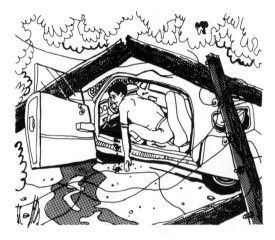

**FIGURE 18.16**
Electric power to a broken utility pole over a wrecked vehicle must be shut off before rescue of the victim can be attempted.

The first-aider must also have the ability to size up the hazards posed by the scene and to determine whether and how it can be entered safely. For example, if a person is found trapped in a motor vehicle on which electric power lines have fallen (Figure 18.16), the first-aider will make sure the power is shut off before attempting to gain access to the person.

In gaining access to an injured or ill person, an array of tools may be needed. Tools useful for most emergencies are a screwdriver, chisel, hammer, pliers, crowbar, knife, heavy duty work gloves, goggles, shovel, tire iron, wrenches, vehicle jack, rope, and chain (Figure 18.17). Learning to be proficient with these tools enhances the first-aider's ability to gain access to and remove an injured person.

Time is crucial in reaching a victim trapped in a motor vehicle wreck, as it often is in other situations as well. In the case of a wreck, the first-aider should attempt to gain access to the vehicle and remove the victim from it in the position in which the vehicle is found. Using anything available, he or she makes sure the vehicle is stabilized. The door should then be tried. If the door is jammed, access is next attempted through the front or rear window. (Side windows should not be used unless life-threatening circumstances require immediate action and the victim cannot be reached through the front or rear window.)

To gain access through a front or rear window, the chrome trim is first extracted. The rubber molding is then cut with a knife and removed (normally this can be accomplished by pulling the rubber out of the molding into which it has been pressed). Next the glass is either pushed or pulled away in one piece. During this process the victim should be shielded with something against broken glass.

If the victim cannot be reached through the front or rear window, there are two avenues. If the vehicle is a pre-1967 model, it might be possible to open the jammed door with a jackhandle. In post-1967 vehicle models, however, doors must be cut open (a cut is made around the lock). If cutting into the vehicle is the only means of reaching the victim, the roof is the easiest part to cut. Cutting with the simple tools that might be

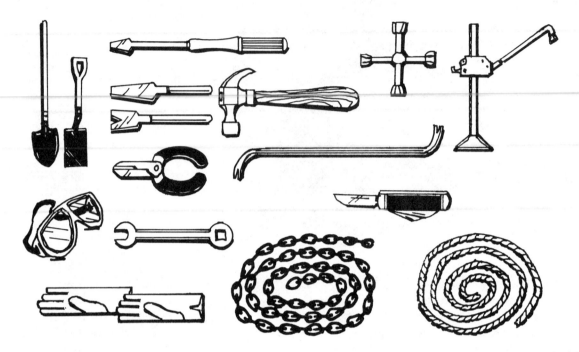

**FIGURE 18.17**

Tools useful for gaining access to persons injured in vehicle wrecks

available to the first-aider is a lengthy process. If the victim's condition and other circumstances allow it, it is wiser for the first-aider to call the fire department or another rescue organization that has the proper equipment.

Gaining access to an individual pinned beneath a vehicle calls for some ingenuity. A jack or any sturdy object capable of creating leverage (e.g., blocks) or the strength of bystanders, or a combination of whatever is available, can be used to lift and secure the vehicle.

Once reached, the injured person is often found with one or more parts of the body needing special attention. For example, an arm or leg may be protruding through the windshield. Such an extruded part should be well padded with bandaging materials. A tool, such as a pair of pliers or a knife, may be used to fold or cut the glass, freeing the body part. Whenever working with broken glass, the first-aider should remember to wear gloves if possible and to protect the victim with a covering.

For a victim jammed within a vehicle, a simple solution such as cutting the seatbelt, removing a shoe, or removing the front or back seat may allow removal. Power tools may be needed, however, in more serious situations. *The first-aider must plan the course of action before beginning extrication.* Time is often a critical factor in victim survival, and a great deal of time can be lost in choosing the wrong path to reach the victim.

# ___PREPARING THE VICTIM FOR REMOVAL: GENERAL FIRST AID PROCEDURES

Once the victim has been reached, first aid for life-threatening conditions is rendered immediately. (If at all possible, all accident victims should be stabilized before being moved. However, and as repeatedly emphasized in this text, when circumstances pose a serious threat to the victim or first-aider, the victim must be moved to a safe place before this is done.)

The next task is to prepare the person for removal to medical care. Due to the nature of most motor vehicle crashes, as well as diving accidents, cave-ins, and structural collapses, neck and back injuries are common. Again, as repeatedly emphasized, the first-aider always checks for these types of injuries. An unconscious victim is handled as though spinal cord injury is present. If the victim has trouble gripping or wiggling the toes or moving body parts or feels weakness or numbness in the extremities, a neck or spinal cord injury should be suspected and a cervical collar used in combination with a backboard in removing the victim.

To secure the cervical collar, the person's head is raised slightly to accommodate passage of the collar beneath the neck. **Caution: The victim's head and neck are kept aligned and the head is not moved unnecessarily.** The first-aider applies the collar gently, being careful to not place unnecessary pressure on the head that could cause further neck or spinal cord injuries. If a prepared collar is not available, a folded towel can be improvised (Figure 18.18) and secured with two safety pins.

To apply the long backboard, the rescuer eases the victim upward slightly so that the board may be placed underneath him or her. Care is taken to keep the body and head stable and aligned. An assistant, if available, secures the board in place. The head is secured to the board first by strapping a cravat across the forehead. Caution must be exercised to avoid tipping the head back. If the cervical support does not sufficiently immobilize the head, a second cravat is applied and tied around the chin. In this case the victim must be watched for possible vomiting and to ascertain that the airway remains unobstructed. Cravats are then placed around the shoulders, the chest, the arms, just below the belt level, the thighs, the knees, the mid-calf area, and the ankles. Another cravat is placed over the ankles and around the board edges. A final cravat secures the feet to the footrest (Figure 18.19). All the cravats are tied at the side. *The cravats should not be used for lifting the victim.*

If the person is found in a sitting position, the short backboard must be applied before the long backboard can be utilized. The cervical collar is applied as already detailed. The victim is then tilted forward enough for the short backboard to be gently eased into place. A cravat is placed across the forehead and another across the chin to secure the head to the board (again with caution that an open airway is maintained). The head must not be moved unnecessarily. The victim's body is then secured to the backboard by cravats at the shoulders, chest, and waist (Figure 18.20). The victim is lifted in the seated position by hands placed under the buttocks. Once lifted, he or she is secured to the long backboard, as described previously.

**FIGURE 18.18**

A cervical collar can be improvised from a folded towel or blanket

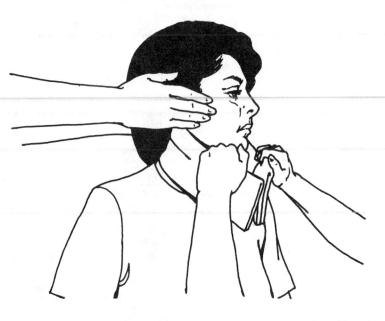

**FIGURE 18.19**

Victim secured to a long backboard

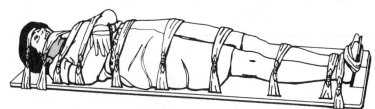

**FIGURE 18.20**

Victim in a sitting position secured to a short backboard

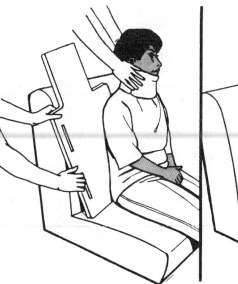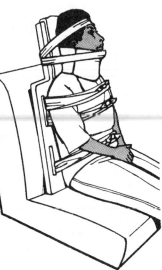

# EXTRICATION FROM MOTOR VEHICLES

## Removal from Vehicle on Its Side

Persons involved in accidents in which the vehicle rests on its side often sustain spinal cord or neck injury. If such injury is suspected, a cervical collar is applied and secured in place and the person is fastened to a short backboard in accordance with the procedures previously outlined. The victim can then be placed on a long backboard (the cravats are not used for lifing). With the aid of two persons in the vehicle, a long backboard is placed at the victim's back as he or she is raised to a vertical position. The victim is then secured to the long backboard and the backboard is hoisted out of the vehicle.

## Removal from Upside-down Vehicle

All loose materials in the vehicle are removed. One first-aider enters the vehicle. The first-aider on the outside assists in controlling the victim's head and neck, if neck or spinal cord injury is suspected. A backboard must be applied, preferably the long backboard. In some situations, however, for example a badly damaged vehicle, the short backboard may have to be used. The victim's feet and legs should be secured (i.e., tied together) with several cravat bandages, to assist in placing the victim on the long backboard. Once the victim is secured, he/she can be moved on to a stretcher (keeping the board in place).

## Removal from Seat of Vehicle

A victim lying on the seat of a wrecked vehicle is probably on his or her side, with the legs hanging off the seat (Figure 18.21). If possible, four persons should be involved in moving the victim. One first-aider holds the head of the victim stable and in line with the body. A second gently moves the victim's feet and legs in line with the body while ensuring that the legs remain extended.

   For a victim in the front seat, two other persons reach over from the back of the front seat and grasp the victim's clothing with both hands, at evenly spaced intervals from the shoulders to the thighs. By gently pulling on the clothes, they roll the victim slightly forward so that a long backboard can be eased into position by one of the first-aiders in front. When the board is in place, the first-aiders working from the back seat gently pull the victim by the clothing to the backboard. They then reach over the victim and grasp the lower edge of the board, holding their arms against the victim. The first-aider at the victim's head holds the head secure and in line with the rest of the body. When the victim is properly aligned, this first-aider also grasps the bottom edge of the board to provide stability during the impending turn. The first-aider at the feet now grasps the bottom edge of the board as well. The first-aider at the head signals the other three when to lift the board and lay it flat on the seat (e.g., "Ready?," "Lift," "Turn," "Lower."). The victim is then secured to the board and removed from the vehicle.

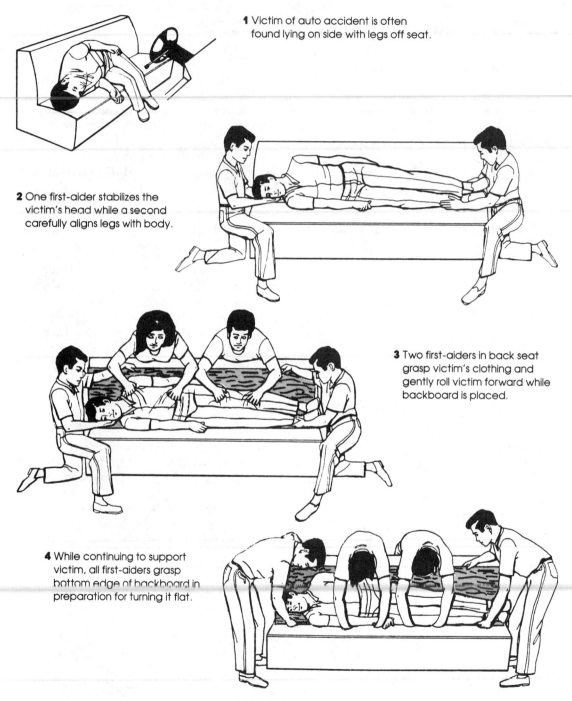

**1** Victim of auto accident is often found lying on side with legs off seat.

**2** One first-aider stabilizes the victim's head while a second carefully aligns legs with body.

**3** Two first-aiders in back seat grasp victim's clothing and gently roll victim forward while backboard is placed.

**4** While continuing to support victim, all first-aiders grasp bottom edge of backboard in preparation for turning it flat.

**FIGURE 18.21**

Application of the long backboard when a victim is found lying on the front seat

## __Removal from Floor of Vehicle

In many accidents the victim is found lying on the front or back floor of the vehicle. For extrication from the front floor (Figure 18.22), the long backboard is placed on the seat next to the victim. As in the case of a victim lying on the seat, the help of four persons is preferable. The first-aider at the victim's head holds the head and neck in line with the body. Another takes a position at the feet and binds the victim's legs together with cravats, tying them at the feet, ankle, and mid-leg area. The remaining first-aiders then work from the back seat, reaching over to grasp the victim's clothing at the thigh, hip, waist, and shoulder. Care should be exercised not to tear the clothes. Pulling on torn clothing could cause jolts leading to further injuries. Care must also be taken to avoid pulling the victim by one or both arms.

Again, the first-aider at the victim's head acts as the signal caller. At the signal, all first-aiders lift the victim, being extremely careful to keep the head and body aligned. When the person has been lifted high enough, he or she is gently settled on the long backboard. The victim is secured on the board, and then the first-aiders in the rear move out of the car to assist with removal of the board and victim from the vehicle.

For a person found lying on the floor in the back of the vehicle, the same extrication procedure is followed, except that the long backboard is laid on the back seat and the two first aiders work from the front seat area instead of the back.

In some instances the victim's clothes are not thick enough to be trusted not to tear if used for lifting or pulling. This problem is solved by placing cravats evenly around the victim's body from the shoulders to the ankles. The cravats are then used for lifting.

# ___EXTRICATION IN OTHER SITUATIONS

## __Elevations or Excavations

In accidents occurring at elevations or in excavations, the victim will often be unconscious. The long backboard should be used if a fracture or other injury necessitates immobilization or if the person is unconscious. If a choice is possible, the rescue should be effected with the person in the horizontal rather than the vertical position, because of the increased support and comfort this provides. Each situation must be evaluated individually, however, to determine which method is most effective for safe rescue of the victim.

As previously noted, if circumstances allow the victim is given first aid care and then placed on a long backboard. The person is secured to the board by cravats strapped through the holes on each side of the board. With an improvised backboard, the cravats may have to go entirely around the board. The knots are placed to one side. The victim's head should be secured by a cushion and two cravats, one placed at the forehead and the other at the chin. If injuries do not preclude it, cravats are placed at the chest, waist, above the knees, and at ankles and feet.

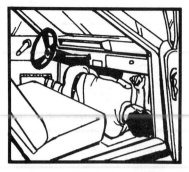 **1** Victim is found lying on front floor of vehicle.

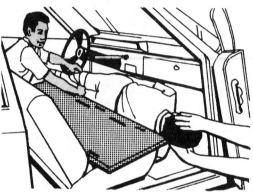

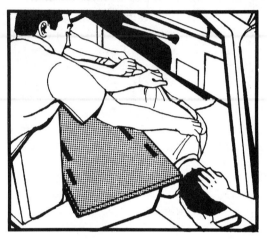

**2** Long backboard is placed on front seat. One first-aider stabilizes victim's head and neck while second ties legs together.

**3** Two more first-aiders grasp victim's clothing from back seat.

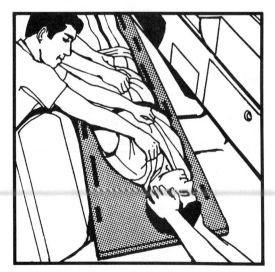

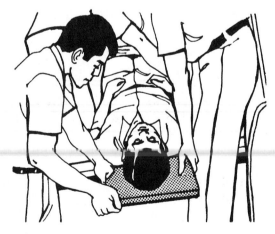

**4** Victim is gently lifted to backboard. Head is kept in alignment.

**5** First-aiders move from rear of car to receive board as it is passed out.

**FIGURE 18.22**

Steps in the removal of a victim from the front floor of a car

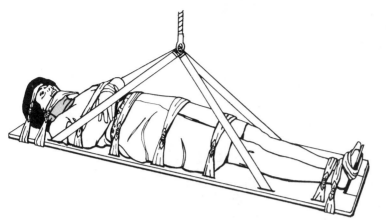

**FIGURE 18.23**

Removal of a victim by means of the horizontal hoist

If a mechanical hoisting device is near and available, removal of the victim may be completed by a technique known as the horizontal hoist (Figure 18.23). The hoisting belts are placed into holes in the long backboard. The rings should be gathered and secured by a hoisting line approximately three fourths of an inch in size. If proper hoisting belts are not available, a three-fourth-inch-wide length of durable material may be used. Any type of raising or lowering equipment can be used.

If a vertical hoist technique is needed, an additional cravat that runs over the chest and under the armpits must be used when securing the victim to the backboard. The other straps remain the same (Figure 18.24). The feet must be well secured to the footrest. However, *the footrest should not be used when vertically hoisting a victim with a leg fracture.* This would place considerable pressure on the leg. In this case the victim is secured by long straps passed around the thighs, across the body, and over the opposite shoulder. The straps are laced through the proper holes on the board.

For hoisting, the hoisting line is laced through the holes in the upper third of the board and secured by a knot at the front of the board in a vertical position (Figure 18.25). Free swinging of the board while being raised or lowered can be prevented by the use of two guidelines extending from either side of the board and controlled by the first-aiders.

It is possible to improvise a board for hoisting a victim if no standard backboard is available. Caution must be taken, however, to assure the security of the cravats holding the victim on the board and particularly to assure the stability of the hoist rope.

## ▬Cave-ins

The site of a cave-in is highly dangerous and must be approached with considerable caution. Since the victim may be hidden from view, the first-aider must be careful to avoid loosening additional material in his or her haste to get to the victim. The situation should be carefully assessed and a plan of action determined. The first objective is to locate the victim and quickly uncover his or her face and head. Once the face and head are free, artificial respiration can be initiated, if indicated. The chest and body are then

**FIGURE 18.24**

Removal of a victim by
means of the vertical hoist

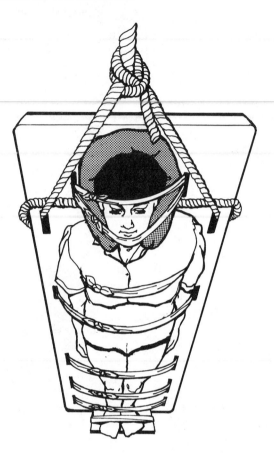

uncovered and other first aid care is rendered as needed. If injuries are severe and removal is necessary, a backboard should be used. Whether the excavation area is shallow or deep, the victim must be secured to the board before removal. In a deep cave-in, a mechanical hoist may be needed.

## __Machine Accidents

An accident in which a person is pinned beneath a machine presents several complexities. Due to the nature of the accident, there may be severe lacerations, avulsions, multiple fractures, burns, and traumatic shock. Initiation of first aid care may be needed simultaneously with the attempt to release the victim. The first step in release is to discontinue power to the machine. If possible, an individual who is familiar with the machine should assist.

In the absence of an automatic releasing device, the machine may have to be dismantled. If this is not possible, an attempt should be made to remove the particular part pinning the victim. In severe accidents, on-the-spot surgery may be the only way to release the victim. Only a physician can decide this and perform the surgery. During the wait for a physician to arrive, the first-aider tries to control bleeding, treats for possible shock, renders psychological assurance, maintains the airway, and provides any other care possible.

## ___Structural Collapse

A structural collapse may present any combination of the following: (1) victim confined, (2) victim confined with atmosphere either lacking oxygen or containing toxic or explosive fumes, (3) victim pinned and injured, and (4) victim located where no means of communication is possible. Extra care must be taken in these situations because the safety of the first-aider is usually also at risk. Of prime importance is determining the exact location of the victim and preparing a plan for reaching and extricating the person. When the victim is reached, first aid care is initiated by stabilizing his or her condition. The person is then prepared for removal. Depending on the severity of the injuries involved, a backboard may or may not have to be used. If the backboard is used, the victim should be properly secured as previously described and all precautions heeded before the removal takes place.

## ___Toxic or Oxygen-Deficient Atmosphere

In an accident in which the victim is in a toxic or oxygen-deficient atmosphere, extrication is not attempted unless the area can be well ventilated or proper respiratory equipment is available. It is recommended that oxygen equipment be used, because there is no way to determine whether oxygen is sufficient. Poisonous gases may be heavier or lighter than air; therefore, ventilation of both high and low areas is required. A lifeline should be established before the first-aider enters a dangerous atmosphere. The lifeline is attended by another first-aider outside. A communications network/signaling system should also be established, so that the first-aider on the outside can keep track of the status of the first-aider inside the emergency area at all times. In a rescue of this nature, it may not be possible to prevent additional injury to the victim during removal. There is no time to care for life-threatening conditions or to place the backboard for spinal cord injury. Further injury can be minimized, however, by moving the victim on the long axis of the body.

_____ **SUMMARY** _____

Accidents and sudden illness happen in all types of environments, and the victim often needs immediate removal from the site or is trapped and needs to be extri-

cated. The first-aider therefore needs skills in transportation and extrication of injured or ill persons, as well as skills in first aid care. The proper moving technique depends on the extent of the injuries sustained. The skilled first-aider should be able to identify a technique that will work effectively in a given situation and satisfactorily perform (or direct) the move. Moving skills can be gained from practice. To gain access to a trapped accident victim, a number of tools, such as a hammer, screwdriver, pliers, and crowbar, may be needed. Proficiency in using these tools enhances the first-aider's usefulness. Many accident situations, such as overturned motor vehicles, present problems in reaching the victim. Knowledge of how to quickly gain access to and remove the victim is essential when hazardous circumstances prevent on-site administration of first aid care.

───────────── **CHAPTER MASTERY: TEST ITEMS** ─────────────

**True and False**                                                          Circle One

1. The extent of injuries has little influence on whether a first-aider       T     F
   chooses the lift or carry technique to move a victim.
2. In the absence of a stretcher, blankets are of little value for transporting  T     F
   a victim with neck or spinal cord injury.
3. A potential problem with improvised stretchers is that the improviser     T     F
   fails to foresee maneuverability obstacles in close quarters.
4. Stability for a victim on a moving stretcher can be accomplished by the    T     F
   method of marching the carriers use.
5. Only professional emergency rescue personnel should remove a victim       T     F
   from a wrecked motor vehicle.
6. In attempting to reach an accident victim, the first-aider should proceed  T     F
   with caution because haste may cause an injury to the first-aider.
7. A wrecked upside-down vehicle should be turned upright before an          T     F
   attempt is made to gain access to the victim.
8. The two most important aids for the first-aider in a case of suspected    T     F
   spinal cord injury are the cervical collar and the backboard.
9. To lift a victim whose clothing is thin, cravats should be placed at even  T     F
   intervals from the shoulders to the ankles.
10. When a vertical hoist is to be used, securing a person with a leg         T     F
   fracture to the footrest of the backboard would be unwise.
11. If a person pinned by a machine cannot be released by ordinary           T     F
   methods, on-the-spot surgery may be the only alternative.

**Fill In the Missing Word(s)**

1. The best transportation technique for a victim in an area of limited space such as
   a tunnel is _____.
2. A good substitute for a litter is _____.

3. Three tools that might be helpful in an extrication attempt are _____, _____, and _____.
4. If it is necessary to care for a neck injury in the absence of a cervical collar, the first-aider should _____.
5. The first objective of the first-aider after gaining access to a victim is to _____.
6. The first objective in an extrication attempt at a cave-in is _____.

## Multiple Choice (Circle the Best Answer)

1. A possible substitute for a blanket as a transportation device when the victim has neck or spinal cord injuries is a (an)
   a. chair.
   b. overcoat.
   c. sheet.
   d. door.
   e. mattress.
2. In attempting to reach a victim trapped in a wrecked motor vehicle, the first effort should be directed at
   a. cutting through the door.
   b. opening the door.
   c. going through the window.
   d. calling the emergency rescue squad.
   e. making sure the victim is alive.
3. An exception to the rule of stabilizing the victim immediately is when
   a. it is raining.
   b. the victim says he or she is okay.
   c. danger is imminent.
   d. other first-aiders are present.
   e. professional emergency personnel have been notified.
4. When extricating a victim from a structural collapse, extra care should be utilized because
   a. the safety of the rescuer is a factor.
   b. the victim probably has multiple injuries.
   c. the victim is unconscious.
   d. the rescuer has little time.
   e. all of the above.
5. The type of extrication situation that requires oxygen equipment and a communications line is a (an)
   a. cave-in.
   b. machine accident.
   c. upside-down vehicle.
   d. oxygen-deficient atmosphere.
   e. overturned motor vehicle.

**Discussion Questions**

1. Identify situations that would necessitate use of the following carries: fore-and-aft carry, fireman's drag, two-hand or four-hand seat carry, direct ground lift carry, and three-person hammock carry.
2. Describe situations in which both the long and the short backboard would be required to move an injured victim.

—————————————— **BIBLIOGRAPHY** ——————————————

American National Red Cross. *Advanced First Aid and Emergency Care.* 2d ed. Garden City, NY: Doubleday, 1979.

Florio, A. E., W. F. Alles, and G. T. Stafford. *Safety Education.* 4th ed. New York: McGraw-Hill, 1979.

Hafen, B. Q. *First Aid for Health Emergencies.* 3d ed. St. Paul: West Publishing, 1985.

Hafen, B. Q., and K. J. Karren. *First Aid and Emergency Care Skills Manual.* 2d ed. Englewood, Colo.: Morton Publishing, 1982.

# INDEX

128572